Hearing Loss: Causes, Symptoms, Diagnosis, and Treatment

Hearing Loss: Causes, Symptoms, Diagnosis, and Treatment

Guest Editor

George K. Psillas

MDPI

Basel • Beijing • Wuhan • Barcelona • Belgrade • Novi Sad • Cluj • Manchester

Guest Editor
George K. Psillas
1st Academic ENT Department
Aristotle University of Thessaloniki
Thessaloniki
Greece

Editorial Office
MDPI AG
Grosspeteranlage 5
4052 Basel, Switzerland

This is a reprint of the Special Issue, published open access by the journal *Audiology Research* (ISSN 2039-4349), freely accessible at: https://www.mdpi.com/journal/audiolres/special_issues/CWSH78AI95.

For citation purposes, cite each article independently as indicated on the article page online and as indicated below:

Lastname, A.A.; Lastname, B.B. Article Title. *Journal Name* **Year**, *Volume Number*, Page Range.

ISBN 978-3-7258-5131-7 (Hbk)
ISBN 978-3-7258-5132-4 (PDF)
https://doi.org/10.3390/books978-3-7258-5132-4

Contents

About the Editor

George K. Psillas

George K. Psillas is a full professor of Otolaryngology, head of the Hearing–Balance Center in the 1st Academic ENT Department of AHEPA Hospital, at the Aristotle University of Thessaloniki. His main interest lies in the field of Otology–Neurotology, where he specializes in ear surgery and oversees outpatient services. His research includes hearing loss restoration, vestibular pathology, vestibular laboratory tests (electro-, videonystagmography, vestibular evoked myogenic potentials, video head impulse test), and facial nerve electrophysiology (nerve excitability test, electroneurography, electromyography). He also has expertise in pediatric otorhinolaryngology, mainly in the investigation of sensorineural hearing loss with the use of specialized hearing tests (auditory brainstem responses, otoacoustic emissions) and genetic methods for the detection of congenital sensorineural hearing loss. He is also interested in the immune-mediated pathophysiologic mechanisms and therapeutic protocols involving the inner ear, conducting laboratory tests and extended audiological test battery to identify underlying autoimmune processes. Finally, his research encompasses the advancements in cochlear implant technology, focusing on innovations aimed at enhancing auditory performance and improving user experience. He has been member of the Barany Society since 2010 and a member of the Francophone Society of Neurotology since 2008. He has published in many international journals and he has presented his work at many international conferences. His clinical supervision is focused on training students and ENT residents on hearing and vestibular rehabilitation, while his research also extends to broader areas of the medical field.

audiology research

Editorial

Clinical Insights into Hearing Loss

George Psillas * and Petros D. Karkos

1st Academic ENT Department, Aristotle University of Thessaloniki, AHEPA Hospital, 1, Stilponos Kyriakidi St., 546 36 Thessaloniki, Greece
* Correspondence: psill@otenet.gr; Tel.: +30-2310-994-762

We are pleased to present a Special Issue addressing new insights into the causes, symptoms, diagnosis, and treatment of hearing loss.

This Special Issue comprises twelve publications that cover topics relating to hearing aids, auditory neuropathy, implantable auditory devices such as cochlear implants, and middle ear and bone conduction implants. In addition, congenital cytomegalovirus-related hearing loss and cisplatin-induced ototoxicity are discussed in the form of a review. Lastly, the effects of different hyperbaric oxygen therapy profiles on hearing improvement are evaluated in patients suffering from sudden sensorineural hearing loss.

Despite technological advancements, hearing aid users still face difficulty in understanding speech in noise. Research primarily focuses on assessing parameters that contribute to the evaluation of patients prior to hearing aid use. The Acceptable Noise Level is a key factor influencing hearing aid fittings, determining how much background noise can be tolerated before it interferes with speech intelligibility. In a multicenter study conducted by Mark Laureyns and colleagues [1], the authors evaluated the influence of the masker multi-talker babble on the Acceptable Noise Level; it was concluded that high-frequency environmental noise is the most important condition affecting Acceptable Noise Level results, regardless of the grade of hearing impairment.

It is recognized that better unaided speech-in-noise performance is associated with greater perceived benefit from hearing aids. The association between unaided speech-in-noise performance and hearing aid use, mediated through perceived benefit, had not been previously studied. Anthony Marcotti and colleagues [2] found no direct association between unaided speech-in-noise performance and hearing aid use; however, unaided speech-in-noise performance, particularly in the left ear, should be considered during the hearing aid fitting process.

Although the correct fitting of hearing aids may be achieved, this is not sufficient; consistent and effective use is essential for success in elderly adults. Abdolhakim Jorbonyan and colleagues [3] demonstrated in Persian adult participants that the use of questionnaires, such as MARS-HA, may provide a better understanding of the level of self-efficacy in using hearing aids; higher self-efficacy in the technical-auditory and psychosocial field was associated with greater hearing aid acceptance and successful use.

In general, hearing-impaired people prefer hearing aids that match their skin color to be less noticeable in their environment. However, over-the-counter hearing aids are only widely available in relatively lighter beige colors, with limited availability for BIPOC (Black, Indigenous, and People of Color) individuals with darker skin colors; this fact may contribute to a relatively inequitable over-the-counter hearing aid device offering to individuals who have mild-to-moderate hearing loss and darker skin colors [4].

Auditory processing disorder in children is a condition in which the brain has difficulty processing and interpreting sounds, particularly speech. Questionnaires and behavioral checklists have been reported in the international literature to pinpoint those children who may be susceptible to auditory processing disorder. The Greek version of these questionnaires has been applied in Greek Cypriot-speaking children [5], and they have aided in identifying children at risk of auditory processing disorder, providing a valuable tool for family counselling.

Congenital cytomegalovirus-related hearing loss is the most prevalent non-genetic cause of pediatric sensorineural hearing loss [6]. Nicoleta Gana and colleagues [7], in a detailed review, described the diagnostic approaches and management strategies employed for congenital cytomegalovirus-related hearing loss; they underlined the need for prompt detection of hearing loss and interdisciplinary care for treatment.

Up to 93% of patients undergoing cisplatin chemotherapy may develop hearing loss, which may result in a decreased quality of life in cancer survivors [8]. In their study, Alexandru Orasan and colleagues [9] reported on otoprotective substances, including antioxidants, anti-inflammatory agents, apoptosis inhibitors, intratympanic injection of N-acetylcysteine, and nanoparticle-based systems; sound conditioning and epigenetic drugs may be used to prevent hearing loss and modulate gene expression.

The treatment of hearing loss is one of the main challenges addressed in this Special Issue, and five papers are devoted specifically to this topic. First, Pawel Rozbicki and colleagues [10] underlined the beneficial effect of the early initation (less than 10 days) of hyperbaric oxygen in up to 15 cycles for the treatment of sudden sensorineural hearing loss. Joan Lorente-Piera and colleagues [11] demonstrated the effectiveness of Vibrant Soundbridge for the treatment of conductive, mixed, or sensorineural hearing loss, especially at higher frequencies; notable hearing amplification was achieved with the placement of the floating mass transducer in the coupling of round and oval windows, ensuring the more efficient transmission of vibrations to the cochlear fluids. Oana Astefanei and colleagues [12] in their comprehensive article concluded that both cochlear implants and bone conduction implants may have a beneficial effect in children and adults with single-sided deafness and asymmetric hearing loss. Mastoid cavity obliteration with the use of a temporoparietal fascial flap injected using injectable platelet-rich fibrin in patients who underwent subtotal petrosectomy for cochlear implantation was first described by Aleksander Zwierz and colleagues [13]. Using a mouse model, David Bächinger and colleagues [14] reported electrophysiological findings that may help to enhance hearing preservation during cochlear implantation; they provided evidence indicating that the more basally a cochlear trauma is located, the larger the cochlear microphonic amplitude drops.

There are a number of gaps in our knowledge in the field of audiology and otology, requiring continued research into early diagnosis, intervention, and individualized strategies. We hope that the articles published in this Special Issue advance our understanding of hearing loss and provide an update on new aspects of clinical practices, novel therapeutic approaches, and surgical techniques.

Conflicts of Interest: The authors declare no conflicts of interest.

References

1. Laureyns, M.; Pugliese, G.; Freyaldenhoven Bryan, M.; Willekens, M.; Gasbarre, A.M.; Zanetti, D.; Gilson, J.; Van Doren, P.; Di Berardino, F. Multicenter Study on the Impact of the Masker Babble Spectrum on the Acceptable Noise Level (ANL) Test. *Audiol. Res.* **2024**, *14*, 1075–1083. [CrossRef] [PubMed]
2. Marcotti, A.; Silva-Letelier, C.; Galaz-Mella, J.; Ianiszewski, A.; Vargas, N.B.; Fuentes-López, E. Association Between Unaided Speech Perception in Noise and Hearing Aid Use Mediated by Perceived Benefit. *Audiol. Res.* **2025**, *15*, 50. [CrossRef] [PubMed]

3. Jorbonyan, A.; Momtaz, Y.A.; Foroughan, M.; Mehrkian, S. Translation, Cross-Cultural Adaptation, and Psychometric Properties of the Persian Version of the Measure of Audiologic Rehabilitation Self-Efficacy for Hearing Aids (P-MARS-HA). *Audiol. Res.* **2025**, *15*, 31. [CrossRef] [PubMed]
4. Kirjava, S.A.; Faulkner, S.J. Over-the-Counter (OTC) Hearing Aid Availability across the Spectrum of Human Skin Colors. *Audiol. Res.* **2024**, *14*, 293–303. [CrossRef] [PubMed]
5. Drosos, K.; Tafiadis, D.; Voniati, L.; Papanicolaou, A.; Thodi, C. Preliminary Validation of the Children's Auditory Performance Scale (CHAPS) and the Auditory Processing Domain Questionnaire (APDQ) in Greek Cypriot Children. *Audiol. Res.* **2024**, *14*, 625–639. [CrossRef] [PubMed]
6. Belcher, R.; Virgin, F.; Duis, J.; Wootten, C. Genetic and Non-genetic Workup for Pediatric Congenital Hearing Loss. *Front Pediatr.* **2021**, *9*, 536730. [CrossRef] [PubMed]
7. Gana, N.; Huluță, I.; Cătănescu, M.-Ș.; Apostol, L.-M.; Nedelea, F.M.; Sima, R.-M.; Botezatu, R.; Panaitescu, A.M.; Gică, N. Congenital Cytomegalovirus-Related Hearing Loss. *Audiol. Res.* **2024**, *14*, 507–517. [CrossRef] [PubMed]
8. Waissbluth, S.; Daniel, S.J. Cisplatin-induced ototoxicity: Transporters playing a role in cisplatin toxicity. *Hear Res.* **2013**, *299*, 37–45. [CrossRef] [PubMed]
9. Orasan, A.; Negru, M.-C.; Morgovan, A.I.; Fleser, R.C.; Sandu, D.; Sitaru, A.M.; Motofelea, A.-C.; Balica, N.C. Strategies to Mitigate Cisplatin-Induced Ototoxicity: A Literature Review of Protective Agents, Mechanisms, and Clinical Gaps. *Audiol. Res.* **2025**, *15*, 22. [CrossRef] [PubMed]
10. Rozbicki, P.; Usowski, J.; Krzywdzińska, S.; Jurkiewicz, D.; Siewiera, J. Assessing the Effectiveness of Different Hyperbaric Oxygen Treatment Methods in Patients with Sudden Sensorineural Hearing Loss. *Audiol. Res.* **2024**, *14*, 333–341. [CrossRef] [PubMed]
11. Lorente-Piera, J.; Manrique-Huarte, R.; Lima, J.P.; Calavia, D.; Manrique, M. Middle Ear Active Implant Indications, Comparative Audiometric Results from Different Approaches, and Coupling with the Vibrant Soundbridge®: A Single Center Experience over More Than 20 Years. *Audiol. Res.* **2024**, *14*, 721–735. [CrossRef] [PubMed]
12. Astefanei, O.; Martu, C.; Cozma, S.; Radulescu, L. Cochlear and Bone Conduction Implants in Asymmetric Hearing Loss and Single-Sided Deafness: Effects on Localization, Speech in Noise, and Quality of Life. *Audiol. Res.* **2025**, *15*, 49. [CrossRef]
13. Zwierz, A.; Masna, K.; Burduk, P.; Hackenberg, S.; Scheich, M. Renewed Concept of Mastoid Cavity Obliteration with the Use of Temporoparietal Fascial Flap Injected by Injectable Platelet-Rich Fibrin after Subtotal Petrosectomy for Cochlear Implant Patients. *Audiol. Res.* **2024**, *14*, 280–292. [CrossRef]
14. Bächinger, D.; Schär, M.; Kunut, A.; Bertschinger, R.; Dobrev, I.; Sijgers, L.; Eckhard, A.H.; Dalbert, A. Impact of Cochlear Trauma Degree and Localization on Intracochlear Electrocochleographic Recordings. *Audiol. Res.* **2025**, *15*, 74. [CrossRef] [PubMed]

audiology research

MDPI

Article

Multicenter Study on the Impact of the Masker Babble Spectrum on the Acceptable Noise Level (ANL) Test

Mark Laureyns [1,2], Giorgia Pugliese [3,4,*], Melinda Freyaldenhoven Bryan [5], Marieke Willekens [1], Anna Maria Gasbarre [4], Diego Zanetti [3,4], Julien Gilson [6], Paul Van Doren [2] and Federica Di Berardino [3,4]

1 Audiology Department, Thomas More University College, 2800 Antwerp, Belgium; mark.laureyns@amplifon.com (M.L.)
2 Amplifon Centre for Research & Studies, 20141 Milan, Italy
3 Department of Clinical Sciences and Community Health, University of Milan, 20122 Milan, Italy; diego.zanetti@unimi.it (D.Z.); federica.diberardino@unimi.it (F.D.B.)
4 Department of Surgical Sciences, Audiology Unit, Fondazione IRCCS Ca' Granda, Ospedale Maggiore Policlinico, 20122 Milan, Italy; annamaria.gasbarre@policlinico.mi.it
5 School of Communication Science & Disorders, Louisiana Tech University, Ruston, LA 71272, USA; melinda@latech.edu
6 Audiology Department, Marie Haps University College, 1050 Brussels, Belgium
* Correspondence: giorgia.pugliese@unimi.it

Abstract: Introduction: Acceptable Noise Level (ANL) is defined as the most comfortable level (MCL) intensity for speech and is calculated by subtracting the maximum noise tolerable by an individual. The ANL test has been used over time to predict hearing aid use and the impact of digital noise reduction. This study analyzes this impact by using different masker babble spectra when performing the ANL test in both hearing-impaired and healthy subjects in three different languages (Dutch, French, and Italian). Materials and Methods: A total of 198 patients underwent the ANL test in their native language using a standardized protocol. The babble file was speech-weighted to match the long-term spectrum of the specific ANL language version. ANL was proposed in three different masking conditions: with multitalker Matched babble speech noise, with the same masking signal with the spectrum reduced from 2 kHz onwards (High Cut), and with the spectrum increased from 2 kHz onwards (High Boost). Results: In all of the comparisons among the three languages, ANL with High Boost noise gave significantly higher (worse) scores than ANL with Matched noise (p-value S1: <0.0001, S2: <0.0001, S3: 0.0003) and ANL with High Cut noise (p-value S1: 0.0002, S2: <0.0001, S3: <0.0001). The ANL values did not show any significant correlation with age and gender. In French, a weak correlation was found between ANL with High Cut noise and the Fletcher index of the worst ear. In Italian, a weak correlation was found between both ANL with Matched and High Boost noise and the Fletcher index of the best ear. Conclusions: ANL with High Boost added to noise stimuli was less acceptable for all patients in all of the languages. The ANL results did not vary in relation to the patients' characteristics. This study confirms that the ANL test has potential application for clinical use regardless of the native language spoken.

Keywords: acceptable noise level; ANL test; noise tolerance in hearing impairment; hearing impairment ANL; ANL test masker babble spectrum

1. Introduction

The first version of the Acceptable Noise Level (ANL) test was developed in 1991 by Nabelek et al. [1]. ANL is calculated by defining the most comfortable level (MCL) intensity for continuous speech selected by an individual and subtracting the maximum background noise level (BNL) that the individual is willing to put up with while listening to the speech. The first objective of the ANL test was to predict hearing aid use [2]. In 2013, Eddins et al. and, in 2019, Shetty et al. demonstrated that ANL is also a predictor of the impact of digital noise reduction (DNR) when using hearing aids [3,4]. Aided ANLs were significantly better (lower) with DNR for subjects with high (poor) ANLs but not for subjects with low (good) ANLs.

Most of the literature regarding ANL shows that ANL does not relate to the grade of hearing loss, age, and gender. In 2012, Olsen et al. [5] investigated the Danish version of ANL, demonstrating its correlation with hearing loss (Pure Tone Audiometry—PTA—in the best ear). Despite this, the correlation was weak, it only occurred in the first ANL session, and the ANL procedure was not standardized; in fact, the test was conducted with the aid of headphones, analyzing each ear independently, and it was striking that the ANL masker babble spectrum did not match the spectrum of the Danish ANL running speech.

We therefore conducted a multicenter study to evaluate the impact of the masker babble spectrum on the ANL test with a specific focus on the relationship between hearing loss and ANL results. The aim of the study is to define if the variations observed in ANL test results has a correlation with the type of masking babble speech noise used during the test, which was performed in three different languages in order to define if this masking effect could be modified by the different speech spectra of the different languages.

2. Materials and Methods

2.1. ANL Speech Material

Francart, Wouters et al. (KU–Leuven University—Belgium) developed 8 ANL files for the Amplifon Centre for Research and Studies, in which standard content was used as running speech and translated into 8 languages, read by a professional native speaker. The recording was performed at 25 dB FS (dB full scale) to ensure a good dynamic range and sound quality, and the average energy was kept at a constant speed. As ANL masker babble, "Auditec multitalker matched babble 20 talkers" was used. This babble file was speech-weighted to match the long-term spectrum of the specific ANL language version [6].

For this study, we created two extra masker babble signals for each language version, one where the spectrum was reduced from 2 kHz onwards (High Cut) and one version where the spectrum was increased from 2 kHz onwards (High Boost). This was performed for the Dutch (S1), French (S2), and Italian (S3) ANL versions; see Figure 1.

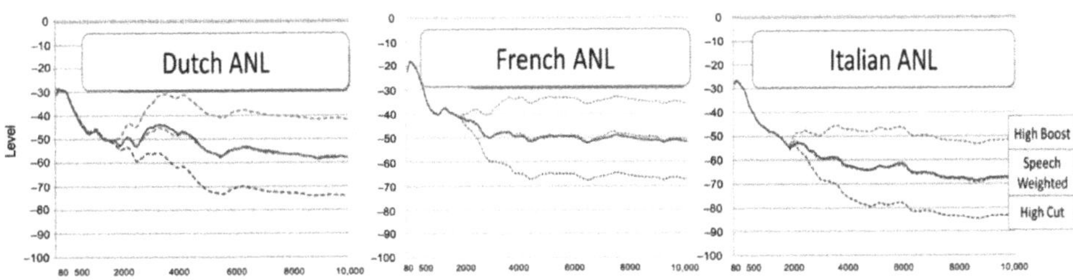

Figure 1. The long-term spectrum of the 3 language versions of the ANL test. High Boost masker babble files: top dotted lines; High Cut masker babble files: bottom dotted lines; speech-weighted masker babble files: middle dotted lines; running speech files: full lines. dBFS: dB Full Scale.

2.2. Equipment and Procedures

Audiometric thresholds, age, gender, and ANLs with 3 different masker babble files were collected for each listener in each of the three medical centers involved in the study.

ANL was performed in Free-Field, using one loudspeaker at 0° and at a one-meter distance from the listeners. The audiometer, Otometrics Aurical Aud, was calibrated according to ISO 8253-3:2012 [7], Acoustics—Audiometric test methods—Part 3: Speech audiometry, and calibration was checked at the listener's position before the experiment.

Participants were given the same instructions across the three centers. Instructions for the MCL level were written as follows: "I will play a story for you. I want you to signal me to increase/decrease the story to determine your most comfortable listening level. I will instruct you along the way. Ask me to increase or decrease the level of the story to a comfortable listening level for you. Imagine I am the volume control of your television set, and you want the volume to be adjusted so you can hear the television at a comfortable level all evening".

The instructions for assessing the BNL level were: "You will listen to the same story with background noise of several people talking at the same time. Tell us to adjust the noise to the MAXIMUM level that you would be willing to "put up with" for a long time while following the story".

Pure-tone audiometry was tested using an Optometric Aurical Aud with TDH 39 headphones with Silent Caps. The audiometers were calibrated according to ISO 8253-1:2010 standard [7],: Pure-tone air and bone conduction audiometry.

2.3. Study Population

This study involved three medical centers: Thomas More University College, Antwerp, Belgium (Dutch), Marie Haps University College, Brussels, Belgium (French), and the University of Milan, Milan, Italy (Italian). A total of 198 patients were involved in the study, subdivided as follows:

Dutch: 73 native Dutch (S1)-speaking subjects, divided into 3 subgroups:

- Group A: 25 hearing-impaired, aged subjects, reporting a "hearing problem", with a Fletcher index higher than 20 dBHL. The average age was 61.4 $\pm$ 18.08 s.d. years, with 40% being female and the average Fletcher index of the best ear being 35 $\pm$ 11.5 s.d. dBHL;
- Group B: 24 control subjects, with the same age and gender as group A, reporting "no hearing problems". The average age was 62.1 $\pm$ 16.52 s.d. years, with 40% being female and the average Fletcher index of the best ear being 11 $\pm$ 8.82 s.d. dBHL;
- Group C: 24 young normal hearing subjects, with a Fletcher index lower than 20 dBHL for each ear; the average age was 22.8 $\pm$ 10.7 s.d. years, with 80% being female and the average Fletcher index of the best ear being 6 $\pm$ 9.1 s.d. dBHL.

French: 90 native French (S2)-speaking subjects, divided into 3 subgroups:

- Group A: 30 hearing-impaired aged subjects, reporting hearing problems, with a Fletcher index higher than 20 dBHL. The average age was 70.9 $\pm$ 11.81 s.d. years, with 53% being female and the average Fletcher index of the best ear equal being 33 $\pm$ 12.19 s.d. dBHL;
- Group B: 30 control subjects, stating that they had no hearing problems. The average age was 57.5 $\pm$ 21.6 s.d. years, with 43% being female and the average Fletcher index of the best ear equal to 16 $\pm$ 3.89 s.d. dBHL;
- Group C: 30 young normal hearing subjects, with a Fletcher index that was lower than 20 dBHL for each ear; the average age was 24.8 $\pm$ 14.7 s.d. years, with 47% being female and the average Fletcher index of the best ear being 7 $\pm$ 12.3 s.d. dBHL.

Italian: 36 native Italian (S3)-speaking, hearing-impaired, aged subjects. They all reported having a hearing problem, and they all had a Fletcher index higher than 20 dBHL; the average age was 73.5 $\pm$ 14.9 s.d. years, with 50% being female and the average Fletcher index of the best ear equal to 50 dBHL (Group A). Group B and C were not included because they had been tested previously in another setting which is not comparable to providing the same results as Group A.

2.4. Statistical Procedures

For the statistical analysis, we used Graph Pad Prism 6 for Windows. The median ANL values were utilized to perform a comparison among the three centers, given that the data distribution was uneven at multiple sites. In order to take into account the unevenness of the ANL test results given the different masker babble spectra used, we used the paired t-test for data with a normal distribution and the Wilcoxon matched-pairs signed rank test for data that did not have a normal distribution. To evaluate the normality of the distribution, we used the D'Agostino and Pearson omnibus normality test. The correlation was calculated with the Pearson correlation test for data with a normal distribution and with the non-parametric Spearman correlation test for data that did not have a normal distribution.

This study received approval from the Ethical Committee of Fondazione IRCCS Ca' Granda Ospedale Maggiore Policlinico of Milan, Italy. Informed consent was obtained from all subjects involved in the study. (Protocol N. 478-2016bis). Patients' anonymity has been guaranteed.

3. Results

3.1. ANL for the Different Masker Babble Types

As reported in Figure 2, considering the total population for the 3 centers, ANL with High Boost noise was significantly higher (worse) than ANL with Matched noise median ANL values: 14 (Dutch), 12 (French), and 4 (Italian); (p-value S1: <0.0001, S2: <0.0001, and S3: 0.0003). The overall median ANL values and the Inter-Quartile Range (IQR) of each sub-group are reported in Table 1.

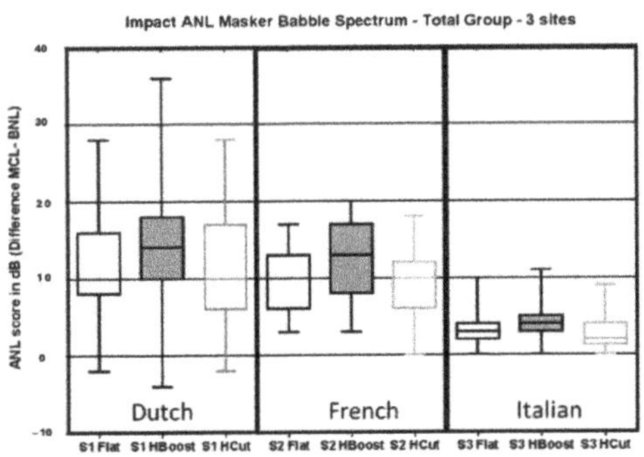

Figure 2. Box and whisker plot (representing the median value, the 25th and 75th percentiles, and the max and minimum values) with the ANL results for the total population at the 3 sites with different ANL masker types (Matched noise: black line with white filling; High Boost noise: black line with grey filling; High Cut noise: grey line with white filling).

Table 1. The median values and Inter-Quartile Range of the ANL in dB for the different sites, the different ANL masker types, and the different subgroups: A: hearing-impaired subjects; B: controls; C: normal hearing subjects.

		Median ANL (dB) (IQR)		
Group	**Masker Babble Spectrum**	**Dutch**	**French**	**Italian**
Total	Matched	10 (8–16)	9 (5–13)	3 (2–4)
	High Boost	14 (10–18)	12 (8–16)	4 (3–5)
	High Cut	10 (6–17)	8.5 (6–12)	2 (1.25–4)
A	Matched	10 (8–16)	10 (3–10)	
	High Boost	16 (8–18)	12.5 (3–12.5)	
	High Cut	12 (7–18)	10 (6.75–13)	

Table 1. *Cont.*

Group	Masker Babble Spectrum	Median ANL (dB) (IQR)		
		Dutch	French	Italian
B	Matched	11 (8–16)	8.5 (5–13)	
	High Boost	13 (8.5–16)	9.5 (7–17)	
	High Cut	11 (6–21.5)	8 (4.75–12)	
C	Matched	10 (8–18)	9.5 (4–13.25)	
	High Boost	16 (10.5–23.5)	12 (7.75–15.25)	
	High Cut	8 (6–14)	7.5 (4.75–12.25)	

ANL with High Boost noise was also significantly higher (worse) than ANL with High Cut noise in all languages (p-values < 0.05). ANL with High Cut noise provided similar results to the Matched noise in Dutch and French (p-values > 0.05), whereas in the Italian language, ANL with High Cut noise provided significantly lower (better) results than ANL with Matched noise (p-value 0.002).

Considering the subgroups, we found that in Dutch and French:

In Group A, ANL with High Boost noise was significantly higher than ANL with Matched noise (p-values < 0.05) and was significantly higher than ANL with High Cut noise (p-values < 0.05); in contrast, there was no difference between ANL with High Cut noise and ANL with Matched noise (p-value > 0.05).

In Group B, ANL with High Boost noise was also significantly higher than ANL with Matched noise (p-values < 0.05) and significantly higher than ANL with High Cut noise in French (p-value < 0.0001), while there was no difference between ANL with High Cut noise and ANL with Matched noise (p-values > 0.05).

In Group C, ANL with High Boost noise was significantly higher than ANL with Matched noise (p-values < 0.0001) and was significantly higher than ANL with High Cut noise (p-values < 0.0001). Furthermore, ANL with High Cut noise was significantly lower (better) than ANL with Matched noise (p-values < 0.05). See Table 2 for the detailed p-values.

Table 2. Statistical comparison of the different ANL results based on the masker type for the different sites and for the different subgroups: A: hearing-impaired subjects; B: controls; C: normal hearing subjects. HB: High Boost; HC: High Cut; ns: not statistically significant (p-value > 0.05).

Group	Masker Babble Spectrum	*p*-Value		
		Dutch	French	Italian
Total	HB vs. Matched	0.0001	0.0001	0.0003
	HB vs. HC	0.0002	<0.0001	<0.0001
	HC vs. Matched	Ns	ns	0.02

Table 2. *Cont.*

		p-Value		
Group	**Masker Babble Spectrum**	**Dutch**	**French**	**Italian**
A	HB vs. Matched	0.03	<0.0001	
	HB vs. HC	0.008	<0.0001	
	HC vs. Matched	Ns	ns	
B	HB vs. Matched	0.06	<0.0001	
	HB vs. HC	Ns	<0.0001	
	HC vs. Matched	Ns	ns	
C	HB vs. Matched	<0.0001	<0.0001	
	HB vs. HC	<0.0001	<0.0001	
	HC vs. Matched	0.008	0.02	

3.2. ANL and Age

For the total population, none of the ANL values correlated with age at any of the centers, as shown in detail in Table 3.

Table 3. Correlation *p*-values for the 3 sites between the 3 types of ANL and age, gender, and hearing loss (Fletcher index and Fletcher high index) for the best (B) and the worst (W) ear. Black font: Pearson *p*; grey font: Spearman *p*. Note that the *p*-values * that are underlined and in bold font represent significant *p*-values.

		Correlation (*p*-Value)		
	Masker Bubble Spectrum	**Dutch**	**French**	**Italian**
Age	Matched	0.92	0.64	0.09
	High Boost	0.15	0.83	0.21
	High Cut	0.26	0.43	0.32
Gender	Matched	0.64	0.64	0.27
	High Boost	**0.047 ***	0.83	0.19
	High Cut	0.97	0.43	0.31
Fletcher Index B	Matched	0.69	0.81	**0.038 ***
	High Boost	0.38	0.85	**0.029 ***
	High Cut	0.72	0.16	0.08
Fletcher High B	Matched	0.67	0.89	0.27
	High Boost	0.12	0.88	0.41
	High Cut	0.63	0.28	0.72
Fletcher Index W	Matched	0.77	0.32	0.22
	High Boost	0.47	0.42	0.21
	High Cut	0.75	**0.034 ***	0.44
Fletcher High W	Matched	0.85	0.24	0.46
	High Boost	0.24	0.56	0.66
	High Cut	0.56	0.05	0.97

3.3. ANL and Gender

For the total population, a weak correlation (Spearman $p = 0.047/r = 0.24$) was found in Dutch (Antwerp—Site 1) for ANL with High Boost and gender. The other ANLs did not correlate with gender. At the other two sites, no correlation was found (Table 3).

3.4. ANL and Hearing Loss

In Dutch, no correlation between ANL and hearing loss was found. In French, a weak correlation was found between ANL with High Cut noise and the Fletcher index of the worst ear (Spearman $p = 0.034/r = 0.22$). In Italian, a weak correlation was found between ANL with Matched noise and the Fletcher index of the best ear (Pearson $p = 0.038/r = 0.35$) and between ANL with High Boost noise and the Fletcher index of the best ear (Pearson $p = 0.029/r = 0.36$). See Table 2 for details.

4. Discussion

The primary application of the ANL test is to objectively quantify noise tolerance in hearing-impaired patients. This feature makes it a valuable parameter in the evaluation of patients prior to hearing aid use [2,8]. Evaluation of the background noise level in these patients is important when setting the parameters in hearing aids, such as noise reduction circuit, microphone sensitivity, and gain [9,10]. This is especially true for those patients who are unwilling to accept noise, helping to reduce the rejection rate of hearing aids; therefore, it can predict the impact of digital noise reduction (DNR) when using hearing aids [3,4,11].

For as much as it is known in the literature at present, ANL results do not seem to be influenced by listener characteristics such as gender, pure-tone average, or language spoken [12,13]. The results of our study are consistent with these data: ANL values did not show any correlation with gender, hearing acuity, and language. Recently, Shetty et al. observed that listening effort increases with age, especially in noisy environments. Despite this, our data did not show any correlation between ANL and age [14].

In 2006, Freyaldenhoven et al. investigated how the type of background noise affects ANL outcomes in normal hearing patients [15]. In accordance with their findings, we observed that the type of masking noise influenced the ANL outcome in all three different languages analyzed. In particular, High Boost noise showed higher values of ANL, regardless of any other patient characteristic considered. The worsening of High Boost noise could be attributed to the difficulties of consonant detection in noise in all of the languages. Likewise, High Cut noise provided significantly better values compared to the Matched noise in the Italian language. Since the Italian speaking frequency is much more targeted on the 2–4 kHz frequencies, we could speculate that this difference is attributable to the different speaking frequency ranges of these three languages. With High Cut noise, in French and Dutch, only young, normal hearing subjects (Group C), who are those more able to detect high frequencies, slightly performed better than with Matched noise, thus supporting this hypothesis.

To the authors' knowledge, this is the first study analyzing the different masking noise effects on ANL values in normal hearing and impaired subjects. The results highlight the ever-worsening contribution of high frequencies in masking noise in all subjects.

Conversely, in 2007, Pyler et al. varied the speech and noise stimuli in ANL with a low-pass filter at 2.0 kHz and 6.0 kHz, showing that ANL was significantly poorer when the speech and noise stimuli were low-pass filtered at 2.0 kHz in relation to the 6.0 kHz condition [16]. Furthermore, the results show that ANL values were not significantly affected by the hearing sensitivity of the listeners. These data are in contrast with what was previously reported in the literature, which showed the sensitivity of ANL in diagnosing hearing loss [5]. Recruitment differences could be a possible explanation for this finding.

The preliminary results of this study may allow us to think that the introduction of high frequencies in noise is the most important condition affecting ANL results, regardless of the grade of hearing impairment. The burden brought by high frequencies in making noise less tolerable by patients, and thus in compromising the ANL value, should be taken into account considering that environmental noise can widely differ in frequency range. This could be a point for further investigation when talking about the noise reduction circuits of hearing aids.

5. Conclusions

Acceptable Noise Level is an objective test to quantify noise tolerance in both hearing-impaired patients and healthy patients. The results do not vary in relation to patient characteristics such as age or gender. As long as standardized protocols and speech-weighted babble files are used, the language spoken does not influence ANL values; thus, its application can provide objective results in predicting hearing aid use worldwide. Varying the spectrum of the masker babble on the ANL significantly influences the test values when high frequencies are introduced to the noise stimuli. Further investigations should focus on the weight brought by high frequencies in making noise less tolerable for patients who are willing to use hearing aids.

Author Contributions: Conceptualization, M.L., F.D.B., M.F.B., M.W., J.G. and P.V.D.; methodology, M.L., F.D.B. and M.F.B.; software, M.W. and A.M.G.; validation, D.Z.; formal analysis, M.W. and A.M.G.; investigation, M.L., F.D.B. and M.F.B.; resources, F.D.B., M.F.B. and M.W.; data curation, G.P., M.W. and A.M.G.; writing—original draft preparation, M.L., G.P. and M.F.B.; writing—review and editing, F.D.B. and G.P.; visualization, M.L., F.D.B., M.W. and D.Z.; supervision, M.L. and M.F.B.; project administration, J.G. and P.V.D. All authors have read and agreed to the published version of the manuscript.

Funding: This research received no external funding.

Institutional Review Board Statement: The study was conducted in accordance with the Declaration of Helsinki and approved by the Ethics Committee of FONDAZIONE IRCCS CA' GRANDA OSPEDALE MAGGIORE POLICLINICO of Milan, Italy (Protocol N. 478-2016bis).

Informed Consent Statement: Informed consent was obtained from all subjects involved in the study.

Data Availability Statement: The data presented in this study are available from the corresponding author upon request due to our privacy policy.

Conflicts of Interest: The authors declare no conflicts of interest.

References

1. Nabelek, A.K.; Tucker, F.M.; Letowski, T.R. Toleration of background noises: Relationship with patterns of hearing aid use by elderly persons. *J. Speech Hear. Res.* **1991**, *34*, 679–685. [CrossRef] [PubMed]
2. Nabelek, A.K.; Freyaldenhoven, M.C.; Tampas, J.W.; Burchfiel, S.B.; Muenchen, R.A. Acceptable noise level as a predictor of hearing aid use. *J. Am. Acad. Audiol.* **2006**, *17*, 626–639. [CrossRef] [PubMed]
3. Eddins, D.; Klein, A.; Arnold, M.; Ellison, J. Acceptable Noise Level: Effect of Presentation Level, Digital Noise Reduction, and Stimulus Type. Poster Presented at the American Auditory Society. 2013. Available online: https://starkeypro.com/pdfs/research-briefs/Acceptable-Noise-Level-poster.pdf (accessed on 2 October 2024).
4. Shetty, H.N.; Nanjundaswamy, N.B. The Effect of Digital Noise Reduction on Annoyance and Speech Perception in Low and High Acceptable Noise Level Groups. *Int. Arch. Otorhinolaryngol.* **2019**, *23*, e433–e439. Available online: https://www.thieme-connect.com/products/ejournals/abstract/10.1055/s-0039-1688811 (accessed on 2 October 2024). [CrossRef] [PubMed]
5. Olsen, S.Ø.; Lantz, J.; Nielsen, L.H.; Brännström, K.J. Acceptable noise level (ANL) with Danish and non-semantic speech materials in adult hearing-aid users. *Int. J. Audiol.* **2012**, *51*, 678–688. [CrossRef] [PubMed]
6. Koch, X.; Dingemanse, G.; Goedegebure, A.; Janse, E. Type of Speech Material Affects Acceptable Noise Level Test Outcome. *Front. Psychol.* **2016**, *7*, 186. [CrossRef] [PubMed]
7. ISO 8253-1:2010 Standard, Acoustics—Audiometric Test Methods—Part 1. Available online: https://www.iso.org/obp/ui/#iso:std:iso:8253:-3:ed-2:v1:en (accessed on 2 October 2024).
8. Walravens, E.; Keidser, G.; Hartley, D.; Hickson, L. An Australian version of the acceptable noise level test and its predictive value for successful hearing aid use in an older population. *Int. J. Audiol.* **2014**, *53*, S52–S59. [CrossRef] [PubMed]
9. Shetty, H.N.; Subbanna, S. Acceptable noise level as a deciding factor for prescribing hearing aids for older adults with cochlear hearing loss—A scoping review. *J. Otol.* **2015**, *10*, 93–98. [CrossRef] [PubMed] [PubMed Central]
10. Plyler, P.N.; Hausladen, J.; Capps, M.; Cox, M.A. Effect of Hearing Aid Technology Level and Individual Characteristics on Listener Outcome Measures. *J. Speech Lang. Hear. Res.* **2021**, *64*, 3317–3329. [CrossRef] [PubMed]

11. Kim, J.H.; Lee, J.H.; Lee, H.K. Advantages of Binaural Amplification to Acceptable Noise Level of Directional Hearing Aid Users. *Clin. Exp. Otorhinolaryngol.* **2014**, *7*, 94–101. [CrossRef] [PubMed]
12. Rogers, D.S.; Harkrider, A.W.; Burchfield, S.B.; Nabelek, A.K. The influence of listener's gender on the acceptance of background noise. *J. Am. Acad. Audiol.* **2003**, *14*, 372–382. [CrossRef] [PubMed]
13. Ho, H.C.; Wu, Y.H.; Hsiao, S.H.; Stangl, E.; Lentz, E.J.; Bentler, R.A. The equivalence of acceptable noise level (ANL) with English, Mandarin, and non-semantic speech: A study across the U.S. and Taiwan. *Int. J. Audiol.* **2013**, *52*, 83–91. [CrossRef] [PubMed]
14. Shetty, H.N.; Raju, S.; Singh, S.S. The relationship between age, acceptable noise level, and listening effort in middle-aged and older-aged individuals. *J. Otol.* **2023**, *18*, 220–229. [CrossRef] [PubMed] [PubMed Central]
15. Freyaldenhoven, M.; Fisher Smiley, D.; Muenchen, R.; Konrad, T. Acceptable Noise Level: Reliability Measures and Comparison to Preference for Background Sounds. *J. Am. Acad. Audiol.* **2006**, *17*, 640–648. [CrossRef] [PubMed]
16. Plyler, P.N.; Madix, S.G.; Thelin, J.W.; Johnston, K.W. Contribution of high-frequency information to the acceptance of background noise in listeners with normal and impaired hearing. *Am. J. Audiol.* **2007**, *16*, 149–156. [CrossRef] [PubMed]

audiology research

MDPI

Article

Association Between Unaided Speech Perception in Noise and Hearing Aid Use Mediated by Perceived Benefit

Anthony Marcotti [1], Catherine Silva-Letelier [2], Javier Galaz-Mella [3], Alejandro Ianiszewski [1], Nicole B. Vargas [4] and Eduardo Fuentes-López [5,*]

1 Escuela de Fonoaudiología, Facultad de Ciencias de la Rehabilitación y Calidad de Vida, Universidad San Sebastián, Santiago 7510157, Chile; anthony.marcotti@uss.cl (A.M.); alejandro.ianiszewsk@uss.cl (A.I.)
2 Magister en Epidemiología, Escuela de Salud Pública, Facultad de Medicina, Pontificia Universidad Católica de Chile, Santiago 8330023, Chile; cpsilva5@uc.cl
3 Faculty of Rehabilitation Sciences, School of Speech Therapy, Exercise and Rehabilitation Sciences Institute, Universidad Andres Bello, Santiago 7591538, Chile; jigalaz@alumni.uc.cl
4 Facultad de Salud y Ciencias Sociales, Universidad de Las Américas, Viña del Mar 2531098, Chile; nvargas9@edu.udla.cl
5 Departamento de Fonoaudiología, Escuela de Ciencias de la Salud, Facultad de Medicina, Pontificia Universidad Católica de Chile, Santiago 7820436, Chile
* Correspondence: eduardo.fuentes@uc.cl; Tel.: +56-2-2354-1345

Abstract: Background/Objectives: The conventional strategy for addressing age-related hearing loss is hearing aid (HA) use, yet many individuals underutilize their devices. Despite the positive effects of HA use, adherence remains low, highlighting the importance of studying associated variables. We hypothesize that better unaided speech perception in noise (SPiN) would be associated with greater perceived benefit from HAs, which, in turn, would be linked to increased HA use. **Methods**: A cross-sectional study design was used, including 114 older adults ($\geq$65 years) who were HA users. HA use and perceived benefit were assessed using questions 1 and 2 of the International Outcome Inventory for Hearing Aids (IOI-HAs), while unaided SPiN performance was measured monaurally with a speech-in-noise test. In the mediation analysis, SPiN performance was the predictor, perceived benefit the mediator, and HA use the outcome. Direct and indirect effects were evaluated using generalized structural equation modeling. **Results**: No significant total effect was found for the right ear. For the left ear, there was a significant indirect effect of SPiN performance on HA use through perceived benefit (OR = 1.26, 95% CI 1.06–1.57, $p = 0.019$) but no direct effect ($p = 0.563$). In addition, a significant total effect of left ear SPiN performance on HA use was observed ($p = 0.041$). **Conclusions**: The findings suggest that unaided SPiN performance—particularly in the left ear—may be indirectly associated with HA use through its effect on perceived benefit. These results underscore the potential value of including SPiN assessments in the HA fitting process and counseling strategies for older adults.

Keywords: hearing aids; speech perception in noise; perceived benefit; older adults; auditory rehabilitation; mediation analysis

1. Introduction

The World Health Organization (WHO) estimates that 25% of older adults worldwide have disabling hearing loss [1]. Age-related hearing loss (ARHL) is a prevalent and potentially modifiable risk factor for adverse health outcomes. It is among the leading contributors to disability-adjusted life years (DALYs) [2] and is associated with increased social isolation [3], higher odds of depression [4], increased risk of falls [5], cognitive impairment [6], and dementia [6,7].

The conventional strategy for addressing ARHL is the use of hearing aids (HAs) [8–10]. Consistent utilization of HAs over time has been significantly associated with improvements in communication [11], generic and specific quality of life [12], and delayed onset of cognitive decline among individuals at risk [13]. Despite these benefits, the proportion of individuals prescribed HA who choose not to use them varies widely, ranging from 1% to 57% [14]. Furthermore, among those who do use them, up to 15% wear them for less than an hour a day [15]. Therefore, investigating the variables associated with HA non-use remains highly relevant.

The hours per day that a person uses their HA is commonly referred to as HA use [16]. Longer usage time is associated with a reduction in participation restrictions, better quality of life, and increased satisfaction and benefits with HA [17]. However, not all older adults who use HAs perceive benefits from their use [18]. Perceived benefit with HAs refers to the subjective assessment of a change in hearing function or communication ability obtained with the HAs [19]. Perceived benefit is associated with HA use [20,21], and, specifically among older adults, the lack of perceived benefit has been identified as one of the main reasons for HA abandonment [22–24].

Both HA use and perceived benefit with HAs are determined by a complex interplay of factors, as highlighted in a recent systematic review by Mothemela et al. [25]. This review identified several audiological factors, such as degree of hearing loss and type of HA fitting, and non-audiological factors, including age, cognitive status, social support, and self-efficacy with HA. Some of the variables identified, such as the degree of hearing loss, show associations with both HA use and perceived benefit with HAs, while others, for example, HA self-efficacy, have been linked only to HA use. Overall, these findings underscore the need to account for a broad range of factors when assessing and optimizing HA outcomes.

Among the various factors influencing HA use and perceived benefit, speech recognition ability is particularly noteworthy [25]. In older adults, difficulties in speech perception tend to increase with age, irrespective of ARHL severity [26]. Several studies have linked better unaided speech perception in quiet conditions to better perceived benefit and increased HA use [20,21,27,28]. Houmøller et al. [20], Wang et al. [21], and Chang et al. [27] demonstrated that higher word recognition scores (WRS)—that is, better speech perception—were associated with higher total scores on the International Outcome Inventory for Hearing Aids (IOI-HAs), which includes questions to assess both use and perceived benefit. Higher IOI-HAs scores indicate better outcomes in the domains evaluated by the instrument. In Wang et al.'s [18] study, the same association was found between WRS and Factor 1 of the IOI-HAs, which includes questions on use, perceived benefit, satisfaction, and quality of life. Additionally, Wu et al. [28] found that the better results of a speech recognition test were associated with both the Factor 1 score and the total score of the IOI-HAs.

However, despite the associations observed with speech perception tests conducted in quiet conditions, some studies have found that these relationships with HA use and perceived benefit outcomes are not sustained over time. Chang et al. [27] found this association in new HA users only one-month post-fitting but not after three months. A possible explanation for this is that speech perception measured in quiet conditions has low ecological validity and does not account for the complexities of real-world listening situations, such as background noise [29].

Older adults experience a decline in hearing performance as they age, which is particularly noticeable in their ability to understand speech in noisy environments [30]. Although the severity of ARHL is a key predictor of performance on tasks involving speech perception in noise (SPiN), research shows that age independently influences these outcomes [31]. In fact, even when controlling for the degree of ARHL, older adults perform significantly worse on behavioral SPiN tasks and report greater difficulties in noisy settings compared to younger adults [32]. These difficulties persist even with the use of HAs [33]. Given that challenges in SPiN can substantially impact daily communication, SPiN tests may offer a more accurate reflection of the real-world benefits that users could perceive with their HAs.

Walden and Walden [34] found that better performance on the unaided QuickSIN test in free-field conditions was associated with higher scores on the Hearing Aid Usefulness Scale (HAUS), an instrument that assesses patients' overall perception of the usefulness of their HAs in daily life, where higher scores indicate greater perceived usefulness. The QuickSIN test is a speech-in-noise measure that presents sentences embedded in fixed levels of multi-talker babble, allowing for the estimation of signal-to-noise ratio (SNR) loss based on the number of key words correctly repeated, where a lower SNR loss reflects better speech-in-noise perception [35].

On the other hand, in Mendel's [36] study, better performance on unaided SPiN measures—specifically, the Revised Speech Perception in Noise (R-SPIN), the Hearing in Noise Test (HINT), and the QuickSIN—was correlated with higher scores in certain dimensions of the Hearing Aid Performance Inventory (HAPI), an instrument designed to evaluate perceived benefit with HAs in various listening situations. Higher scores on the HAPI indicate greater perceived benefit. The R-SPIN test evaluates speech perception in noise by presenting sentences with high- and low-predictability contexts, where high-predictability sentences provide contextual cues to aid in understanding, while low-predictability sentences rely more on auditory processing [37]. In contrast, the HINT is an adaptive test that determines the signal-to-noise ratio (SNR) at which 50% of sentences are correctly repeated, using spectrally matched noise presented at a fixed level from different azimuth angles while adjusting speech intensity [38]. Together, these tests provide a comprehensive evaluation of speech perception in noise, which appears to be closely linked to the perceived benefits of HA.

The findings of Walden and Walden's [34] and Mendel's [36] studies suggest that unaided SPiN performance may predict the perceived benefits of HA. Walden and Walden [34] studied HA users with 2 months to 20 years of experience (mean = 5.3 years). Mendel [36], on the other hand, examined users with 6 months to 6 years of experience (mean = 1.7 years), suggesting that this association holds for both new and experienced users. However, the relationship between SPiN performance and actual HA use was not investigated.

Based on the findings described above, better unaided SPiN performance is associated with greater perceived benefit from HAs [34,36]. In turn, greater perceived benefit is associated with increased HA use [20,21]. However, previous research has not explicitly examined the potential mediated relationships among these variables. It is possible to hypothesize that better-unaided SPiN performance could be indirectly associated with increased HA use through greater perceived benefit. Therefore, the primary objective of the present study was to evaluate the direct and indirect associations—through perceived benefit with HAs—between unaided SPiN performance and HA use. Additionally, as observed with speech perception in quiet conditions [21,28], it is possible to hypothesize that there is, in turn, a direct association between SPiN performance and HA use. Consequently, the secondary objective was to examine the direct association between unaided

SPiN performance and HA use. This information could aid clinicians in the HA fitting process, especially when counseling new HA users regarding realistic expectations.

2. Materials and Methods

2.1. Study Design

The present study is a secondary data analysis of the clinical trial ISRCTN54021189 available at https://www.isrctn.com/ISRCTN54021189 (accessed on 3 March 2025). A cross-sectional analysis of the baseline measurements from the clinical trial was conducted. The study protocol received approval from the Ethical Scientific Committees at the Facultad de Medicina of the Pontificia Universidad Católica de Chile (180405001), Servicio de Salud Metropolitano Sur-Oriente (NO2886), and Servicio de Salud Metropolitano Sur (23-25042019) of the Metropolitan Region, Chile. All the participants provided informed consent. This study was reported in accordance with the Strengthening the Reporting of Observational Studies in Epidemiology (STROBE) guidelines [39].

Participants were recruited between October 2019 and October 2020, and evaluations were carried out between December 2019 and December 2020. All the assessments took place at Family Health Centers (CESFAM in Spanish), the most common type of primary health care (PHC) establishment in the Chilean public health system. Four centers from the municipalities of Puente Alto, San Bernardo, and San Joaquín in the Metropolitan Region, and one center from the municipality of Valparaíso in the Valparaíso Region participated in the study. The study anticipated no harm, adverse effects, or risks for the participants.

2.2. Participants

All the participants were older adults aged 65 or above who had received HAs through the Chilean public health system's Explicit Health Guarantees (GES) within the five years preceding the study. To be included in the study, participants needed to possess at least one functional HA. Additionally, they were required to have a normal cognitive status, demonstrated by a score of ≥22 on the Chilean-validated version of the Mini-Mental State Examination (MMSE) [40], which has previously been used in studies with similar populations [41], and no communication disorders of neurological origin.

The GES public policy provides HAs either for free or with a maximum copayment of 20%, depending on the health coverage of the beneficiary, to all adults aged 65 or older with bilateral hearing loss and a pure tone average (PTA) of ≥40 dB HL at the frequencies of 0.5, 1.0, 2.0, and 4.0 kHz [38]. Exceptionally, this policy also includes individuals with a PTA of ≥35 dB HL in the better ear, who have at least mild/moderate hearing difficulty, as evidenced by a score of ≥10 on the Shortened Hearing Handicap Inventory for the Elderly (HHIE-S). Health services operating under this policy are required to procure HAs through public tenders targeted at private companies. The HAs obtained through these tenders are of low range, with an average cost of USD 250 per unit, and have a minimum of 8 channels and up to 4 programs. All the devices are digital behind-the-ear (BTE) models, with no variability in device type or core technology across users. Minor differences, such as silicone or acrylic earmolds, are determined by audiological criteria and do not represent functional heterogeneity. The standard GES program provision includes only one HA, regardless of whether hearing loss is bilateral. However, if after one year the patient demonstrates consistent device usage, the GES program contemplates the provision of a second HA. Despite this regulation, it is common for patients to be unaware that they may qualify for a second device, resulting in continued use of only one HA. Thus, most of the study samples received monaural fittings. In practice, when only one device is provided, it is often placed in the right ear for practical reasons, as most users are right-handed and find it easier to manipulate the device on that side.

The list of beneficiaries of the GES policy from the past five years was accessed at each participating PHC center. Out of a total of 516 potential participants, 261 were assessed for eligibility. The remaining 255 were not evaluated because they could not be contacted (n = 116), declined to participate (n = 57), had moved to another city (n = 44), their families reported their death (n = 17), or for other reasons (n = 21). Of the subjects assessed for eligibility, 147 were excluded due to cognitive impairment (n = 48), malfunctioning HA (n = 39), lost HA (n = 17), and other reasons (n = 12). Additionally, some subjects decided not to participate after being assessed for eligibility (n = 31). Ultimately, 114 subjects participated in this study.

2.3. Variables

2.3.1. Predictor: Speech Perception in Noise (SPiN)

For the evaluation of SPiN, the Speech in Noise (SIN) test from the Santiago APD auditory processing battery [42] was used. This test consists of 4 lists of 25 monosyllabic words presented monaurally with ipsilateral white noise. Each ear was evaluated with 2 lists: one with a signal-to-noise ratio (SNR) of 10 dB and another at 0 dB. The test was administered at an intensity of 40 dB HL above the PTA, and the subject's task was to repeat the words they heard. Each correctly repeated word was scored as 4%, with a maximum performance score of 100%. For each ear, a single SPiN score was calculated as the average of the performances from the 10 dB and 0 dB SNR lists. This test was recorded in mp3 format with a quality of 320 kbps and played on a from Samsung Galaxy Note 10.1 Tablet (Seoul, South Korea), connected to the CD input of the audiometer using a 2 RCA to 3.5 mm Mini Jack cable. A Resonance® r27a audiometer (Gazzaniga, Bergamo, Italy) with Telephonics TDH-39 headphones (Santa Ana, CA, USA) was used. Calibration was performed according to the instructions of the Santiago APD battery by Auditec Inc (St. Louis, MO, USA) [42]: a track containing a 1000 Hz pure tone included in the test material was used to adjust the audiometer's VU meter to 0 dB, using channel 1 for the left ear and channel 2 for the right ear. In the absence of a soundproof booth, a consultation room at the participating establishments was designated and exclusively equipped for this study. Evaluations were scheduled during times when the ambient noise level did not exceed 45 dBA, as measured by an Amprobe SM-10 (Everett, WA, USA) sound level meter [43]. All the participants were assessed under these same conditions. Additionally, all the participants had already initiated HA use at the time of the SPiN testing.

Since the evaluations were conducted in PHC facilities rather than in controlled audiological environments, free-field testing was not feasible due to the lack of sound-treated rooms, calibrated speaker systems, and spatial setups typically required for accurate presentation [44]. In this context, monaural testing via headphones allowed for greater control over the presentation and enabled ear-specific performance to be assessed—particularly relevant given the variability in participants' HA configurations (unilateral right, unilateral left, or bilateral). Finally, the SPiN test itself was specifically developed for monaural presentation through headphones [42], further supporting the methodological approach used in this study.

2.3.2. Mediator: Perceived Benefit

To evaluate the perceived benefit with HAs, question 2 from the same IOI-HAs instrument [45] was used: "*Piense en una situación donde usted realmente hubiera querido escuchar mejor antes de obtener su(s) audífono(s) actual(es). En las últimas dos semanas, ¿cuánto le ha ayudado el (los) audífono(s) en esa situación?"* [*Think about the situation where you most wanted to hear better, before you got your present hearing aid*(s). Over the past two weeks, how much *has the hearing aid helped in that situation?*]". On an ordinal scale, the possible answers ranged from *"no ayudó (helped not at all)"*, *"ayudó poco (helped slightly)"*, *"ayudó moderadamente (helped moderately)"*, *"ayudó bastante (helped quite a lot)"*, *"ayudó mucho (helped very much)"*. The answers were coded from 5 points (i.e., *helped very much*) to 1 point (i.e., *helped not at all*).

2.3.3. Outcome: Hearing Aid Use

To evaluate HA use, question 1 of the Spanish version of the IOI-HAs [45] was used: *"Piense cuanto ha utilizado usted su(s) audífono(s) actual(es) en las últimas dos semanas. En un día común, ¿cuántas horas ha usado usted el(los) audífono(s)? [Think about how much you used your present hearing aid(s) over the past two weeks. On an average day, how many hours did you use the hearing aid(s)?]"*. Responses were measured on an ordinal scale ranging from *"ninguna (none)"*, *"menos de una hora al día (less than 1 h a day)"*, *"de 1 a 4 horas al día (1 to 4 h a day)"*, *"de 4 a 8 horas al día (4 to 8 h a day)"*, *to "más de 8 horas al día (more than 8 h a day)"*. The answers were coded from 5 points (i.e., more than 8 h a day) to 1 point (i.e., none).

2.4. *Covariables*

Sociodemographic information, health background, and other audiological variables were also collected to characterize the sample and control for potential confounding variables. The sociodemographic information included age, sex, years of formal education, monthly income, and number of cohabitants. Health background included general health perception, assessed with the following question: *"En general, ¿cómo describiría su salud? [In general, how would you describe your health?]", with response options ranging from "mala (bad)", "regular (alright)", "buena (good)", "muy buena (very good)", to "excelente (excellent)"*; monthly spending on medication; the number of chronic diseases by asking about common health conditions in the national older adult population: hypertension (*"¿Alguna vez un doctor o enfermera le ha dicho que tiene la presión alta, es decir, hipertensión? [Has a doctor or nurse ever told you that you have high blood pressure, that is, hypertension?]"*), diabetes (*"¿Alguna vez un doctor o enfermera le ha dicho que tiene diabetes, es decir, niveles altos de azúcar en la sangre? [Has a doctor or nurse ever told you that you have diabetes, that is, high blood sugar levels?]"*), osteoarticular problems (*"¿Alguna vez un médico le ha dicho que tiene artritis, osteoporosis, arthrosis, o problemas en articulaciones? [Has a doctor ever told you that you have arthritis, osteoporosis, osteoarthritis, or joint problems?]"*), and cardiac problems (*"¿Alguna vez un doctor o enfermera le ha dicho que ha tenido un ataque al corazón, una enfermedad coronaria, angina, o insuficiencia cardíaca? [Has a doctor or nurse ever told you that you have had a heart attack, coronary artery disease, angina, or heart failure?]"*).

All this information was collected using questions from the Chilean National Survey of Dependency in Older Adults (ENADEAM in Spanish) [46], an instrument previously utilized in similar studies [22,23,41,47,48]. Additionally, the risk of depression was assessed through the 15-item Yesavage Geriatric Depression Scale (GDS-15) [49]. This scale comprises 15 dichotomous (yes/no) questions designed to evaluate various dimensions of mental health, including mood, life satisfaction, energy levels, and anxiety. Higher scores on the GDS indicate a greater likelihood of depression.

Audiological variables included the PTA for frequencies 500, 1000, 2000, and 4000 Hz, HA implementation laterality, months of experience using HAs, and self-efficacy with HAs. The PTA, HA implementation laterality, and months of experience were obtained from clinical records. For the PTA, the record of the latest audiometric exam was considered. No subject had an audiometric exam older than one year. Self-efficacy was measured using the basic handling (7 items) and advanced handling (5 items) subscales from the Spanish version of the Measure of Audiologic Rehabilitation Self-Efficacy for Hearing Aids (S-MARS-HA) [47]. These subscales assess the individual's confidence in performing different tasks related to HA use. The S-MARS-HA responses were measured on a continuous scale from 0% (unable to perform the task) to 100% (completely confident in performing the task).

Additionally, although all the participants had a normal MMSE, the Addenbrooke's Cognitive Examination Revised (ACE-R) was used to provide a more detailed cognitive profile. All the questionnaires and instruments that needed to be completed directly by the participants were provided in printed format, with large, easy-to-read fonts. If necessary, an evaluator read the questions and their possible answers aloud, after which the participants responded verbally or indicated their response by pointing with their hand.

2.5. Statistical Analysis

The following variables were analyzed as categorical variables: HA use, perceived benefit with HAs, self-perception of health status, sex, and HA implementation laterality. Descriptive statistics for these variables included absolute and relative frequencies. The variables analyzed as numerical variables were SPiN, age, years of education, monthly income, number of cohabitants, number of chronic diseases, monthly spending on medication, risk of depression, months of experience using HAs, self-efficacy with HAs, cognitive profile, and PTA. Descriptive statistics were reported as absolute and relative frequencies for categorical variables, and median (p50) with interquartile range (p25–p75) for numerical variables. The Mann-Whitney U test was used for comparisons between the ears for PTA, SPiN, and experience using HAs.

To identify potential confounders related to HA use and perceived benefit with HAs, univariate ordinal regression models were estimated, and odds ratios (OR) were obtained as measures of association. Variables that showed a statistically significant association ($p < 0.1$) were included in a multivariate ordinal generalized structural equation model (GSEM). This GSEM consisted of two multivariate ordinal regression models: one for HA use and one for perceived benefit with HAs. These models were integrated into the GSEM framework to evaluate an indirect or mediated effect between SPiN performance and HA use, with perceived benefit as the mediating factor. Additionally, the variables of age, PTA, and cognitive status were incorporated into this model because, according to the literature, they are associated with both SPiN performance [31] and HA use and perceived benefit with HAs [25] and thus were controlled for in the analysis.

The mediation analysis included a direct path from SPiN (predictor) to HA use (outcome), as well as an indirect path from SPiN to perceived benefit with HAs (mediator), which then led to HA use (outcome). The total effect of SPiN on HA use was estimated by summing the direct and indirect effects. These estimations were conducted independently for the SPiN performance of each ear. The details of the model can be seen in Figure 1.

In the multivariate GSEM, the ordinal family and logit link were used, and the standard error was adjusted for clustering. An indirect (mediated) effect was considered present if the non-linear combination of the estimators—that is, the product of the path coefficient from SPiN performance to perceived benefit with HAs, and the path coefficient from perceived benefit with HAs to HA use—was statistically significant ($p < 0.05$) [46]. This procedure was conducted separately for each ear. The mediation model was carried out to avoid the presence of overadjustment bias in the total effect when the predictor and mediator variables are included in the multivariate ordinal regression model. Additionally, the mediated model allows for the decomposition of direct and indirect effects.

Effect sizes were reported as odds ratios with corresponding confidence intervals for both the direct and indirect pathways, as well as for the predictor–mediator and mediator–outcome pathways, following the recommendations outlined in the Guideline for Reporting Mediation Analyses of Randomized Trials and Observational Studies [50]. The guideline also indicates that reporting the proportion mediated is not always advisable, as there can be considerable uncertainty around it, especially in small samples. Thus, the focus should be on the indirect and direct effects. Additionally, VanderWeele [51] noted that the proportion mediated tends to be unstable and imprecise in small samples. In this study, given the limitations in sample size, the proportion mediated was not reported.

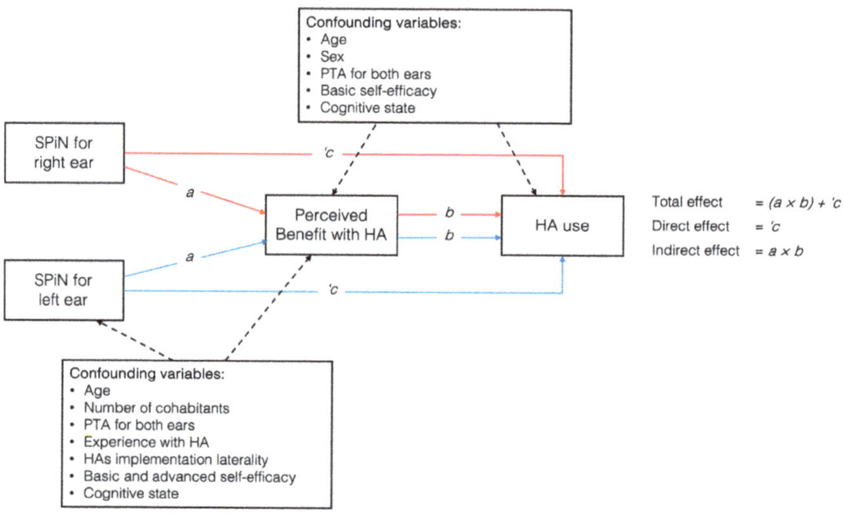

Figure 1. Proposed model of variable relationships between speech perception in noise (SPiN) and hearing aid use, mediated by perceived benefit, with covariates included for both ears. Note: HAs = hearing aids; PTA = pure tone average.

In addition, to conduct a sensitivity analysis of the results, the mediation model was re-estimated using the structural equation model (SEM) with partial least squares (PLS), considering the same variables used in the multivariate ordinal GSEM model. According to Venturini and Mehmetoglu [52], the use of this methodology is recommended for small sample sizes. The Monte Carlo method with 50,000 simulations was used to estimate 95% confidence intervals (95% CI). All the analyses were conducted using STATA v18 software. The "gsem" command of this software was used for GSEM estimation [53].

3. Results

3.1. Sample Description

Of the 114 participants, 57.98% (n = 66) were women. The median age was 79 years (p25–p75 = 73–85). A total of 55.75% (n = 63) of the participants used an HA only in the right ear. No significant differences were observed between the ears for PTA (p = 0.406), SPiN performance (p = 0.085), or months of experience with HA use (p = 0.156). The characteristics of the sample can be found in Table 1.

Table 1. Characteristics of the sample of Chilean older adults (n = 114) who were fitted with hearing aids in the public healthcare sector.

Variable		n (%) or p50 (p25–p75)
Women in the sample		66 (57.89)
Age in years		79 (73–85)
Years of education		6 (4–11)
Number of cohabitants		2 (2–3)
Self-perception of state of health		
	Excellent	5 (4.39)
	Very good	5 (4.39)
	Good	37 (32.46)
	Alright	49 (42.98)
	Bad	18 (15.79)
Number of chronic illnesses		2 (1–3)
Monthly income (in Chilean pesos)		$180,000 ($140,000–220,000)
Monthly spending on medication (in Chilean pesos)		$15,000 ($0–30,000)
Hearing aids implementation laterality		
	Only on right ear	63 (55.75)
	Only on left ear	33 (29.20)
	On both ears	17 (15.04)
Months of experience using hearing aids		24 (12–48)
Pure tone average		
	Right ear	62.5 (52.50–72.50)
	Left ear	61.3 (51.60–69.40)
Self-efficacy with hearing aids (S-MARS-HA)		
	Basic handling scale	77.1 (60–88.60)
	Advanced handling scale	70 (48–80)
Depression (GDS)		4 (2–7)
Cognitive state (ACE-R)		71.50 (59–80)

S-MARS-HA = Spanish version of Measure of Audiologic Rehabilitation Self-Efficacy for Hearing Aids; GDS = Yesavage Geriatric Depression Scale; ACE-R = Addenbrooke's Cognitive Examination—Revised.

3.2. SPiN Performance

In the right ear, the median performance at 10 dB SNR was 72% (p25–p75 = 44–80), while at 0 dB SNR, it was 68% (p25–p75 = 52–84). The median performance of the left ear at 10 dB SNR was 68% (p25–p75 = 48–80), while at 0 dB SNR, it was 68% (p25–p75 = 40–80). The median combined performance was 70% (p25–p75 = 44–82) for the right ear and 66% (p25–p75 = 44–80) for the left ear. The detailed distribution of these performances can be seen in Figure 2.

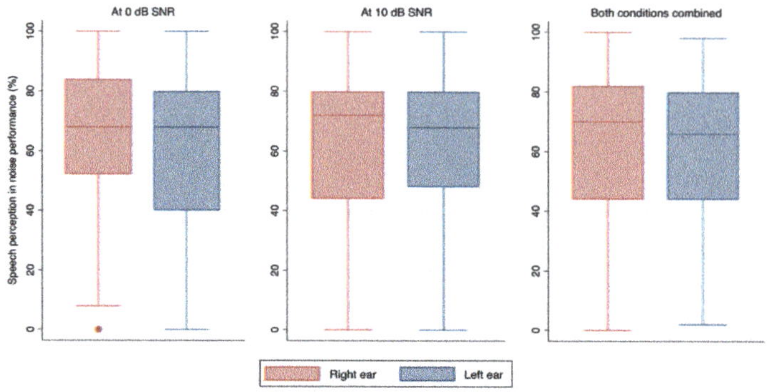

Figure 2. Median and 25th to 75th percentile of speech perception in noise performance at 0 dB and 10 dB SNR, and for both conditions combined for the left and right ears. Note: SNR = signal-to-noise ratio.

3.3. Perceived Benefit with HAs and HA Use

Regarding question 2 of the IOI-HAs, perceived benefit with HAs, the most frequent responses were "helped quite a lot", with 42.11% (n = 48), followed by "helped very much", with 25.44% (n = 29), and "helped moderately", with 13.16% (n = 15). The most frequent responses for question 1 of the IOI-HAs regarding HA use were "use for more than 8 h a day", with 47.37% (n = 54), "1 to 4 h a day", with 19.30% (n = 22), and "4 to 8 h a day", with 15.79% (n = 18). The details of these and other responses can be seen in Table 2.

Table 2. Absolute frequency and percentage of responses for questions 1 and 2 of the Spanish version of the IOI-HAs questionnaire.

Answer Category	Question 2 of IOI-HAs [b] n (%)	Question 1 of IOI-HAs [a] n (%)
1	12 (10.53)	16 (14.04)
2	10 (8.77)	4 (3.51)
3	15 (13.16)	22 (19.30)
4	48 (42.11)	18 (15.79)
5	29 (25.44)	54 (47.37)
Total	114 (100)	114 (100)

IOI-HAs = International Outcome Inventory for Hearing Aids. Statistically significant effects are marked in bold. [a] "Think about how much you used your present hearing aid(s) over the past two weeks. On an average day, how many hours did you use the hearing aids?" with possible answers 1: None, 2: Less than 1 h/day, 3: 1–4 h/day, 4: 4–8 h/day, 5: More than 8 h/day. [b] "Think about the situation where you most wanted to hear better, before you got your present hearing aid(s). Over the past two weeks, how much has the hearing aid helped in that situation?" with possible answers 1: Helped not at all, 2: Helped slightly, 3: Helped moderately, 4: Helped quite a lot, 5: Helped very much.

3.4. Variables Related to Outcome and Mediator

The results of the univariate ordinal regression models can be found in Table 3. Being female was negatively associated with the odds of advancing one category in HA use compared to being male (OR = 0.51, 95% CI 0.26–1.02; $p = 0.056$). Additionally, a positive association with HA use was observed both for each 10-point increase in the basic handling subscale of HA self-efficacy (OR = 1.16, 95% CI 0.97–1.39; $p = 0.097$) and for each category increase in perceived benefit with HAs (OR = 2.13, 95% CI 1.56–2.90; $p < 0.001$). Thus, greater self-efficacy and higher perceived *benefit were positively associated with increased HA use.*

In relation to perceived benefit with HAs, a negative association was observed with age, meaning that each additional year of age was associated with lower odds of reporting increased perceived benefit (OR = 0.93; 95% CI 0.89–0.98; p = 0.006). Conversely, perceived benefit increased significantly with each additional cohabitant in the household (OR = 1.51; 95% CI 1.09–2.08; $p = 0.013$) when using bilateral HAs compared to unilateral right-ear use (OR = 2.88; 95% CI 1.07–7.78; $p = 0.037$) and with each additional month of HA experience (OR = 1.01; 95% CI 1.00–1.01; $p = 0.046$). Higher self-efficacy scores in both basic (OR = 1.36; 95% CI 1.13–1.64; $p = 0.001$) and advanced handling of HAs (OR = 1.43; 95% CI 1.21–1.70; $p < 0.001$) also correlated positively with increased perceived benefit. Additionally, better SPiN performance in both the right ear (OR = 1.08; 95% CI 1.02–1.14; $p = 0.008$) and the left ear (OR = 1.19; 95% CI 1.11–1.27; $p < 0.001$) was associated with greater perceived benefit.

Regarding multivariate ordinal regression models, as the main outcome, HA use was solely and positively associated with perceived benefit with HAs (OR = 2.44; 95% CI 1.47–4.03; $p = 0.001$). This result corroborates that the effect of SPiN performance on HA use is primarily mediated, confirming the presence of overadjustment bias in the total effect when both the predictor and mediator variables are included in the multivariate ordinal regression model. In relation to perceived benefit with HAs, it was negatively associated with age (OR = 0.93; 95% CI 0.87–0.99; $p = 0.022$) and positively associated with SPiN for the left ear (OR = 1.29; 95% CI 1.09–1.48; $p = 0.001$). The rest of the variables that were significantly associated with both HA use and perceived benefit with HAs in the univariate models ceased to be significant.

Table 3. Univariate ordinal regressions for HA use and perceived benefit with HAs.

Variables	Univariate Model for HAs Use OR (95% CI)	*p*-Value	Univariate Model for Perceived Benefit OR (95% CI)	*p*-Value
Being a woman	**0.51 (0.26–1.02)**	**0.056**	1.13 (0.57–2.21)	0.731
Age in years	1.01 (0.97–1.06)	0.581	**0.93 (0.89–0.98)**	**0.006**
Years of education	0.97 (0.89–1.05)	0.428	1.01 (0.93–1.09)	0.885
Number of cohabitants	1.01 (0.75–1.37)	0.952	**1.51 (1.09–2.08)**	**0.013**
Self-perception of state of health				
Excellent	*Reference*	-	*Reference*	-
Very good	0.35 (0.02–5.03)	0.436	1.12 (0.13–9.47)	0.917
Good	0.48 (0.05–4.87)	0.534	1.36 (0.26–7.11)	0.719
Alright	0.19 (0.02–1.90)	0.158	0.79 (0.16–3.99)	0.778
Bad	0.19 (0.02–2.09)	0.175	0.42 (0.07–2.38)	0.327
Number of chronic illnesses	0.83 (0.52–1.30)	0.411	0.85 (0.54–1.35)	0.490
Monthly income (in Chilean pesos)	0.99 (0.99–1.00)	0.570	1.00 (0.99–1.00)	0.938
Months of experience with hearing aids	1.00 (1.00–1.01)	0.660	**1.01 (1.00–1.01)**	**0.046**
Monthly spending on medication (in Chilean pesos)	0.99 (0.99–1.00)	0.789	0.99 (0.99–1.00)	0.616
Hearing aids implementation laterality				
Only on right ear	*Reference*	-	*Reference*	-
Only on left ear	0.63 (0.29–1.40)	0.260	1.90 (0.85–4.22)	0.117
On both ears	2.11 (0.77–5.76)	0.147	**2.88 (1.07–7.78)**	**0.037**
Pure tone average (frequencies 500, 1000, 2000, and 4000 Hz)				
Right ear	1.02 (0.99–1.04)	0.183	1.02 (1.00–1.04)	0.117
Left ear	1.00 (0.97–1.02)	0.910	0.99 (0.96–1.02)	0.447
Self-efficacy with hearing aids (S-MARS-HA)				
Basic handling subscale [a]	**1.16 (0.97–1.39)**	**0.097**	**1.36 (1.13–1.64)**	**0.001**
Advanced handling subscale [a]	1.01 (1.00–1.03)	0.185	**1.43 (1.21–1.70)**	**<0.001**
Depression (Yesavage Geriatric Depression Scale)	1.07 (0.96–1.18)	0.219	0.95 (0.86–1.05)	0.303
Speech perception in noise test (SPIN test)				
On the right ear [b]	0.98 (0.93–1.04)	0.542	**1.08 (1.02–1.14)**	**0.008**
On the left ear [b]	1.02 (0.96–1.08)	0.570	**1.19 (1.11–1.27)**	**<0.001**
Cognitive state (Addenbrooke's Cognitive Examination—Revised)	0.99 (0.97–1.02)	0.485	1.00 (0.98–1.02)	0.966
Perceived benefit (Question N°2 from the IOI-HAs questionnaire)	**2.13 (1.56–2.90)**	**<0.001**	-	-

OR = odds ratio; CI = confidence interval; IOI-HAs: International Outcome Inventory for Hearing Aids; S-MARS-HA= Spanish version of Measure of Audiologic Rehabilitation Self-Efficacy for Hearing Aids. [a] Change expressed per 10-point increase. [b] Change expressed per 4-point increase. Note: Statistically significant variables with $p < 0.1$ are presented in bold.

3.5. Mediation Analysis

Figure 3 presents the mediation model with its respective coefficients. SPiN performance in the right ear did not present a significant total effect (OR = 0.91; 95% CI 0.77–1.05; $p = 0.228$) on HA use. In the left ear, a significant indirect effect (OR = 1.26; 95% CI 1.06–1.57; $p = 0.019$) and a significant total effect (OR = 1.20; 95% CI 1.00–1.41; $p = 0.041$) were observed but not a direct effect (OR = 0.96; 95% CI 0.83–1.09; $p = 0.563$). These findings were replicated through a sensitivity analysis using a SEM model with partial least squares, revealing a positive and significant indirect effect of the SPiN path on the left ear on HA use, through perceived benefit ($p < 0.001$). Similarly, the results for the right ear remained consistent, with SPiN showing no significant direct effect with HA use ($p = 0.095$), aligning with the main results (see Table S1). Thus, participants with better SPiN performance in the left ear had higher odds of advancing in perceived benefit categories, which translated into higher odds of advancing in HA use categories.

Following the recommendations of the Guideline for Reporting Mediation Analyses of Randomized Trials and Observational Studies [50], the proportion mediated was not reported. However, the findings suggest that the observed effect is primarily mediated. This is supported by the fact that once the mediator was included in the multivariate ordinal regression model, the effect of SPiN was no longer statistically significant, indicating that the direct pathway did not reach statistical significance and that the observed effect is primarily attributable to the indirect pathway.

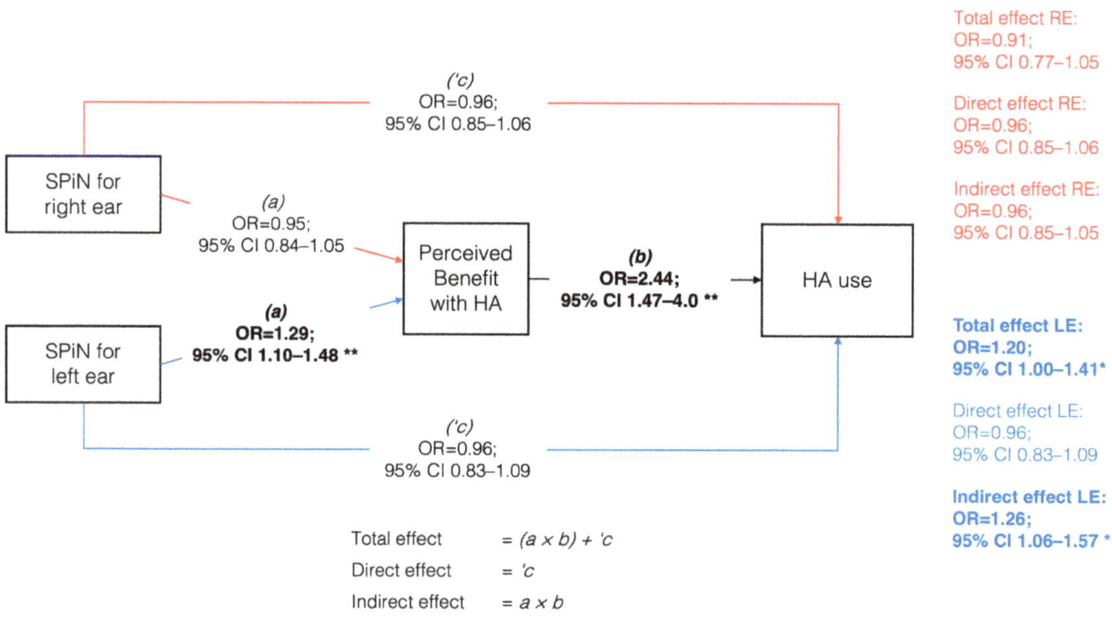

Figure 3. Generalized structural equation model between speech perception in noise (SPiN) for the right and left ear and hearing aids use, mediated by perceived benefit. Odds ratios expressed per 4-point change on SPiN. Note: RE = right ear; LE = left ear; OR = odds ratio; CI = confidence interval. * $p < 0.05$; ** $p < 0.01$. Bolded estimates indicate statistically significant effects.

4. Discussion

4.1. Mediated Association Between Unaided SPiN and HA Use

The primary objective of the present study was to evaluate the direct and indirect associations, through perceived benefit with HAs, between unaided SPiN performance and HA use. In our mediation analysis, SPiN performance was positively associated with perceived benefit, which, in turn, contributed to increased odds of HA use. Ear-specific effects were observed: whereas the SPiN performance in the right ear showed no significant total effect, a significant total effect was observed for the left ear, which was mainly mediated by perceived benefit (significant indirect effect).

The association between unaided SPiN performance and HA use, mediated through perceived benefit, had not been previously studied. However, prior research has demonstrated a relationship between SPiN performance and perceived benefit [34,36]. Mendel [36] examined 21 HA users aged 33 to 75 years, 17 of whom were bilateral users, with HA experience ranging from 6 months to 6 years (mean = 1.7 years). The study found a significant association between unaided SPiN performance and benefit-related questions from the HAPI questionnaire, specifically those assessing the perception of environmental sounds in quiet and noisy conditions, as well as conversations with both familiar and unfamiliar talkers. SPiN performance was measured using the R-SPIN, HINT, and QuickSIN, all presented in a free-field setup. However, Mendel [36] did not investigate potential associations between SPiN performance and HA use.

Walden and Walden [34] studied 50 adults aged 49 to 94 years, 39 of whom were bilateral HA users, with experience ranging from 2 months to 20 years (mean = 5.3 years). They found that better performance on the unaided QuickSIN test was associated with higher scores on the HAUS—that is, better perceived benefit. This scale estimates the patient's overall perception of the usefulness of their HA in daily life on a scale from 1 to 100. A score of 1 indicates, "My hearing aid(s) are of no use to me", while a score of 100 indicates, "My hearing aid(s) are so useful that they meet every need I have for them". Similar to Mendel's [36] study, the association between SPiN performance and HA use was not examined.

Similar to Mendel's [36] and Walden and Walden's [34] works, the participants in the present study had a wide range of experience using HA. Since this variable was significantly associated with perceived benefit with HAs in the univariate model, it was controlled for in the multivariate GSEM model. The association between SPiN performance and perceived benefit with HAs, as well as the indirect effect of SPiN on HA use, remained significant in the multivariate GSEM model. This finding suggests that unaided SPiN measures could serve as a reliable predictor of these HA outcomes in both new and experienced HA users, unlike unaided speech perception measures in quiet conditions, which have demonstrated significant associations only among new HA users [20,27].

In relation to HA experience, the recent systematic review by Mothemela et al. [25] identified only one study examining its association with HA use, and that study reported no significant relationship. Moreover, no studies were found that evaluated the link between HA experience and perceived benefit. In our study, longer-term HA experience—measured as the number of months using the device—was significantly associated with greater perceived benefit in the univariate analysis. This finding suggests that users may perceive more benefit as their experience with the device increases, potentially due to improved adaptation, greater familiarity with its features, or more effective integration into everyday communication. However, this relationship may also reflect reverse causality, whereby individuals who perceive greater benefit are more likely to continue using their HA consistently, thereby accumulating more months of use. Future longitudinal studies are needed to clarify whether extended HA use enhances perceived benefit or, conversely, whether perceived benefit encourages continued device use over time.

In contrast to the findings of this study, and those reported by Mendel [36] and Walden and Walden [34], Grunditz and Magnusson [54] did not find an association between SPiN performance and perceived benefit with HAs. These authors studied 102 subjects aged 24 to 91 years, 96 of whom were bilateral HA users, and all of whom were new users with 12 to 16 weeks of experience. The study employed a free-field SPiN test using monosyllabic words presented in the presence of an artificial noise signal. This noise had the same modulation properties as natural speech but was completely unintelligible and exhibited a speech-like spectrum, with an SNR of +6 dB. The SPiN performance in the unaided condition was not associated with Item 2 (perceived benefit with HAs) of the IOI-HAs. However, it was significantly associated with Item 3 (residual activity restriction), Item 5 (residual participation restriction), and Item 6 (impact on others), as well as with the total IOI-HAs score.

The discrepancy between the findings of Grunditz and Magnusson [54] and those of the present study, as well as Mendel [36] and Walden and Walden [34], may be attributed to differences in the type of SPiN test used. Grunditz and Magnusson used a speech recognition in noise test with a fixed, favorable SNR of +6 dB, which likely reduced the overall difficulty of the task. In contrast, Mendel [36] and Walden and Walden [34] utilized tests designed to determine the speech reception threshold, reaching more challenging SNRs—QuickSIN, for example, includes conditions as low as 0 dB SNR, and HINT is an adaptive test that adjusts to pinpoint the SNR at which 50% of the speech is correctly understood. In the present study, we used a SPiN test with two conditions—one at +10 dB and another at 0 dB—thus incorporating a more challenging SNR condition. More challenging SNR conditions may have greater ecological validity, given that real-world SNRs are rarely as favorable. In contrast, the relatively easier SNR condition used by Grunditz and Magnusson may have limited the test's sensitivity to variations in perceived benefit, contributing to the absence of an association between SPiN performance and perceived benefit with HAs.

On the other hand, the relationship between perceived benefit with HAs and HA use has also been demonstrated in previous studies [20,21]. In the study by Houmøller et al. [20], two groups were examined: 1090 new HA users and 417 experienced users (with more than 4 years of experience). In both groups, daily hours of HA use were significantly associated with Factor 1 of the IOI-HAs, which includes a question on perceived benefit. Similarly, Wang et al. [21] found that daily HA use was associated with better scores on Factor 1 of the IOI-HAs in a sample of 235 adult HA users with usage experience ranging from 3 months to 20 years.

Additionally, a lack of perceived benefit with HAs has been identified as one of the main reasons for discontinuation of HA use among older adults [22–24]. In a first retrospective cohort study, Fuentes-López et al. [22] investigated 355 older adult HA users. At 30 months post-fitting, the cumulative incidence of HA discontinuation was 21.7%, and among those who discontinued, 18.2% reported little or no perceived benefit. In a subsequent study with similar characteristics, Fuentes-López et al. [23] examined 455 older adult HA users with at least one year of HA use. Within this cohort, 18% of the participants had discontinued use of their devices; notably, among these individuals, 26.3% reported little or no perceived benefit. In both studies, the lack of perceived benefit was the most common reason for HA abandonment.

Iwahashi et al. [24] investigated two groups of adult HA users, subjects who had received their devices one year earlier and were invited to a follow-up and control session.

The first group comprised 200 subjects who attended the session, while the second group consisted of 108 who did not. In the first group, 13% discontinued HA use, and among those, 17% cited a lack of perceived benefit—the second most frequent reason for discontinuation. In the second group, 30.6% discontinued use, with 13.2% reporting a lack of perceived benefit, making it the third most common cause of HA discontinuation.

An unexpected finding in the present study was that the mediated relationship between unaided SPiN performance and HA use differed by ear. Specifically, only the SPiN performance in the left ear was significantly associated with HA use, even after adjusting for HA configuration (i.e., whether subjects used right unilateral, left unilateral, or bilateral adaptations). Previous studies examining the association between SPiN performance and perceived benefit with HAs [34,36,54], and between SPiN performance and HA use [54] employed psychoacoustic tests presented binaurally in a free-field setup. In contrast, the SPiN test used in the present study was administered monaurally via headphones, allowing for independent scoring for each ear.

Some studies have proposed that the auditory pathway responsible for left ear input may be more affected by aging than the right ear pathway, resulting in earlier and more pronounced declines in speech processing [55]. This hypothesis is supported by psychoacoustic [56,57] and electrophysiological studies [58–60], which show a weaker left ear for speech processing among older adults in both unaided and aided conditions [61]. Furthermore, research conducted on older adults has found that left ear SPiN scores tend to be lower than those for the right ear, particularly in the presence of background noise [61–63]. These interaural processing differences may compromise older adults' ability to use binaural cues for analyzing the spatial characteristics of complex acoustic environments [64], potentially leading to binaural interference. Such interference could reduce the actual benefits provided by HA and may ultimately contribute to decreased HA use [65,66].

Our study showed no significant differences in SPiN performance between the ears, suggesting reduced interaural asymmetry. We hypothesize that this balanced auditory processing led to improved binaural integration, which, in turn, enhanced the perceived benefit of HAs and ultimately increased their use, even when the device was not specifically used in the left ear. However, with our previous data, we cannot confirm this hypothesis because SPiN was not assessed before HA fitting, thus it is not possible to determine whether the similar auditory processing between the ears was a result of HA utilization or reflects a pre-existing condition [67].

Although only left ear SPiN performance was significantly associated with HA use in the mediation analysis, more than half of the participants were fitted with an HA in the right ear only. In addition, within the GES program, when only one device is provided, it is commonly placed in the right ear for practical reasons, as most users are right-handed [68]. Consequently, the aided ear is not necessarily the one with better residual hearing or superior SPiN performance. Interestingly, bilateral HA fitting was significantly associated with higher perceived benefit in our univariate model. This is a noteworthy finding, as the recent systematic review by Mothemela et al. [25] did not identify any studies that explicitly examined the association between HA laterality and perceived benefit. While the review reported mixed results regarding bilateral fitting and HA use, the relationship with perceived benefit remains largely unexplored in the literature. Nonetheless, in our analyses, HA laterality was included as a covariate and adjusted for in the multivariate mediation model. As such, the indirect association between left ear SPiN performance and HA use—mediated through perceived benefit—remained statistically independent of the laterality of HA implementation.

4.2. Direct Association Between Unaided SPiN and Hearing Aid Use

The secondary objective of the present study was to assess the direct association between unaided SPiN performance and HA use. In this analysis, the SPiN performance in neither ear showed a direct association with HA use. This result aligns with the findings of Grunditz and Magnusson [54], who found no association between their SPiN test and HA use (as measured by question 1 of the IOI-HAs), although they did observe associations between unaided SPiN performance and Factor 2 items (residual activity limitations, residual participation restriction, and impact on others), as well as the total IOI-HAs score. These results suggest that SPiN performance may be indirectly related to HA use via its influence on other outcome variables, consistent with Houmøller et al. [20], who reported that higher Factor 2 scores were linked to increased daily HA use.

The lack of a direct association between unaided SPiN performance and HA use observed in the present study may be attributable to the underlying mechanisms influencing HA utilization. It is likely that decreases in HA use occur predominantly when individuals explicitly perceive an insufficient benefit or encounter substantial communication challenges, rather than being directly driven by their objective SPiN performance. In other words, lower unaided SPiN performance alone might not lead to decreased HA use unless it translates into noticeable dissatisfaction or significant limitations in everyday listening situations. Future studies could explore specific SPiN thresholds at which the perceived benefit meaningfully decreases, thus directly impacting HA use. Identifying these thresholds would enable clinicians to proactively manage perceived communication difficulties and potentially prevent HA abandonment through tailored interventions and individualized counseling strategies.

4.3. Clinical Implications

The present findings have relevant implications for audiological assessment and rehabilitation. First, the observed indirect association between unaided SPiN performance and HA use—mediated through perceived benefit—suggests that SPiN measures can provide clinically meaningful information about potential HA outcomes. This information could be used to support realistic expectation management regarding the perceived benefit patients may experience with HA. Effectively managing expectations may help prevent disappointment and disengagement, particularly by addressing patients' attitudes, beliefs, and motivation—factors that have been associated with HA use and perceived benefit [25,69].

The potential clinical utility of SPiN testing lies in its ecological validity—that is, its ability to reflect the complex auditory demands of real-world listening environments [29]. Binaural SPiN tests are particularly valuable in this regard, as they account for binaural integration and spatial hearing—fundamental skills for speech perception in noise [70,71], which are known to decline with age [72]. However, monaural SPiN tests also offer important clinical information by isolating ear-specific performance. In the present study, the fact that the relationship between unaided SPiN and HA use was significant only for the left ear, despite adjusting for HA configuration, underscores the relevance of ear-specific assessment in older adults. Audiologists may benefit from combining monaural and binaural SPiN measures to obtain a more complete understanding of functional hearing and guide individualized rehabilitation.

Importantly, SPiN performance is not a static ability but a modifiable auditory function. Evidence from recent studies indicates that both monaural and binaural SPiN outcomes can improve through targeted auditory training programs [73]. These interventions may focus on bottom-up mechanisms, such as pitch, spatial, or temporal cue processing, as well as top-down cognitive functions, like working memory and attention. Patients with limited unaided SPiN abilities may benefit from structured training protocols aimed at improving these underlying mechanisms. Tailoring follow-up and rehabilitation strategies based on individual SPiN profiles may contribute to more effective, targeted, and responsive care.

4.4. Limitations

A major limitation of this study design is that it does not allow for a clear determination of the temporal relationship between SPiN performance and HA outcomes. In the review by Lavie et al. [67], some findings suggest that HA use may induce neuronal plasticity changes that improve unaided SPiN performance. Although the evidence has not been entirely consistent, it is possible that SPiN performance measured prior to HA fitting may be modified by subsequent HA use. In the present study, all the participants had already initiated HA use at the time of SPiN testing. The median duration of HA use was 24 months (interquartile range: 12–48 months), which indicates that participants had varying levels of auditory experience prior to SPiN assessment. While the results reported in the review by Lavie et al. suggest amplification-induced improvements in speech perception over time, these findings should be interpreted with caution, as the observed improvements were small, and the methodological quality of the studies was moderate. Future research using longitudinal designs is needed to better understand the directionality and potential causality of these relationships.

As a second limitation, it should be noted that HA use was measured via self-reporting using question 1 of the IOI-HAs. Some research has indicated that self-reports tend to overestimate actual HA use measured by data-logging [74,75]; however, one previous study has shown minimal discrepancies between self-reported HA usage and data-logging, with an average overestimation of only 1.2 h [74]. Additionally, the IOI-HAs is a standardized and widely used tool for assessing HA use in the literature [76], which facilitates comparisons with other studies. Nonetheless, these estimates may be influenced by the structure of the response options. The IOI-HAs includes broad categorical intervals (e.g., "1 to 4 h", "4 to 8 h") that likely minimize the impact of small reporting discrepancies in moderate-use ranges. However, ceiling effects have been reported for IOI-HAs question 1, with a large proportion of users selecting "more than 8 h per day" [74]. In our sample, 47.37% chose this option, reducing variability at the upper end of the scale. This may attenuate associations with other variables and underestimate effect sizes or indirect effects in mediation models. Over-reporting also appears more pronounced in the lowest usage categories. Solheim and Hickson [75] found that participants who did not use their HA at all (per data-logging) reported nearly two hours of daily use. Such misreporting may increase misclassification risk in models examining minimal use. These potential biases should be considered when interpreting associations involving self-reported HA use, and future studies would benefit from including both subjective and objective usage measures.

Despite the limitations of the present study, the use of a mediation model represents a strength, as it provides a deeper understanding of the relationships between unaided SPiN performance, perceived benefit, and HA use. Unlike previous studies that analyzed these variables independently, mediation analysis identified indirect pathways, explicitly highlighting the mediating role of perceived benefit with HAs. Furthermore, mediation analysis helps mitigate the risk of overadjustment bias inherent in conventional multivariate models. For instance, SPiN performance in the left ear was significantly associated with perceived benefit but ceased to be significant in the multivariate ordinal regression model. This suggests that mediation analysis helps mitigate the risk of overadjustment bias inherent in conventional multivariate models. Thus, the conclusions would have been biased if a conventional analysis strategy based on multivariate regression models had been used.

5. Conclusions

In the present study, a mediated or indirect association was observed between unaided SPiN performance and HA use through perceived benefit with HAs. This association was independent of HA experience and bilateral or unilateral adaptations, yet it was observed only for the left ear. Additionally, no direct association between unaided SPiN performance and HA use was observed. These findings suggest that psychoacoustic measures of SPiN may serve as a useful tool for guiding the HA fitting process, providing counseling on realistic expectations for new HA users, and planning potential interventions.

Supplementary Materials: The following supporting information can be downloaded at: https://www.mdpi.com/article/10.3390/audiolres15030050/s1, Table S1: Estimation of the indirect effect of SPIN on HA use mediated by the perceived benefit of using a HA [a].

Author Contributions: Conceptualization, A.M. and E.F.-L.; methodology, A.M. and E.F.-L.; data curation, A.M. and C.S.-L.; formal analysis, A.M., C.S.-L. and E.F.-L.; investigation, A.M. and N.B.V.; writing—original draft preparation, A.M., C.S.-L., J.G.-M., A.I. and E.F.-L.; writing—review and editing, A.M., A.I., N.B.V. and E.F.-L.; visualization, A.M., C.S.-L. and E.F.-L.; supervision, A.M. and J.G.-M.; project administration, A.M. and E.F.-L.; funding acquisition, A.M. and E.F.-L. All authors have read and agreed to the published version of the manuscript.

Funding: This research was financed by the National Commission for Scientific and Technological Research (CONICYT in Spanish), the Fund for Encouraging Scientific and Technological Development (FONDEF in Spanish), and the Government of Chile's Ministry of Health (MINSAL in Spanish) through the Fund for Health Research and Development (FONIS in Spanish, SA18I0138, 2018 and FONIS SA20I0120, 2020). It also received funding from the National Research and Development Agency (ANID, Chile), through the National Fund for Scientific and Technological Development (FONDECYT in Spanish), grant number: FONDECYT N°11201327. The funders had no role in the study design, data collection and analysis, decision to publish, or preparation of the manuscript.

Institutional Review Board Statement: This study was conducted in accordance with the Declaration of Helsinki. The study protocol received approval from the following Ethical Scientific Committees: the Facultad de Medicina at the Pontificia Universidad Católica de Chile (protocol code 180405001, approved on 3 April 2018), Servicio de Salud Metropolitano Sur-Oriente (protocol code NO2886, approved on 23 May 2019), and Servicio de Salud Metropolitano Sur (protocol code 23-25042019, approved on 4 May 2019), all within the Metropolitan Region of Chile.

Informed Consent Statement: Informed consent was obtained from all the subjects involved in this study. Written informed consent for publication was secured from each participant to ensure that any potentially identifiable information is released with their approval.

Data Availability Statement: The dataset used and analyzed during the current study is available from the corresponding author upon reasonable request.

Acknowledgments: We thank those who volunteered their time to participate in the study and those who reviewed drafts of this paper.

Conflicts of Interest: The authors declare no conflicts of interest. The funders had no role in the design of the study; in the collection, analyses, or interpretation of data; in the writing of the manuscript; or in the decision to publish the results.

Abbreviations

The following abbreviations are used in this manuscript:

SPiN	Speech perception in noise
HA	Hearing aid

References

1. World Health Organization (WHO). Deafness and Hearing Loss. Available online: https://www.who.int/news-room/fact-sheets/detail/deafness-and-hearing-loss (accessed on 10 March 2025).
2. Kassebaum, N.J.; Arora, M.; Barber, R.M.; Bhutta, Z.A.; Brown, J.; Carter, A.; Casey, D.C.; Charlson, F.J.; Coates, M.M.; Coggeshall, M.; et al. Global, regional, and national disability-adjusted life-years (DALYs) for 315 diseases and injuries and healthy life expectancy (HALE), 1990–2015: A systematic analysis for the Global Burden of Disease Study 2015. *Lancet* **2016**, *388*, 1603–1658. [CrossRef]
3. Shukla, A.; Harper, M.; Pedersen, E.; Goman, A.; Suen, J.J.; Price, C.; Applebaum, J.; Hoyer, M.; Lin, F.R.; Reed, N.S. Hearing Loss, Loneliness, and Social Isolation: A Systematic Review. *Otolaryngol. Head. Neck Surg.* **2020**, *162*, 622–633. [CrossRef] [PubMed]
4. Lawrence, B.J.; Jayakody, D.M.P.; Bennett, R.J.; Eikelboom, R.H.; Gasson, N.; Friedland, P.L. Hearing Loss and Depression in Older Adults: A Systematic Review and Meta-analysis. *Gerontologist* **2020**, *60*, e137–e154. [CrossRef]
5. Jiam, N.T.L.; Li, C.; Agrawal, Y. Hearing loss and falls: A systematic review and meta-analysis. *Laryngoscope* **2016**, *126*, 2587–2596. [CrossRef]
6. Loughrey, D.G.; Kelly, M.E.; Kelley, G.A.; Brennan, S.; Lawlor, B.A. Association of Age-Related Hearing Loss With Cognitive Function, Cognitive Impairment, and Dementia: A Systematic Review and Meta-analysis. *JAMA Otolaryngol. Head Neck Surg.* **2018**, *144*, 115–126. [CrossRef] [PubMed]
7. Yeo, B.S.Y.; Song, H.J.J.M.D.; Toh, E.M.S.; Ng, L.S.; Ho, C.S.H.; Ho, R.; Merchant, R.A.; Tan, B.K.J.; Loh, W.S. Association of Hearing Aids and Cochlear Implants with Cognitive Decline and Dementia: A Systematic Review and Meta-analysis. *JAMA Neurol.* **2023**, *80*, 134–141. [CrossRef]
8. Hanratty, B.; Lawlor, D. Effective management of the elderly hearing impaired—A review. *J. Public. Health Med.* **2000**, *22*, 512–517. [CrossRef] [PubMed]
9. Huang, Q.; Tang, J. Age-related hearing loss or presbycusis. *Eur. Arch. Oto-Rhino-Laryngol.* **2010**, *267*, 1179–1191. [CrossRef]
10. Zheng, Q.; Xu, Z.; Li, N.; Wang, Y.; Zhang, T.; Jing, J. Age-related hearing loss in older adults: Etiology and rehabilitation strategies. *Front. Neurosci.* **2024**, *18*, 1428564. [CrossRef]
11. Dornhoffer, J.R.; Meyer, T.A.; Dubno, J.R.; McRackan, T.R. Assessment of Hearing Aid Benefit Using Patient-Reported Outcomes and Audiologic Measures. *Audiol. Neurotol.* **2020**, *25*, 215–223. [CrossRef]
12. Ferguson, M.A.; Kitterick, P.T.; Chong, L.Y.; Edmondson-Jones, M.; Barker, F.; Hoare, D.J. Hearing aids for mild to moderate hearing loss in adults. *Cochrane Database Syst. Rev.* **2017**, *9*, CD012023. [CrossRef]
13. Lin, F.R.; Pike, J.R.; Albert, M.S.; Arnold, M.; Burgard, S.; Chisolm, T.; Couper, D.; Deal, J.A.; Goman, A.M.; Glynn, N.W.; et al. Hearing intervention versus health education control to reduce cognitive decline in older adults with hearing loss in the USA (ACHIEVE): A multicentre, randomised controlled trial. *Lancet* **2023**, *402*, 786–797. [CrossRef] [PubMed]
14. Dillon, H.; Day, J.; Bant, S.; Munro, K.J. Adoption, use and non-use of hearing aids: A robust estimate based on Welsh national survey statistics. *Int. J. Audiol.* **2020**, *59*, 567–573. [CrossRef]
15. Aazh, H.; Prasher, D.; Nanchahal, K.; Moore, B.C.J. Hearing aid use and its determinants in the UK National Health Service: A cross-sectional study at the Royal Surrey County Hospital. *Int. J. Audiol.* **2015**, *54*, 152–161. [CrossRef]
16. Cox, R.M. Assessment of subjective outcome of hearing aid fitting: Getting the client's point of view. *Int. J. Audiol.* **2003**, *42* (Suppl. S1), 90–96. [CrossRef] [PubMed]
17. Jilla, A.M.; Johnson, C.E.; Danhauer, J.L.; Anderson, M.; Smith, J.N.; Sullivan, J.C.; Sanchez, K.R. Predictors of Hearing Aid Use in the Advanced Digital Era: An Investigation of Benefit, Satisfaction, and Self-Efficacy. *J. Am. Acad. Audiol.* **2020**, *31*, 87–95. [CrossRef]
18. Stark, P.; Hickson, L. Outcomes of hearing aid fitting for older people with hearing impairment and their significant others. *Int. J. Audiol.* **2004**, *43*, 390–398. [CrossRef] [PubMed]
19. Cox, R.M.; Alexander, G.C. Amplification and Aural Rehabilitation Maturation of Hearing Aid Benefit: Objective and Subjective Measurements. *Ear Hear.* **1992**, *13*, 131–141. [CrossRef]
20. Houmøller, S.S.; Wolff, A.; Möller, S.; Narne, V.K.; Narayanan, S.K.; Godballe, C.; Hougaard, D.D.; Loquet, G.; Gaihede, M.; Hammershøi, D.; et al. Prediction of successful hearing aid treatment in first-time and experienced hearing aid users: Using the International Outcome Inventory for Hearing Aids. *Int. J. Audiol.* **2022**, *61*, 119–129. [CrossRef]
21. Wang, X.; Zheng, Y.; Liu, Y.; Lu, J.; Cui, Z.; Li, Z. Effects of demographic, audiologic, and hearing-aid-related variables on the outcomes of using hearing aids. *Eur. Arch. Oto-Rhino-Laryngol.* **2022**, *279*, 3857–3865. [CrossRef]
22. Fuentes-López, E.; Fuente, A.; Valdivia, G.; Luna-Monsalve, M. Effects of auditory and socio-demographic variables on discontinuation of hearing aid use among older adults with hearing loss fitted in the Chilean public health sector. *BMC Geriatr.* **2019**, *19*, 245. [CrossRef] [PubMed]

23. Fuentes-López, E.; Galaz-Mella, J.; Ayala, S.; De la Fuente, C.; Luna-Monsalve, M.; Nieman, C.; Marcotti, A. Association be-tween the home-to-healthcare center distance and hearing aid abandonment among older adults. *Front. Public. Health* **2024**, *12*, 1364000. [CrossRef] [PubMed]
24. Jardim, I.d.S.; Shirayama, Y.; Yuasa, M.; Bento, R.F.; Iwahashi, J.H. Hearing aid use and adherence to treatment in a publicly-funded health service from the city of São Paulo, Brazil. *Int. Arch. Otorhinolaryngol.* **2015**, *19*, 210–215. [CrossRef] [PubMed]
25. Mothemela, B.; Manchaiah, V.; Mahomed-Asmail, F.; Knoetze, M.; Swanepoel, D.W. Factors influencing hearing aid use, benefit and satisfaction in adults: A systematic review of the past decade. *Int. J. Audiol.* **2024**, *63*, 661–674. [CrossRef]
26. Hoppe, U.; Hocke, T.; Iro, H. Age-Related Decline of Speech Perception. *Front. Aging Neurosci.* **2022**, *14*, 891202. [CrossRef]
27. Chang, Y.S.; Choi, J.; Moon, I.J.; Hong, S.H.; Chung, W.H.; Cho, Y.S. Factors associated with self-reported outcome in adaptation of hearing aid. *Acta Otolaryngol.* **2016**, *136*, 905–911. [CrossRef]
28. Wu, X.; Ren, Y.; Wang, Q.; Li, B.; Wu, H.; Huang, Z.; Wang, X. Factors associated with the efficiency of hearing aids for patients with age-related hearing loss. *Clin. Interv. Aging* **2019**, *14*, 485–492. [CrossRef]
29. Billings, C.J.; Olsen, T.M.; Charney, L.; Madsen, B.M.; Holmes, C.E. Speech-in-Noise Testing: An Introduction for Audiologists. *Semin. Hear.* **2024**, *45*, 55–82. [CrossRef]
30. Weissgerber, T.; Müller, C.; Stöver, T.; Baumann, U. Age Differences in Speech Perception in Noise and Sound Localization in Individuals With Subjective Normal Hearing. *Front. Psychol.* **2022**, *13*, 845285. [CrossRef]
31. Kocabay, A.P.; Aslan, F.; Yüce, D.; Turkyilmaz, D. Speech in Noise: Implications of Age, Hearing Loss, and Cognition. *Folia Phoniatr. Logop.* **2022**, *74*, 345–351. [CrossRef]
32. Heidari, A.; Moossavi, A.; Yadegari, F.; Bakhshi, E.; Ahadi, M. Effects of age on speech-in-noise identification: Subjective ratings of hearing difficulties and encoding of fundamental frequency in older adults. *J. Audiol. Otol.* **2018**, *22*, 134–139. [CrossRef] [PubMed]
33. Lavie, L.; Banai, K.; Attias, J.; Karni, A. How difficult is difficult? Speech perception in noise in the elderly hearing impaired. *J. Basic. Clin. Physiol. Pharmacol.* **2014**, *25*, 313–316. [CrossRef] [PubMed]
34. Walden, T.C.; Walden, B.E. Predicting success with hearing aids in everyday living. *J. Am. Acad. Audiol.* **2004**, *15*, 342–352. [CrossRef] [PubMed]
35. Killion, M.C.; Niquette, P.A.; Gudmundsen, G.I.; Revit, L.J.; Banerjee, S. Development of a quick speech-in-noise test for measuring signal-to-noise ratio loss in normal-hearing and hearing-impaired listeners. *J. Acoust. Soc. Am.* **2004**, *116*, 2395–2405. [CrossRef]
36. Mendel, L.L. Objective and Subjective Hearing Aid Assessment Outcomes. *Am. J. Audiol.* **2007**, *16*, 118–129. [CrossRef]
37. Wilson, R.H.; McArdl, R.; Watt, K.L.; Smith, S.L. The revised speech perception in noise test (R-SPIN) in a multiple signal-to-noise ratio paradigm. *J. Am. Acad. Audiol.* **2012**, *23*, 590–605. [CrossRef]
38. Nilsson, M.; Soli, S.D.; Sullivan, J.A. Development of the Hearing in Noise Test for the measurement of speech reception thresholds in quiet and in noise. *J. Acoust. Soc. Am.* **1994**, *95*, 1085–1099. [CrossRef]
39. on Elm, E.; Altman, D.G.; Egger, M.; Pocock, S.J.; Gøtzsche, P.C.; Vandenbroucke, J.P.; Initiative, S. The Strengthening the Reporting of Observational Studies in Epidemiology (STROBE) statement: Guidelines for reporting observational studies. *Lancet* **2007**, *370*, 1453–1457. [CrossRef]
40. Quiroga, P.; Albala, B.C.; Klaasen, G. Validación de un test de tamizaje para el diagnóstico de demencia asociada a edad, en Chile Validation of a screening test for age associated cognitive impairment, in Chile. *Rev. Med. Chil.* **2004**, *132*, 467–478. [CrossRef]
41. Fuentes-López, E.; Fuente, A.; Cardemil, F.; Valdivia, G.; Albala, C. Prevalence and associated factors of hearing aid use among older adults in Chile. *Int. J. Audiol.* **2017**, *56*, 810–818. [CrossRef]
42. Fuente, A.; McPherson, B. Auditory processing tests for Spanish-speaking adults: An initial study. *Int. J. Audiol.* **2006**, *45*, 645–659. [CrossRef] [PubMed]
43. Lankford, J.E.; Perrone, D.C.; Ma, T.D.; Thunder, M.A. Ambient Noise Levels in Mobile Audiometric Testing Facilities: Compliance with Industry Standards. *AAOHN J.* **1999**, *47*, 163–167. [CrossRef] [PubMed]
44. British Society of Audiology. Practice Guidance: The Acoustics of Sound Field Audiometry in Clinical Audiological Applications. 2019. Available online: www.thebsa.org.uk (accessed on 3 March 2025).
45. Cox, R.M.; Stephens, D.; Kramer, S.E. Translations of the International Outcome Inventory for Hearing Aids (IOI-HA): Traducciones del Inventario Internacional de Resultados para Auxiliares Auditivos (IOI-HA). *Int. J. Audiol.* **2002**, *41*, 3–26. [CrossRef] [PubMed]
46. Servicio Nacional del Adulto Mayor. Estudio Nacional de Dependencia en las Personas Mayores. Available online: https://www.senama.gob.cl/storage/docs/Dependencia-Personas-Mayores-2009.pdf (accessed on 15 March 2025).
47. Fuentes-López, E.; Fuente, A.; Valdivia, G.; Luna-Monsalve, M. Does educational level predict hearing aid self-efficacy in experienced older adult hearing aid users from Latin America? Validation process of the Spanish version of the MARS-HA questionnaire. *PLoS ONE* **2019**, *14*, e0226085. [CrossRef]

48. Fuentes-López, E.; Luna-Monsalve, M.; Silva-Letelier, C.; Marcotti, A. Interaction effect of self-efficacy and joint problems on hearing aid abandonment among older adults. *Int. J. Audiol.* **2024**, 1–11. [CrossRef]
49. Gallardo-Peralta, L.P.; Rodríguez-Blázquez, C.; Ayala-García, A.; Forjaz, M.J. Multi-ethnic validation of 15-item Geriatric Depression Scale in Chile. *Psicol. Reflex. E Critica* **2020**, *33*, 7. [CrossRef]
50. Lee, H.; Cashin, A.G.; Lamb, S.E.; Hopewell, S.; Vansteelandt, S.; Vanderweele, T.J.; MacKinnon, D.P.; Mansell, G.; Collins, G.S.; Golub, R.M.; et al. A Guideline for Reporting Mediation Analyses of Randomized Trials and Observational Studies: The AGReMA Statement. *JAMA* **2021**, *326*, 1045–1056. [CrossRef]
51. VanderWeele, T. *Explanation in Causal Inference: Methods for Mediation and Interaction*; Oxford University Press: New York, NY, USA, 2015.
52. Venturini, S.; Mehmetoglu, M. Plssem: A stata package for structural equation modeling with partial least squares. *J. Stat. Softw.* **2019**, *88*, 1–35. [CrossRef]
53. Kenny, D.A. MedPower: An Interactive Tool for the Estimation of Power in Tests of Mediation. 2017. Available online: https://davidakenny.shinyapps.io/MedPower/ (accessed on 16 June 2024).
54. Grunditz, M.; Magnusson, L. Validation of a speech-in-noise test used for verification of hearing aid fitting. *Hear. Balance Commun.* **2013**, *11*, 64–71. [CrossRef]
55. Jerger, J.; Chmiel, R.; Allen, J.; Wilson, A. Effects of Age and Gender on Dichotic Sentence Identification. *Ear Hear.* **1994**, *15*, 274–286. [CrossRef]
56. Roup, C. Dichotic Word Recognition in Noise and the Right-Ear Advantage. *J. Speech Lang. Hear. Res.* **2011**, *54*, 292–297. [CrossRef] [PubMed]
57. Roup, C.M.; Wiley, T.L.; Wilson, R.H. Dichotic Word Recognition in Young and Older Adults. *J. Am. Acad. Audiol.* **2006**, *17*, 230–240. [CrossRef] [PubMed]
58. Ianiszewski, A.; Fuente, A.; Gagné, J.-P. Association Between the Right Ear Advantage in Dichotic Listening and Interaural Differences in Sensory Processing at Lower Levels of the Auditory System in Older Adults. *Ear Hear.* **2021**, *42*, 1381–1396. [CrossRef]
59. Weihing, J.; Musiek, F. The influence of aging on interaural asymmetries in middle latency response amplitude. *J. Am. Acad. Audiol.* **2014**, *25*, 324–334. [CrossRef] [PubMed]
60. Ianiszewski, A.; Fuente, A.; Gagné, J.-P. Auditory brainstem response asymmetries in older adults: An exploratory study using click and speech stimuli. *PLoS ONE* **2021**, *16*, e0251287. [CrossRef]
61. Behtani, L.; Fuente, A.; Ianiszewski, A.; Al Osman, R.; Hickson, L. Right-ear advantage for unaided and aided speech perception in noise in older adults. *J. Int. Adv. Otol.* **2021**, *17*, 115–120. [CrossRef]
62. Mukari, S.Z.-M.S.; Wahat, N.H.A.; Mazlan, R. Effects of ageing and hearing thresholds on speech perception in quiet and in noise perceived in different locations. *Korean J. Audiol.* **2014**, *18*, 112–118. [CrossRef]
63. Tadros, S.F.; Frisina, S.T.; Mapes, F.; Kim, S.; Frisina, D.R.; Frisina, R.D. Loss of peripheral right-ear advantage in age-related hearing loss. *Audiol. Neurootol.* **2005**, *10*, 44–52. [CrossRef]
64. Derleth, P.; Georganti, E.; Latzel, M.; Courtois, G.; Hofbauer, M.; Raether, J.; Kuehnel, V. Binaural Signal Processing in Hearing Aids. *Semin. Hear.* **2021**, *42*, 206–223. [CrossRef]
65. Jerger, J.; Silman, S.; Silverman, C.; Emmer, M. Binaural interference: Quo vadis? *J. Am. Acad. Audiol.* **2017**, *28*, 266–270. [CrossRef]
66. McArdle, R.A.; Killion, M.; Mennite, M.A.; Chisolm, T.H. Are two ears not better than one? *J. Am. Acad. Audiol.* **2012**, *23*, 171–181. [CrossRef]
67. Lavie, L.; Shechter Shvartzman, L.; Banai, K. Plastic changes in speech perception in older adults with hearing impairment following hearing aid use: A systematic review. *Int. J. Audiol.* **2022**, *61*, 975–983. [CrossRef] [PubMed]
68. Ministerio, S. Hipoacusia bilateral en personas de 65 años y más que requieren uso de audífono. In *Ministerio de Salud*; Gobierno de Chile: Santiago, Chile, 2013.
69. Fuentes-López, E.; Galaz-Mella, J.; Nieman, C.L.; Luna-Monsalve, M.; Marcotti, A. Effect of Attitudes Toward Hearing Loss and Hearing Aids on the Risk of Device Abandonment Among Older Adults With Hearing Loss Fitted in the Chilean Public Health Sector. *Ear Hear.* **2025**. [CrossRef]
70. Ellinger, R.L.; Jakien, K.M.; Gallun, F.J. The role of interaural differences on speech intelligibility in complex multitalker environments. *J. Acoust. Soc. Am.* **2017**, *141*, 170–176. [CrossRef] [PubMed]
71. Cameron, S.; Dillon, H.; Newall, P. Development and Evaluation of the Listening in Spatialized Noise Test. *Ear Hear.* **2006**, *27*, 30–42. [CrossRef] [PubMed]
72. Ghahraman, M.A.; Ashrafi, M.; Mohammadkhani, G.; Jalaie, S. Effects of aging on spatial hearing. *Aging Clin. Exp. Res.* **2020**, *32*, 733–739. [CrossRef]

73. Gohari, N.; Dastgerdi, Z.H.; Rouhbakhsh, N.; Afshar, S.; Mobini, R. Training Programs for Improving Speech Perception in Noise: A Review. *J. Audiol. Otol.* **2023**, *27*, 1–9. [CrossRef]
74. Laplante-Lévesque, A.; Nielsen, C.; Jensen, L.D.; Naylor, G. Patterns of hearing aid usage predict hearing aid use amount (data logged and self-reported) and overreport. *J. Am. Acad. Audiol.* **2014**, *25*, 187–198. [CrossRef]
75. Solheim, J.; Hickson, L. Hearing aid use in the elderly as measured by datalogging and self-report. *Int. J. Audiol.* **2017**, *56*, 472–479. [CrossRef]
76. Perez, E.; Edmonds, B.A. A systematic review of studies measuring and reporting hearing aid usage in older adults since 1999: A descriptive summary of measurement tools. *PLoS ONE* **2012**, *7*, e31831. [CrossRef]

audiology research

MDPI

Article

Translation, Cross-Cultural Adaptation, and Psychometric Properties of the Persian Version of the Measure of Audiologic Rehabilitation Self-Efficacy for Hearing Aids (P-MARS-HA)

Abdolhakim Jorbonyan [1], Yadollah Abolfathi Momtaz [2,3,*], Mahshid Foroughan [3] and Saeideh Mehrkian [4]

1 Department of Geriatric Health, School of Health, Mazandaran University of Medical Sciences, Sari 48157-33971, Iran; a.jourbonian@mazums.ac.ir
2 Malaysian Research Institute on Ageing, University Putra Malaysia, Serdang 43400, Malaysia
3 Iranian Research Center on Aging, The University of Social Welfare and Rehabilitation Sciences, Tehran 19857-13871, Iran; ma.foroughan@uswr.ac.ir
4 Department of Audiology, The University of Social Welfare and Rehabilitation Sciences, Tehran 19857-13871, Iran; sa.mehrkian@uswr.ac.ir
* Correspondence: ya.momtaz@uswr.ac.ir; Tel.: +98-21-22180083 (ext. 92); Fax: +98-21-22180109

Abstract: Objectives: This study aimed to translate, cross-culturally adapt, and evaluate the psychometric properties of the Persian version of the Measure of Audiologic Rehabilitation Self-Efficacy for Hearing Aids (MARS-HA) in elderly Iranian adults. Methods and Materials: This cross-sectional study was conducted in Tehran, 2021. Following translation and cross-cultural adaptation, the face validity, content validity, and reliability of the questionnaire were assessed. The Satisfaction with Amplification in Daily Life (SADL) questionnaire was used to assess concurrent validity. Study participants included 300 hearing-aid users aged 60 years and older who completed the research instruments. Data were analyzed using Confirmatory Factor Analysis (CFA), Cronbach's alpha coefficient, Pearson correlation coefficient, independent t-tests, and analysis of variance (ANOVA) in SPSS and AMOS version 24. The significance level was set at $p \leq 0.05$ for all tests. Results: The mean (SD) age of the participants was 71.38 (8.05) years. The face and content validity of the questionnaire were confirmed by ten experts (CVI > 0.91). The CFA supported the four-factor structure of the questionnaire, and the goodness-of-fit indices indicated that the final model had a good fit. The Cronbach's alpha for the total questionnaire was 0.93, and for the subscales, it ranged between 0.83 and 0.93. The Pearson's correlation analysis results showed a positive and significant correlation between MARS-HA and SADL scores ($r = 0.61$, $p < 0.05$), supporting criterion validity. Conclusions: The P-MARS-HA questionnaire demonstrates good validity and reliability and can be used as an appropriate tool for assessing self-efficacy in hearing-aid use among elderly Iranian adults.

Keywords: hearing aids; self-efficacy; cross-cultural adaptation; psychometric properties; elderly

1. Introduction

Aging is a complex and dynamic process characterized by physical, psychological, and social changes over time. These changes are deeply interconnected, reflecting a continuous process of growth, development, and adaptation until the time of death [1,2]. Many elderly adults experience declines in health and physical function during aging, which can affect their psychological and social well-being and, ultimately, their quality of life [3–5]. Age-related hearing loss (ARHL) is one such physical change in aging, typically starting in early adulthood and approximately doubling in prevalence with each decade of life. Epidemiological studies have shown that more than two-thirds of individuals aged 60 and older suffer from Presbycusis. This type of hearing loss results from a combination of physiological changes related to the aging process and other external risk factors, characterized by a gradual loss of sensory hair cells in the inner ear, which are responsible for converting sound into neural signals [6,7]. Research indicates that hearing loss is associated with significant consequences in aging, including dementia, increased risk of falls, reduced physical activity, and other adverse health conditions. These associations may arise through the effects of hearing loss on individuals' socio-emotional status, such as depression, social isolation, and feelings of loneliness due to communication limitations and barriers [6,8].

Therefore, based on expert recommendations, the use of hearing aids, as the most common approach to compensate for and enhance hearing ability, can significantly control or reduce the negative consequences of presbycusis. Studies have shown that hearing aids not only improve hearing outcomes and health-related quality of life but may also have a protective effect on adverse aging outcomes, including cognitive dysfunction and depressive symptoms [9,10]. However, adopting hearing aids alone is not sufficient; effective and consistent use is essential for success in auditory rehabilitation. Numerous studies have indicated that a significant number of elderly adults do not use their hearing aids regularly or effectively or discontinue their use altogether after some time [11]. One study noted that only about 20% to 50% of elderly adults with hearing impairment use their hearing aids optimally [12].

Studies indicate that adherence to hearing-aid use among older adults is influenced by two categories of factors: (1) technical–auditory factors, including the severity of hearing loss, speech clarity, type of hearing aid, presence of tinnitus, side effects, and environmental noise; and (2) psychosocial factors, such as individual attitudes, motivation, ability to manage hearing aids, and particularly self-efficacy (an individual's belief in their capacity to address challenges related to hearing aids) [13–16]. Higher self-efficacy is associated with greater hearing-aid acceptance, satisfaction, and successful use, whereas lower self-efficacy may lead to discontinuation. Self-efficacy is recognized as a critical determinant in sustaining health-related behaviors and improving therapeutic outcomes. Therefore, integrating self-management strategies and enhancing self-efficacy could play a vital role in promoting the successful use of hearing aids among older adults [17–19]. To this end, West and Smith (2007), based on Bandura's self-efficacy questionnaire guidelines [20] and considering potential reasons for non-adherence to hearing-aid use, such as not benefiting adequately from hearing aids in the presence of background noise, difficulty becoming used to using hearing aids, and concerns regarding the mismanagement and incorrect use of hearing aids due to age-related issues in elderly adults, designed the MARS-HA instrument to assess current self-efficacy beliefs related to hearing aids. This tool can help audiologists to better identify factors influencing patients' success in using hearing aids and, thereby, provide the necessary support to improve treatment outcomes [21].

The MARS-HA instrument includes 24 items and 4 subscales Aided Listening (AL), Basic Handling (BH), Adjustment (Ad), and Advanced Handling (AH) that assess self-efficacy in the mentioned areas and overall self-efficacy in hearing-aid use. For each question, respondents should use a 10-unit scale to indicate how confident they are that they can do that item from 0% (I cannot do this) to 100% (I am sure I can do this); a higher score on this instrument indicates higher self-efficacy. According to West and Smith, scores of 80 percent or higher indicate adequate levels of self-efficacy. The MARS-HA questionnaire has been used in numerous studies, including research by Kelly-Campbell and McMillan (2015), Johnson CE et al. (2018), and Johnson et al. (2024), in which the association of self-efficacy with successful use and satisfaction with hearing aids has been examined [22–24]. In addition, the questionnaire has been translated into Spanish [25] and French–Canadian [26], and its psychometric properties have been confirmed. Given the emphasis of previous studies on the point that the MARS-HA instrument can assist in clinical settings during the auditory rehabilitation process, planning training sessions for hearing-aid use, and monitoring the correct and successful use of hearing aids in different time periods, it is necessary to enable its use in other countries as well. However, to date, there is no evidence that a Persian version of this tool is available. Therefore, the objective of the present study is to translate, cross-culturally adapt, and psychometrically evaluate the Persian version of the MARS-HA. This study seeks to create a valid and reliable tool that can be effectively used in assessing hearing-aid self-efficacy among Persian-speaking users and to help improve the quality of life of elderly adults.

2. Materials and Methods

2.1. Study Design

This cross-sectional study was conducted in 2021 with the aim of cross-cultural adaptation and evaluation of the psychometric properties of the Persian version of the Measure of Audiologic Rehabilitation Self-Efficacy for Hearing Aids (P-MARS-HA).

2.2. Participants

In this study, 300 hearing-aid users, aged 60 years or older, residing in Tehran, Iran, were selected as participants. For sampling, the city of Tehran was divided into four areas based on socio-economic development levels: low, low–middle, high–middle, and high. Several audiology clinics were then randomly selected in each area to collect contact information for elderly adults who had received hearing aids from these clinics. Participants were divided into four groups based on their place of residence, and ultimately, 75 individuals from each group were randomly selected (via lottery) as the study sample.

2.3. Inclusion Criteria

At least 6 months post-hearing fitting (unilateral and bilateral hearing aids), ability to communicate and sufficient fluency in Persian to answer the questions, voluntary consent to participate in the study, and normal cognitive ability (AMT ≥ 7) [27]. Exclusion Criteria: Unwillingness to continue participation in the study and incomplete questionnaires.

2.4. Research Instruments

In this study, data were collected using a demographic information form, the Measure of Audiologic Rehabilitation Self-Efficacy for Hearing Aids (MARS-HA) questionnaire, the Satisfaction with Amplification in Daily Life (SADL) questionnaire (for criterion validity), and the participants' most recent audiograms.

a. Measure of Audiologic Rehabilitation Self-Efficacy for Hearing Aids Questionnaire (MARS-HA)
   West and Smith (2007) designed the Measure of Audiologic Rehabilitation Self-Efficacy for Hearing Aids (MARS-HA) to assess current self-efficacy beliefs related to hearing aids [21]. This scale consists of 24 questions and 4 subscales: 1. Aided Listening (9 items): This subscale assesses an individual's self-efficacy when listening with a hearing aid in a specific listening situation; for example, "I could understand a one-on-one conversation in a quiet place if I wore hearing aids". 2. Basic Handling (7 items): This includes questions assessing an individual's self-efficacy in the basic management of a hearing aid, for example, "I can insert a battery into a hearing aid with ease". 3. Adjustment (3 items): Questions assessing an individual's self-efficacy

in adjusting to the hearing aid, for example, "I could get used to the sound quality of hearing aids". 4. Advanced Handling (5 items): Questions assessing a hearing-aid user's self-efficacy in performing advanced hearing aid tasks, for example, "I can troubleshoot a hearing aid when it stops working". For scoring the questions, respondents should report how much confidence they have in their ability on a 10-unit interval scale (0, 10, 20...100 percent) for each question. If they feel they do not have the ability or skill, they score zero, and if they are completely confident in performing that skill, they consider a score of 100 for themselves. A higher score on this questionnaire indicates greater self-efficacy. According to West and Smith, if the average score of the questionnaire is higher than 80 percent, it indicates a sufficient level of self-efficacy. West and Smith reported the reliability of this instrument for experienced hearing-aid users, using Cronbach's alpha coefficient for the total scale as 0.91, and for the subscales "Basic Handling", "Advanced Handling", "Adjustments", and "Aided Listening" as 0.88, 0.67, 0.73, and 0.91, respectively. In addition, using the test–retest method, the reliability of the instrument was obtained as 0.88 [21].

b. Satisfaction with Amplification in Daily Life (SADL)
The Satisfaction with Amplification in Daily Life questionnaire is a valid instrument designed by Cox and Alexander (1999) [28]. This instrument assesses an individual's satisfaction in various aspects of hearing-aid use and consists of 15 items and four subscales: Positive Effects, Services and Costs, Negative Features, and Personal Image. The average score obtained from each subscale assesses the individual's range of satisfaction and forms the overall questionnaire score. The method of responding to questions is based on a 7-option Likert scale (from completely agree to completely disagree), such that in four questions (2, 4, 7, 13), scoring is reversed. In the research by Faraji Khiavi et al. (2014), the face and content validity of the Persian version of this tool were reviewed and confirmed by five experts, and its internal reliability was obtained as 0.8 through the calculation of Cronbach's alpha index [29].

2.5. Description of the Procedure

Phase (1): Translation and Localization

In the translation and localization process, initial approval was obtained from the original designers of the questionnaire by sending an email explaining the purpose of the psychometric evaluation and the preparation of the Persian version of the instrument. In the next step, using the forward–backward translation method, the original (English) version of the questionnaire was translated into Persian by two Persian-speaking translators, one of whom was proficient in the terminology and translation of audiology texts. Subsequently, the translations were compared, and the questions were reconciled in terms of meaning and concept. By selecting the best options, a Persian version of this instrument was ultimately prepared. To ensure the complete alignment of the Persian translation with the original text and the fluency of the sentences, the final version of the questionnaire was back-translated into the original language by another translator who was fluent in English and had not previously seen the original questionnaire. At this stage, the English versions were compared, and necessary corrections were applied to the Persian version of the questionnaire under the supervision of translators and experts (including five audiologists and five gerontologists, all holding Ph.D. degrees). Finally, the final Persian version of the questionnaire was obtained.

Phase (2): Psychometric Properties

After translating and preparing the Persian version of The Measure of Audiologic Rehabilitation Self-Efficacy for Hearing Aids Questionnaire (P-MARS-HA), the psychometric properties of the questionnaire, including face and content validity, floor and ceiling effects, reliability (internal consistency and stability), construct validity (confirmatory factor analysis), and criterion validity, were evaluated and examined.

2.6. Data Analysis

In this study, descriptive statistics, including frequency distribution (percentage), mean, and standard deviation, were used to describe the demographic characteristics of the study sample. For inferential data analysis, considering the normal distribution of data based on skewness and kurtosis tests (in the range of −2 to +2), independent *t*-tests (to compare the means of two groups), one-way analysis of variance (ANOVA) (to examine differences between means in multiple groups), and Pearson correlation coefficient (to examine the relationship between variables) were used. Data analysis was performed using SPSS (version 24) and AMOS (version 24) software, and the statistical significance level was set at $p < 0.05$ for all tests.

3. Results

3.1. Floor and Ceiling Effects

The results indicated that a small percentage of participants were at the extreme ends of the score range; specifically, only 2% achieved the lowest score, and 2% achieved the highest score. This balanced distribution of scores suggests that the questionnaire used did not have significant floor or ceiling effects.

3.2. Descriptive Results

In this study, 300 elderly hearing-aid users participated. The mean (SD) age of the participants was 71.38 (±8.05) years. Regarding gender, half of the participants were female (50.7%). Most participants were married (70.3%), and 81% of them used digital hearing aids (Table 1). The mean (SD) overall P-MARS-HA scale score was 65.24 (±15.94). The lowest mean score was for the Advanced Handling (AH) subscale, and the highest mean score was for the Basic Handling (BH) subscale (Table 2). The correlation of all subscales with the overall questionnaire mean was positive and significant using Pearson's correlation coefficient ($p < 0.05$) (Table 2). The correlation between the P-MARS-HA scale and participants' age was negative and significant ($r = -0.26$, $p < 0.05$), meaning that as age increases, the self-efficacy of elderly adults in using hearing aids decreases. Independent *t*-test results showed that In-The-Ear (ITE) hearing-aid users had significantly higher self-efficacy compared to Behind-The-Ear (BTE) hearing-aid users ($p < 0.05$), but this difference was not significant for gender and type of hearing-aid prescription (unilateral or bilateral) ($p > 0.05$).

Analysis of variance results showed that the mean P-MARS-HA questionnaire score differed significantly across groups based on education, marital status, and degree of hearing loss in the worse ear (WEA), and type of hearing aid ($p < 0.05$) (Table 3). The Scheffe post hoc test results showed that mean self-efficacy was significantly higher in married individuals compared to single individuals, in individuals with a university education level compared to illiterate and elementary-educated individuals, in individuals with mild to moderate hearing loss compared to severe to profound hearing loss, and in digital hearing-aid users compared to analog and programmable hearing-aid users ($p < 0.05$).

Table 1. Demographic characteristics of the participants (N = 300).

Variables		Frequency (%)
Age	Mean (SD):	71.38 (8.05)
Gender	Female	152 (50.7%)
	Male	148 (49.3%)
Education status	Illiterate	45 (15%)
	Primary	66 (22%)
	Secondary	65 (21.7%)
	Diploma	77 (25.7%)
	Higher education	47 (15.6%)
Marital Status	Married	211 (70.3%)
	Widow	71 (23.7%)
	Divorced	18 (6%)
Types of Hearing Aids	Digital	243 (81%)
	Programmable	37 (12.3%)
	Analog	20 (6.7%)
Degree of hearing impairment (WEA)	<26 dB HL	0
	26–40 dB HL	9 (3%)
	41–55 dB HL	82 (27.3%)
	56–70 dB HL	149 (49.7%)
	71 dB HL	60 (20%)
Hearing aid fitting	Unilateral	98 (32.7%)
	Bilateral	202 (67.3%)
Style of hearing aid	Behind the ear (BTE)	203 (67.7%)
	In-the-ear (ITE)	97 (32.3%)

WEA = worse ear average (averaged over 0.5, 1, 2, and 4 kHz).

Table 2. Correlation coefficients and reliability of P-MARS-HA scores (n = 300).

Variables	Mean (SD)	Basic Handling	Advanced Handling	Adjustment	Aided Listening	Overall Score
Basic handling	73.76 (21.94)	1				
Advanced handling	40.03 (23.05)	0.67 *	1			
Adjustment	67.01 (24.97)	0.46 *	0.45 *	1		
Aided listening	72.03 (17.39)	0.29 *	0.30 *	0.48 *	1	
Overall score	65.24 (15.94)	0.81 *	0.78 *	0.71 *	0.71 *	1
Reliability (Cronbach's Alpha)	-	0.90	0.83	0.87	0.93	0.93

$p < 0.05$ *.

Table 3. Statistical comparison of sociodemographic subgroups (n = 300).

Variables.		Mean (SD)	T/F Statistic	p-Value
Gender	Male	64.77 (14.45)	−0.49	0.62
	Female	65.69 (17.30)		
Marital status	Single	60.40 (17.05)	4.75	0.009 *
	Married	66.48 (15.21)		
	Divorced or widowed	69.76 (16.54)		

Table 3. *Cont.*

Variables.		Mean (SD)	T/F Statistic	*p*-Value
Education	Illiterate	60.37 (18.25)	5.36	0.001 *
	Primary	60.19 (14.24)		
	Secondary	67.05 (15.78)		
	Diploma	66.94 (15.25)		
	Higher education	71.70 (14.15)		
Degree of hearing impairment (WEA)	26–40 dB HL	66.88 (21.56)	4.91	0.002 *
	41–55 dB HL	67.44 (13.34)		
	56–70 dB HL	66.74 (16.03)		
	71 dB HL	58.34 (16.63)		
Hearing-aid fitting	Unilateral	66.17 (16.92)	0.7	0.48
	Bilateral	64.79 (15.42)		
Types of hearing aids	Digital	66.61 (15.21)	4.91	0.008 *
	Programmable	60.13 (18.54)		
	Analog	58.12 (17.50)		
Style of hearing aid	Behind the ear (BTE)	62.14 (16.30)	25.74	0.001 *
	In-the-ear (ITE)	71.73 (12.99)		

$p < 0.05$ *.

3.3. Face Validity

To assess the face validity of the P-MARS-HA questionnaire, 10 experts in the fields of gerontology and audiology were asked to evaluate the clarity, comprehensibility, and relevance of each question to the main objective of the questionnaire. The results indicated that all questions, from the perspective of these experts, had sufficient clarity and relevance and adequately covered the objective of the questionnaire. Additionally, the impact score of all questions was reported to be higher than 1.5, which is another confirmation of the favorable face validity of the questionnaire. Based on these findings, no need was identified to remove or modify the questionnaire questions at this stage.

3.4. Content Validity

The content validity of the questionnaire was assessed by evaluating ten experts in the fields of gerontology and audiology. Experts evaluated each of the questionnaire's items based on the criteria of necessity and importance, and then the content validity ratio (CVR) and content validity index (CVI) were calculated. The CVR and CVI values for all items were higher than 0.80 and 0.91, respectively, indicating that the P-MARS-HA instrument has acceptable content validity.

3.5. Construct Validity (Confirmatory Factor Analysis)

The construct validity of the questionnaire was assessed using a confirmatory factor analysis (CFA). After performing modifications, the final model had an acceptable fit. Factor loadings are within the acceptable range (>0.5) (Table 4), and the final model is presented in the diagram (Figure 1). In this study, the goodness-of-fit index of the chi-squared per the number of degrees of freedom (χ^2/df) was 4.02, indicating an acceptable model fit. The values of other fit indices are also reported in Table 5. Another noteworthy point is that the correlation between the items of the instrument was significant and positive ($p < 0.05$).

Table 4. Goodness-of-fit indices for the measured model of the P-MARS-HA.

Model	χ^2/df	CFI	PCFI	RMSEA	GFI	IFI
Recommended value	<5	≥0.9	>0.5	<0.1	≥0.9	0–1
P-MARS-HA	4.02	0.93	0.67	0.09	0.901	0.89

χ^2/df: Chi-square test; CFI: comparative fit index; PCFI: parsimony comparative fit index; RMSEA: root mean square error of approximation; IFI: incremental fit index; GFI: goodness-of-fit index.

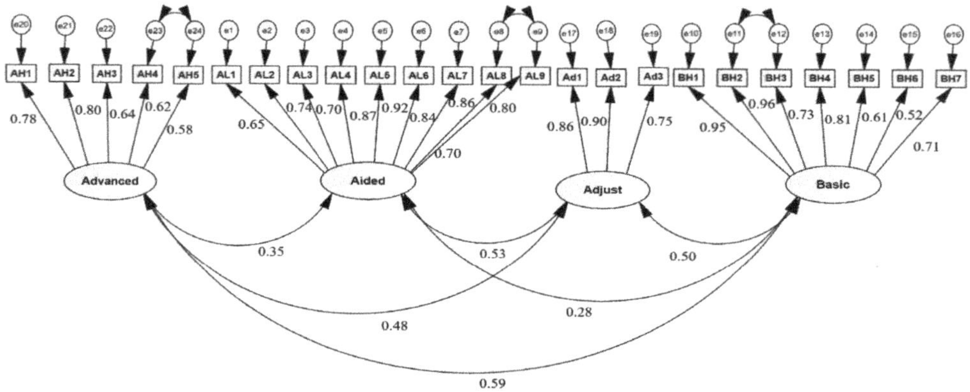

Figure 1. The final measurement model of the research and its parameters using standardized coefficients. AH: Advanced Handling, AL: Aided Listening, Ad: Adjustment, BH: Basic Handling.

Table 5. Regression coefficients of the paths.

	Path	Standardized Regression Coefficient	Standard Error	C.R Statistic	*p* Value
1	AL1<— Aided listening	0.64			
2	AL2<— Aided listening	0.74	0.10	11.36	0.001 *
3	AL3<— Aided listening	0.69	0.12	10.76	0.001 *
4	AL4<— Aided listening	0.87	0.13	12.90	0.001 *
5	AL 5<— Aided listening	0.92	0.14	13.45	0.001 *
6	AL 6<— Aided listening	0.84	0.13	12.58	0.001 *
7	AL 7<— Aided listening	0.85	0.13	12.73	0.001 *
8	AL8<— Aided listening	0.79	0.13	12.09	0.001 *
9	AL 9<— Aided listening	0.69	0.12	10.74	0.001 *
10	BH1<— Basic handling	0.94			0.001 *
11	BH2<— Basic handling	0.95	0.02	34.38	0.001 *
12	BH3<— Basic handling	0.72	0.05	16.32	0.001 *
13	BH4<— Basic handling	0.80	0.03	20.68	0.001 *
14	BH5<— Basic handling	0.61	0.04	12.61	0.001 *
15	BH6<— Basic handling	0.51	0.05	10.03	0.001 *
16	BH7<— Basic handling	0.71	0.04	16.05	0.001 *
17	Ad1<— Adjustment	0.86			0.001 *
18	Ad2<— Adjustment	0.90	0.06	18.40	0.001 *

Table 5. *Cont.*

	Path	Standardized Regression Coefficient	Standard Error	C.R Statistic	p Value
19	Ad3<— Adjustment	0.74	0.05	14.74	0.001 *
20	AH1<— Advanced handling	0.77			0.001 *
21	AH2<— Advanced handling	0.79	0.07	12.76	0.001 *
22	AH3<— Advanced handling	0.63	0.06	10.38	0.001 *
23	AH4<— Advanced handling	0.62	0.08	10.31	0.001 *
24	AH5<— Advanced handling	0.58	0.05	9.37	0.001 *

AH: Advanced Handling, AL: Aided Listening, Ad: Adjustment, BH: Basic Handling, $p < 0.05$ *.

3.6. Criterion Validity

To assess criterion validity, the concurrent validity method was used, whereby the correlation between the MARS-HA questionnaire and Satisfaction with Amplification in Daily Life (SADL) was evaluated. Pearson's correlation analysis results showed that there is a positive and significant correlation between MARS-HA and SADL scores ($r = 0.61$, $p < 0.05$). This finding indicates that individuals with higher self-efficacy in using hearing aids have greater satisfaction with their hearing aids. Given that the correlation of 0.61 is in the medium to strong range, it can be concluded that the P-MARS-HA questionnaire has predictive criterion validity and can be used as a tool to predict the level of satisfaction of individuals with hearing aids.

3.7. Reliability

The internal reliability of the P-MARS-HA questionnaire was assessed by calculating the Cronbach's alpha coefficient. The Cronbach's alpha value for the entire questionnaire was 0.93, indicating good reliability. The alpha values for the subscales were slightly different: Basic Handling: 0.90, Advanced Handling: 0.83, Adjustment: 0.87, and Aided Listening: 0.93 (Table 2). The analysis of the correlation of each question with the rest of the questions also showed that all questions correlate higher than 0.4 with each other. Therefore, the reliability of this questionnaire seems desirable.

4. Discussion

Assessing self-efficacy in hearing-aid use can help identify psychological and practical barriers to hearing-aid use. Additionally, it can provide strategies to increase the acceptance and effective use of hearing aids in elderly adults. Therefore, the present study aimed to translate, cross-culturally adapt, and examine the psychometric properties of the Persian version of The MARS-HA. A total of 300 hearing-aid users aged 60 years and older participated in this study. The results of this study indicated that the Persian version of the MARS-HA scale has a favorable translation and acceptable psychometric properties in elderly adult Persian-speaking hearing-aid users.

In the descriptive–analytical findings of the study, the mean (SD) of the Persian version of the MARS-HA was 65.24 (±15.94), and there was a positive and significant relationship between all subscales. Consistent with this finding, the original version and the Spanish and French–Canadian versions also showed a positive and significant relationship between the subscales. The obtained mean was equal to the mean of the original questionnaire and lower than the mean of other versions of the questionnaire [21,25,26]. Among the subscales, the lowest mean was related to Advanced Handling, and the highest mean was related to Basic Handling. Consistent with this finding, other versions of this questionnaire also showed that Advanced Handling had the lowest mean [21,25,26]. It seems that the self-efficacy of elderly adults in performing tasks that require more complex knowledge, greater cognitive ability, and finer motor skills, such as troubleshooting, cleaning, and caring for the hearing aid, is lower than that for simpler and more repetitive tasks, such as inserting the battery into the hearing aid and placing the hearing aid on the ear. In this regard, strengthening self-efficacy through technical training, support services, and encouraging elderly adults to practice and perform these tasks can be effective.

The findings of the study showed that individuals with older age, individuals with lower education, individuals who are single, and individuals with a greater degree of hearing loss had lower self-efficacy. Consistent with our study, in the study by Fuentes et al. (2019), individuals with higher education and a lower PTA (Pure tone average) had greater self-efficacy in hearing-aid use. However, in that study, age was not significantly associated with self-efficacy in hearing-aid use and was contrary to the findings of our study [25]. Individuals with higher education usually have high activity and social participation, and their access to information is greater. In addition, they have a greater ability to understand the technical instructions of hearing aids. These factors can increase self-efficacy in individuals with higher education. In the study by Johnson & Sarangi (2023), it was reported that factors such as family encouragement and social support can have a significant impact on self-efficacy in hearing-aid use [22]. In our study, it was also found that married individuals, compared to single individuals who are usually deprived of receiving direct support from their spouse, have greater self-efficacy in hearing-aid use. Studies have shown that with increasing age, elderly adults, due to a decline in cognitive abilities (memory, attention) and physical abilities (fine motor skills), may have difficulty performing complex tasks [30,31]. Therefore, their self-efficacy in performing more complex hearing-aid tasks may be lower. On the other hand, concern about damaging the hearing aid and lack of access to appropriate training can also exacerbate this issue. In terms of the degree of hearing loss, it seems that individuals with more severe hearing loss, due to the functional limitations of hearing aids in noisy environments, technical challenges and more complex settings of more powerful hearing aids, and the lower participation of individuals with severe hearing loss in activities, have less self-efficacy in using hearing aids.

The validity and reliability of the Persian version of MARS-HA in this study were approximately like the original version and other versions of this questionnaire. In terms of reliability, the Cronbach's alpha coefficient obtained from the Persian version of the MARS-HA questionnaire was 0.93, and for the subscales, it was higher than 0.8, which was similar to the original version and slightly higher than the Spanish and French–Canadian versions [21,25,26].

The results of the present study provide strong evidence in support of the construct validity of the Persian version of the MARS-HA questionnaire. Confirmatory factor analysis (CFA) showed that the factor structure of the original version was also preserved in the Persian sample. The values of the fit indices also indicate that the constructs of the questionnaire are understood and experienced in the cultural context of Iran in the same way as they are defined in the original culture of the questionnaire. Factor loadings higher than 0.5 and significant for all items in the relevant factor indicate that items well measure their intended construct. Also, the significant and expected correlations between the different factors of the questionnaire confirm the convergent validity of this instrument. Regarding predictive criterion validity, a positive and significant relationship was obtained in this study between P-MARS-HA and SADL. In confirmation of this finding, in the studies of Kelly et al. (2015) and Ferguson et al. (2016), MARS-HA had a positive and significant relationship with SADL [18,24]. It seems that people who have high self-efficacy in using hearing aids are better able to cope with challenges, such as adjusting the device, adapting to noisy environments, or communicating in groups. This confidence increases the feeling of control over life and enhances satisfaction with the hearing aid. In summary, the MARS-HA questionnaire is recognized as an instrument with high potential in clinical and research settings. This questionnaire can be useful in guiding the auditory rehabilitation process, planning initial hearing-aid familiarization sessions, and determining the goals of subsequent visits for patients using hearing aids [21]. The use of P-MARS-HA as a clinical tool can lead to better outcomes in hearing-aid use, including increased self-efficacy in hearing-aid use. Finally, successful use of hearing aids can lead to an improved quality of life for elderly adults.

5. Conclusions

According to the results of the study, the Persian version of the MARS-HA scale has acceptable validity and reliability in the Iranian community, and it can be used to assess self-efficacy in hearing-aid use in elderly adults using hearing aids. This instrument, with its four subscales, covers various dimensions of self-efficacy related to hearing-aid use, which include Advanced Handling, Basic Handling, Aided Listening, and Adjustment. The use of this tool enables hearing specialists to gain a better understanding of level of self-efficacy of elderly adults in using hearing aids, and based on that, design and implement more appropriate auditory rehabilitation programs.

6. Clinical Applications

The P-MARS-HA facilitates optimized hearing-aid outcomes by assessing self-efficacy across four domains: Basic Handling, Adjustment, Aided Listening, and Advanced Handling. Administration of the tool is recommended 2–4 weeks post-fitting to identify challenges during initial acclimatization, with follow-up assessments suggested at 3- and 6-month intervals. Low self-efficacy scores guide targeted interventions, such as hands-on training, scenario-based counseling, communication strategy practice, and psychosocial support. Integrating MARS-HA into clinical workflows—through pre-visit screenings, SMART goal-setting, and multidisciplinary care—establishes a personalized, data-driven approach. Clinical studies demonstrate that this integration enhances hearing-aid adherence, reduces device abandonment, and improves patients' quality of life by addressing practical and psychosocial barriers to successful rehabilitation.

7. Limitations

This study has some limitations that should be considered. First, the cross-sectional design of the study does not allow for examining changes in self-efficacy over time and their impact on related outcomes. Second, while other versions of the questionnaire have compared the self-efficacy of experienced and novice hearing-aid users, the present study only examined users who had been using hearing aids for at least six months. This may limit the generalizability of some of the results to all hearing-aid users, particularly in the early stages of hearing-aid use.

Author Contributions: A.J. and Y.A.M.: Study design, data collection, data analysis, manuscript drafting/revision. M.F.: Research consultation, manuscript design/review (with Y.A.M.). S.M.: Statistical analysis, manuscript editing (with A.J.). All authors have read and agreed to the published version of the manuscript.

Funding: This research received no external funding.

Institutional Review Board Statement: This study received approval from the Ethics Committee of the University of Social Welfare and Rehabilitation Sciences in Tehran (USWR) (IR.USWR.REC.1399.027, 25 February 2020). The committee adheres to the ethical principles outlined in the Declaration of Helsinki.

Informed Consent Statement: Informed consent was obtained from all subjects involved in the study. Written informed consent has been obtained from the patients to publish this paper.

Data Availability Statement: Since this paper is extracted from a thesis, open access to the raw data is not permitted by the Medical University. If necessary, the authors can provide access to the data with the permission of the university.

Acknowledgments: The source of the data used in this paper was the Ph.D. thesis of Abdolhakim Jorbonyan, a student at the Department of Gerontology in the Social Welfare and Rehabilitation Sciences University. We deeply appreciate the elderly and the audiology clinics that fully cooperated on this research project.

Conflicts of Interest: The authors declare no conflicts of interest.

References

1. Younis, N.M.; Ibrahim, R.M.; Ahmed, M.M. Health problems related to Quality of Life among Aging in Iraq. *J. Curr. Med. Res. Opinion.* **2024**, *7*, 3015–3024.
2. Hajizadeh, A.; Albelbeisi, A.H.; Tajvar, M. Impacts of Population Ageing on the Functions of the Health System: A Systematic Review. *Iran. J. Ageing.* **2024**, *19*, 328–361. [CrossRef]
3. Velaithan, V.; Tan, M.-M.; Yu, T.-F.; Liem, A.; Teh, P.-L.; Su, T.T. The association of self-perception of aging and quality of life in older adults: A systematic review. *Gerontologist* **2024**, *64*, gnad041. [CrossRef] [PubMed]
4. Naseh, L.; Mohammadi-Shahboulaghi, F.; Khankeh, H.R.; Norouzi Tabrizi, K. Successful Aging: Concept Analysis with Walker and Avant's Approach. *Iran. J. Ageing.* **2024**, *19*, 158–175. [CrossRef]
5. Afrashteh, M.Y.; Majzoobi, M.R.; Janjani, P.; Forstmeier, S. The relationship between the meaning of life, psychological well-being, self-care, and social capital, with depression and death anxiety in the elderly living in nursing homes: The mediating role of loneliness. *Heliyon* **2024**, *10*, e30124. [CrossRef]
6. Lin, F.R. Age-related hearing loss. *N. Engl. J. Med.* **2024**, *390*, 1505–1512. [CrossRef]
7. Haile, L.M.; Orji, A.U.; Reavis, K.M.; Briant, P.S.; Lucas, K.M.; Alahdab, F.; Bärnighausen, T.W.; Bell, A.W.; Cao, C.; Dai, X.J.E.; et al. Hearing loss prevalence, years lived with disability, and hearing aid use in the United States from 1990 to 2019: Findings from the global burden of disease study. *Ear Hear.* **2024**, *45*, 257–267.
8. Shukla, A.; Reed, N.S.; Armstrong, N.M.; Lin, F.R.; Deal, J.A.; Goman, A.M. Hearing Loss, Hearing Aid Use, and Depressive Symptoms in Older Adults-Findings from the Atherosclerosis Risk in Communities Neurocognitive Study (ARIC-NCS). *J. Gerontol. Ser. B* **2021**, *76*, 518–523. [CrossRef]
9. Sanders, M.E.; Kant, E.; Smit, A.L.; Stegeman, I. The effect of hearing aids on cognitive function: A systematic review. *PLoS ONE* **2021**, *16*, e0261207. [CrossRef] [PubMed]
10. Committee on Accessible and Affordable Hearing Health Care for Adults; Board on Health Sciences Policy; Health and Medicine Division; National Academies of Sciences, Engineering, and Medicine; Blazer, D.G.; Domnitz, S.; Liverman, C.T. (Eds.) The National Academies Collection: Reports funded by National Institutes of Health. In *Hearing Health Care for Adults: Priorities for Improving Access and Affordability*; National Academies Press (US): Washington, DC, USA, 2016.
11. Lisan, Q.; Goldberg, M.; Lahlou, G.; Ozguler, A.; Lemonnier, S.; Jouven, X.; Zins, M.; Empana, J.-P. Prevalence of hearing loss and hearing aid use among adults in France in the CONSTANCES study. *JAMA Netw. Open* **2022**, *5*, e2217633. [CrossRef]
12. Oosthuizen, I.; Manchaiah, V.; Launer, S.; Swanepoel, D.W. Hearing aid experiences of adult hearing aid owners during and after fitting: A systematic review of qualitative studies. *Trends Hear.* **2022**, *26*, 23312165221130584. [CrossRef] [PubMed]
13. Houmøller, S.; Wolff, A.; Möller, S.; Narne, V.; Narayanan, S.; Godballe, C.; Hougaard, D.; Loquet, G.; Gaihede, M.; Hammershøi, D.J. Prediction of successful hearing aid treatment in first-time and experienced hearing aid users: Using the International Outcome Inventory for Hearing Aids. *Int. J. Audiol.* **2022**, *61*, 119–129. [CrossRef]
14. Knoetze, M.; Manchaiah, V.; Mothemela, B.; Swanepoel, D.W. Factors influencing hearing help-seeking and hearing aid uptake in adults: A systematic review of the past decade. *Trends Hear.* **2023**, *27*, 23312165231157255. [CrossRef]
15. Franks, I.; Timmer, B.H. Reasons for the non-use of hearing aids: Perspectives of non-users, past users, and family members. *Int. J. Audiol.* **2024**, *63*, 794–801. [CrossRef]
16. Tavanai, E.; Khalili, M.E.; Shahidipour, Z.; Jalaie, S.; Ghahraman, M.A.; Rouhbakhsh, N.; Rahimi, V. Hearing handicaps, communication difficulties and depression in the older adults: A comparison of hearing aid users and non-users. *Eur. Arch. Oto-Rhino-Laryngol.* **2023**, *280*, 5229–5240. [CrossRef]
17. Sarangi, L.; Johnson, J. An exploration of associations between hearing aid self-efficacy and other measurable characteristics of naïve and experienced hearing aid users. *Int. J. Audiol.* **2023**, *62*, 343–349. [CrossRef]

18. Ferguson, M.A.; Woolley, A.; Munro, K.J. The impact of self-efficacy, expectations, and readiness on hearing aid outcomes. *Int. J. Audiol.* **2016**, *55* (Suppl. 3), S34–S41. [CrossRef] [PubMed]
19. Meyer, C.; Hickson, L.; Fletcher, A. Identifying the barriers and facilitators to optimal hearing aid self-efficacy. *Int. J. Audiol.* **2014**, *53* (Suppl. 1), S28–S37. [CrossRef] [PubMed]
20. Bandura, A. Guide for constructing self-efficacy scales. *Self-Effic. Beliefs Adolesc.* **2006**, *5*, 307–337.
21. West, R.L.; Smith, S.L. Development of a hearing aid self-efficacy questionnaire. *Int. J. Audiol.* **2007**, *46*, 759–771. [CrossRef]
22. Johnson, J.; Sarangi, L. Shared experiences among successful hearing aid users with high hearing aid self-efficacy. *Int. J. Audiol.* **2024**, *63*, 579–586. [CrossRef] [PubMed]
23. Johnson, C.E.; Jilla, A.M.; Danhauer, J.L.; Sullivan, J.C.; Sanchez, K.R. (Eds.) Benefits from, satisfaction with, and self-efficacy for advanced digital hearing aids in users with mild sensorineural hearing loss. In *Seminars in Hearing*; Thieme Medical Publishers: New York, NY, USA, 2018.
24. Kelly-Campbell, R.J.; McMillan, A. The relationship between hearing aid self-efficacy and hearing aid satisfaction. *Am. J. Audiol.* **2015**, *24*, 529–535. [CrossRef]
25. Fuentes-López, E.; Fuente, A.; Valdivia, G.; Luna-Monsalve, M. Does educational level predict hearing aid self-efficacy in experienced older adult hearing aid users from Latin America? Validation process of the Spanish version of the MARS-HA questionnaire. *PLoS ONE* **2019**, *14*, e0226085. [CrossRef]
26. Vincent, C.; Gagné, J.-P.; Leroux, T.; Clothier, A.; Larivière, M.; Dumont, F.S.; Gendron, M. French-Canadian translation and validation of four questionnaires assessing hearing impairment and handicap. *Int. J. Audiol.* **2017**, *56*, 248–259. [CrossRef] [PubMed]
27. Bakhtiyari, F.; Foroughan, M.; Fakhrzadeh, H.; Nazari, N.; Najafi, B.; Alizadeh, M.; Arzaghi, M.; Sharifi, F.; Shoaee, S.; Mostafa, Q.; et al. Validation of the persian version of Abbreviated Mental Test (AMT) in elderly residents of Kahrizak charity foundation. *Iran. J. Diabetes Metab.* **2014**, *13*, 487–494.
28. Cox, R.M.; Alexander, G.C. hearing. Measuring satisfaction with amplification in daily life: The SADL scale. *Ear Hear.* **1999**, *20*, 306–320. [CrossRef] [PubMed]
29. FarajiKhiavi, F.; Bayat, A.; Dashti, R.; Sameni, S.J. Hearing aid-related satisfaction based on type and degree of hearing loss in elderly. *Bimon. Audiol.-Tehran Univ. Med. Sci.* **2015**, *23*, 114–122.
30. Mahomed-Asmail, F.; Graham, M.A.; Swanepoel, W.; Manchaiah, V.; Yerraguntla, K.; Karlsson, E. Predictors of hearing loss disability: A multinational study using the ICF core set. *Int. J. Audiol.* **2025**, 1–8. [CrossRef]
31. Gomez, R.; Ferguson, M. Improving self-efficacy for hearing aid self-management: The early delivery of a multimedia-based education programme in first-time hearing aid users. *Int. J. Audiol.* **2020**, *59*, 272–281. [CrossRef]

audiology research

MDPI

Article

Over-the-Counter (OTC) Hearing Aid Availability across the Spectrum of Human Skin Colors

Shade Avery Kirjava [1,*] and Sam Jones Faulkner [2]

[1] Department of Health, Society, and Behavior, University of California, Irvine, CA 92697, USA
[2] Program in Inclusive Design, OCAD University, Toronto, ON M5T 1W1, Canada; samfaulkner@ocadu.ca
* Correspondence: skirjava@uci.edu

Abstract: Background: Over-the-counter (OTC) hearing aids were recently approved for sale in the United States. Research has shown that consumers prefer hearing devices that match their skin color because these devices are less noticeable. Colorism is discrimination against individuals with relatively darker skin that manifests in "skin-color" product offerings as products being offered primarily in relatively lighter colors. Methods: This study compared images of U.S. Food and Drug Administration (FDA)-registered over-the-counter hearing aids to a range of human skin colors. Results: Most over-the-counter hearing aids are only offered in relatively lighter beige colors. Few over-the-counter hearing aids are available in darker skin colors. Conclusions: These findings may represent structural bias, preventing equitable access to darker skin-color OTC hearing aids for individuals with darker skin.

Keywords: over-the-counter hearing aids; race factors; hearing aids

1. Introduction

Hearing loss is a critical public health concern. It affects about 1.5 billion people globally and costs about $980 billion USD in lost productivity alone annually [1]. The most common types of hearing loss, age-related and noise-induced hearing loss, are irreversible and typically treated with hearing aids prescribed by licensed hearing healthcare providers. In 2022, the FDA approved the sale of over-the-counter (OTC) hearing aids in the United States to reduce barriers in hearing healthcare treatment access [2]. However, unequitable OTC hearing aid device offerings threaten the potential of OTC hearing aids to reduce hearing health inequity. OTC hearing aids are non-prescription hearing aids designed as a more affordable alternative to prescription hearing aids, which are not covered by traditional Medicare and can cost upwards of $5000 [3–5]. The social epidemiologic framework of factors driving hearing health outcomes introduced by Nieman et al. positions OTC hearing aid use as an important factor in reducing hearing health inequity [3–6]. The model by Nieman et al. also suggests that racism and stigma about wearing hearing aids are key structural factors in understanding rates of hearing aid use.

Structural racism in the form of colorism has not been evaluated in the United States OTC hearing aid market. If present, this colorism may potentially limit OTC hearing aid uptake for individuals with relatively darker skin. As OTC hearing aids are an emerging market in the United States, there is room for great improvement in product selection, as hopefully the awareness of colorism with these devices will change future colorway options. Colorism is defined as the additional marginalization of BIPOC (Black, indigenous, and people of color) people with darker skin tones compared to peers with lighter skin tones and the valuing of features akin to euro-centric whiteness causing products in "skin colors" to be offered primarily or solely in relatively lighter colors [7]. Many industries have been reckoning with colorism in their product offerings in the aftermath of the 2020 George Floyd protests [8]. Brands such as Band-aid [9] and Crayola [10] have since launched or re-launched products that give more comprehensive skin tone options in an attempt to develop more equitable product portfolios. While the changes that happened in 2020 across the marketing and product development spheres were the beginning of a broader shift across industries, these more diverse skin-color product offerings were not adopted in all industries.

Hearing aids are one of the many industries that must consider their skin-color product offerings. Traditionally, a hearing aid was designed to blend in with the user's skin or hair color. This design choice was made primarily due to the stigma associated with individuals wearing hearing aids being viewed as elderly or disabled. While the stigma has slowly become less prevalent in recent years, most users still prefer more discreet devices [11–14]. Having the option for hearing aid shells that blend into the user's skin or hair color is an important consideration for hearing aid companies to consider when developing product colorways.

This study examines if OTC hearing aids in skin colors across the spectrum of typical human skin are available for purchase in the United States. It was predicted that there would be more OTC hearing aid offerings in relatively lighter skin colors compared to relatively darker skin colors. The goal of this study is not to perpetuate the stigma that hearing aids should be discreet, invisible, and hidden by means of blending the devices into a user's hair or skin color. Instead, the goal is to highlight the inequitable device offerings that then limit a user's ability to decide for themselves what they feel most comfortable with.

1.1. Colorism

Colorism is a phenomenon that has long been intertwined with the United States' racist history [7]. The issue of preferring lighter skin, especially in marketing, has become more frequently challenged in the wake of the Black Lives Matter protests in 2020 [15]. However, despite the backlash companies like Heineken, Crayola, and Band-Aid have faced, colorism is still prevalent in many industries globally [15]. While this paper will specifically be considering the consequences of colorism in OTC hearing aids, the impact of the effect must be understood to contextualize these consequences, especially as colorism permeates many different aspects of everyday life. The effects of colorism are so far-reaching that it has even been documented that children in South Africa are more likely to use lighter crayons when drawing self-portraits despite them not matching their own darker skin tones [16]. With society often promoting and valuing relatively lighter euro-centric skin, large communities of people can feel unrepresented and can begin to internalize the idea that dark skin is not "pretty" or "worthy" of appreciation [17]. Not only are the effects of colorism attributed to negative self-perception, but there is evidence that people with darker skin tones are more likely to be fired and live in lower socio-economic conditions due to this racial bias [18].

1.2. Healthcare Inequality and Racism

After understanding the impacts of colorism, it is important to build on its specific relationship to healthcare. BIPOC people are often more apprehensive about accessing medical care due to a history of prejudice and discrimination from the healthcare system (that continues in many places to this day) [13]. In hearing care, racial disparities persist and are subject to the same issues as the rest of the healthcare system. For example, white people are more likely to report regular hearing aid use despite Black people having had more recent hearing tests [19]. This is partly due to two race-related factors, one being that white people are more likely to have higher socio-economic status than Black people living in the United States, and hearing tests are covered by Medicare but hearing aids are not [19,20]. Since Black people are more likely to be less affluent than their white peers, their lower hearing aid use rates can be related back to the combination of the high cost of the devices along with the lack of adequate insurance coverage [6].

1.3. Social Perceptions of Hearing Aids

It is now evident that BIPOC people are less likely to have access to hearing aids, so one must next consider perceptions of hearing aids themselves and how that may also influence device uptake rates. Hearing aids are often associated with negative aspects of aging, so much so that the, "Hearing Aid Effect" was coined to describe the stigma that people wearing hearing aids experience [14,21,22]. This stigma can lead to not only a reduced uptake in hearing aids but an increase in social isolation, loneliness, and negative self-perception [11,21]. Notably, a study on perceptions of hearing aids indicated that the "Hearing Aid Effect" is present for brightly colored hearing devices, but not ones matching skin tone [23]. If hearing devices are not available in the participant's skin tone, the Hearing Aid Effect stigma becomes more impactful. This means that BIPOC people who are trying to access hearing aids but are worried about the consequences associated with the device stigma do not have the same ability to mitigate those concerns as white hearing aid users do.

1.4. Consequences of Unmanaged Hearing Loss

Managing hearing loss can look different depending on the kind of loss and the resources the individual has access to, but typically, hearing loss is addressed with the use of hearing aids [24]. So, if an individual cannot afford hearing aids or is too ashamed due to the stigma of wearing them, how will that impact the person's life moving forward? Hearing loss has been linked to an increased risk of dementia and general cognitive decline, at least partly due to the additional processing required to participate in a conversation [24–26]. People who do not have the financial or social security required for hearing aids are at a greater disadvantage when trying to address their hearing loss. Since it has already been established that BIPOC people are less likely to be able to afford care and face additional social scrutiny, a conclusion can be drawn that BIPOC communities with hearing loss are at a greater risk of experiencing cognitive decline.

1.5. Over-the-Counter Hearing Aids

Next, it is important to consider what is being done in the hearing health industry to attempt to reduce some of the barriers like prohibitively high device costs and increased social stigma. When the FDA authorized the sale of OTC devices, they specifically cited both the high cost and the social stigma associated with hearing aids as reasons why OTCs needed to be introduced to the market [2]. These devices are designed to disrupt the high device cost by offering self-testing and fitting, which eliminates the need for going to an audiologist, which, as established above, can be a barrier in and of itself for BIPOC people needing healthcare. While OTCs are not meant to replace the field of audiology, given that the average delay between when someone realizes they have a hearing loss and them attempting to manage it is nine years, they are a good entry point to close that gap and mitigate the effects that can lead to dementia [27]. The same study on the time between hearing aid candidacy and adoption even notes that BIPOC folks tend to have even longer delays than white folks [27]. Given that communicating aurally with unmanaged hearing loss causes increased cognitive effort, which can quickly lead to cognitive decline, it is crucial for the nine-year gap to be minimized as much as possible.

1.6. Knowledge Gap

From reviewing the literature on the intersection of colorism and hearing health, it has become evident to the authors that hearing healthcare services, including access to hearing aids, are not equitably available to all populations, with reduced access to hearing healthcare for some historically marginalized populations, including BIPOC individuals. There is also a lack of information on hearing aid use and acceptability for BIPOC people in the United States. While there exist a few more modern papers, it is challenging to obtain data due to the lack of trust between BIPOC patients and medical personnel, especially after tragedies like the Tuskegee incident [28]. Finally, since OTCs are relatively new at the time of this study, there are relatively sparse data on their usage compared to other medical devices [2]. This research attempts to assess the availability of OTC hearing aids across the range of possible human skin colors.

2. Materials and Methods

For this study, the U.S. Food and Drug Administration Establishment Registration and Device Listing database was used to identify FDA-cleared over-the-counter hearing aids in August 2023, as shown in Figure 1 [29]. The database was searched for devices with product codes QUF, QUG, QUH, and QDD, which identify hearing aids for sale without a prescription [30]. All companies with devices registered with these product codes were extracted from the database in August 2023. Duplicates were defined as the same products being listed by several regional divisions of the same firm (e.g., a single firm registering a device separately with both the firm's South African and Danish divisions). For products with duplicate entries, only a single product was included in the analyses to avoid over-representing duplicates in the analysis.

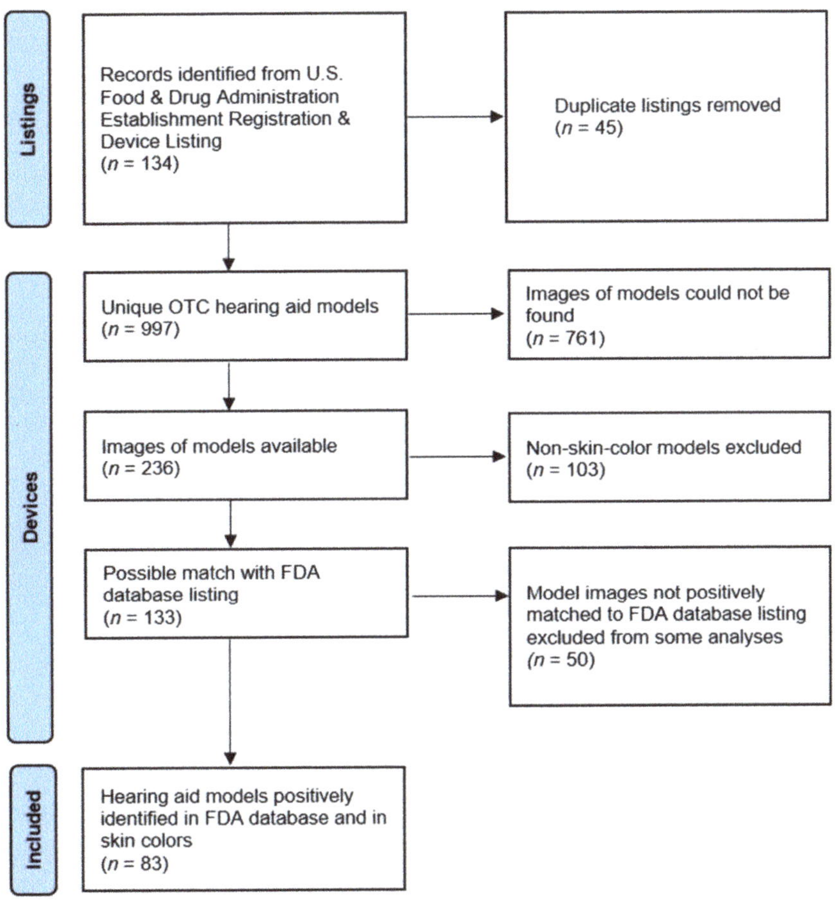

Figure 1. Data collection process.

2.1. Data Collection

Google and Bing search engines were used in August and September 2023 to identify images for the hearing aid models listed in the FDA database. Search strings with various combinations of the company name and hearing aid model name or number were used to identify the company's website or the online marketplace where the hearing aids were listed. These websites were used to identify and download images of each model hearing aid listed in the FDA database. Where a definite match between model name or number and image could not be made due to lack of a model name or model number listed in the FDA database, all potential device matches by that company were downloaded for analysis. Only behind-the-ear (BTE) models were included in the analysis, as in-the-ear (ITE) styles are often made to resemble commercially available Bluetooth headsets designed for phone calls, not to blend into the patient's skin or attempt to make themselves less visible by having a smaller size, instead of matching an individual's skin color.

2.2. Color Extraction

Where multiple images were available for a given hearing aid model, images that displayed the lateral side view of the device, that were real depictions of the device (as opposed to computer-generated renderings), that had frontal lighting, and that were not being worn by a person in the image were chosen. A single pixel was extracted from the central area of the lateral hearing aid casing for each device and was chosen to be representative of the color of the hearing aid casing. The extracted color was not chosen from areas with text, logos, or a casing seam. The single HEX color value for each device was converted to a CIELAB color space value, an international standard for defining the color of an object. Where a single hearing aid model was offered in several colors, the process was repeated for each model color.

An 11-color skin color palette was used to represent the range of possible human skin colors, as shown in Figure 2. The skin color palette was validated for international contexts and the full development of the palette is available elsewhere [31]. HEX color values for each portion of the palate are available in Table 1 CIELAB color space values were also extracted from each of the 11 skin colors in the palette. The color of each hearing aid model was compared to all 11 skin colors using the CIELAB ΔE^* color-difference formula, an international standard and validated formula. The exact formulas used to perform the comparisons are reported in depth elsewhere [32]. The skin color with the smallest difference value for each hearing aid was recorded as that device's most similar skin color.

Table 1. Proportion of hearing aids by skin color.

Palette Color	Hex Color Code	Skin Color Only %	Definite Model Match and Skin Color Only %
1	FBF2F3	6.0	7.2
2	F4D7D9	0.8	0
3	E7C1B8	13.5	15.7
4	E6C8A2	21.1	16.9
5	BEA07E	41.4	42.2
6	9C7953	6.8	6.0
7	81654F	6.8	7.2
8	6F503C	0.8	1.2
9	513B2E	1.5	2.4
10	422811	0	0
11	373028	1.5	1.2

Figure 2. Color palette of possible human skin colors [31].

3. Results

The number of listings in each product code category is shown in Table 2. After duplicate listings were removed, 89 listings were included in the final sample. The listings varied widely in the number of model numbers included in the listings, with most firms registering only 1 device and some firms registering up to 80 unique model numbers, as shown in Figure 3. The countries represented in the sample are shown in Table 3. In total, 997 unique models were listed in the database.

Table 2. Product codes in FDA database.

Product Code	Description	Number of Entries	Number of Entries, Duplicates Excluded
QUF	Preset hearing aids without wireless capability	45	43
QUG	Preset hearing aids with wireless capability	56	38
QUH	Self-fitting hearing aids with user input for sale online or in physical stores	15	4
QDD	Self-fitting hearing aids with user input for sale online	18	4

Table 3. Listings in the database by country of origin.

Country	N	%
Australia	1	1.1
China	55	61.8
Denmark	1	1.1
Mexico	1	1.1
Philippines	1	1.1
South Africa	3	3.4
South Korea	1	1.1
Taiwan	2	2.2
USA	23	25.8
Vietnam	1	1.1

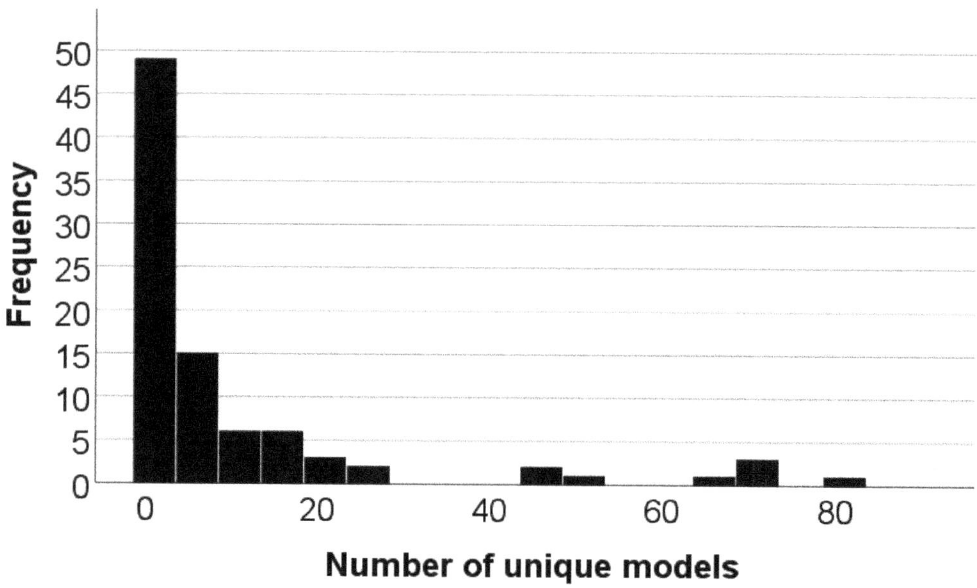

Figure 3. Number of models per listing.

Out of the 997 unique models, images of 236 could be found. A definite match was found between the model number listed in the FDA database and the image listed online for 65.3% (n = 154) of these devices. A total of 61 (25.8%) devices were found for companies that did not list a specific model number on their FDA submission. A total of 103 (43.6%) devices that were clearly not typical skin colors (silver, blue, etc.) were excluded from the skin-color analyses. The final sample of hearing aid models that were meant to represent possible skin colors and were listed in the FDA database comprised 83 unique models.

The proportion of hearing aids most like each skin color palette is shown in Figure 4 and Table 3. The hex color code for each skin color in the palette is also provided. Far more hearing aids in the sample were offered in relatively lighter colors, with few or no options available for darker skin colors. Among skin-color hearing aids that could be conclusively matched to submissions to the FDA database, the five lightest skin colors accounted for 81.9% of devices.

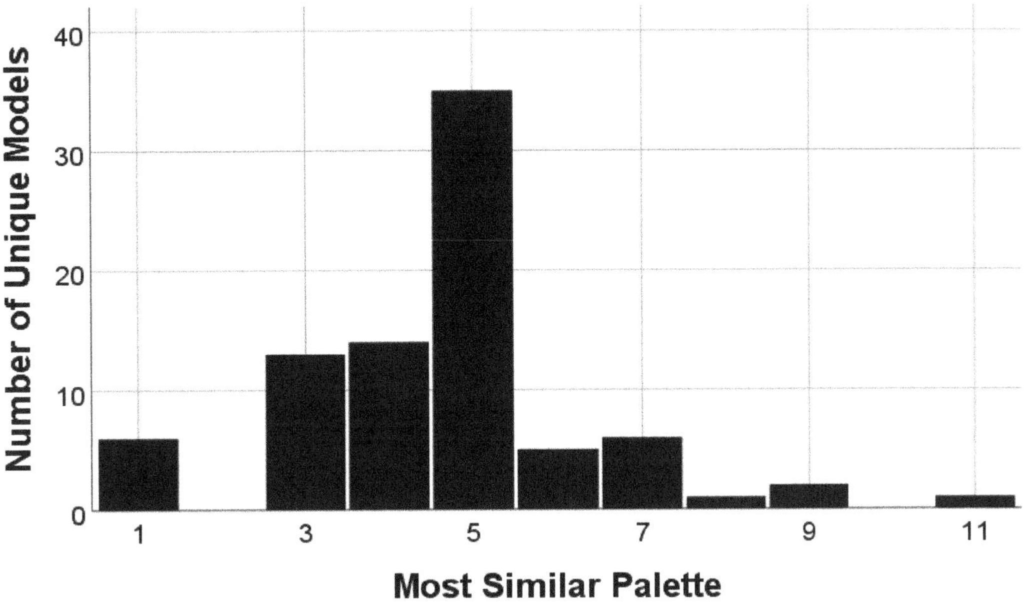

Figure 4. Proportion of hearing aids by skin color.

4. Discussion

4.1. Major Findings

This study has revealed that FDA-cleared OTC hearing aids are 82% more likely to be offered in relatively lighter skin tones aligning with PERLA tones 1–5 vs. relatively darker skin colors (82% vs. 18%, respectively). For the four darkest skin tones, only 4.8% of OTC hearing aids on the market offered a matching product. It is well documented that racism and the priority of product design for lighter skin tones has persisted in Western culture for hundreds of years [33]. This is what informed the initial hypothesis that product offerings would favor lighter skin tones, which, as discovered in Section 3, was determined to be true. This means that BIPOC individuals are much less likely to have access to OTC hearing aids that best reflect their skin tone, which both perpetuates systemic racism in product development and limits more affordable hearing care options due to the stigma that can come with visibly wearing a hearing aid.

4.2. Importance of Findings

BIPOC hearing aid users are subject to increased stigmatization due to their intersectional racialized identity and disability [19]. There are several consequences that may result from the OTC color offering inequity. For example, BIPOC people may opt for an in-the-ear hearing aid to minimize device visibility, but this may not be the best product choice for their type of hearing loss [13]. This group of hearing aid wearers is also at an increased risk of bullying and disability-related harassment in addition to the often-daily hate toward their skin color. One of the most devastating implications is that OTCs were intended to be an affordable introduction into receiving support for hearing loss. With BIPOC people already more likely to be living in a lower income bracket, OTCs could have been a better option to help mitigate the consequences of untreated hearing loss, such as dementia and social isolation [11,13].

In noting the disparity between product offerings for different skin tones, further implications arise. There is a history of inequity for BIPOC people attempting to access healthcare in the United States that continues to be pervasive in the present day [33]. Hearing care is a form of healthcare, and it is not immune to the institutional racism existing in all levels of healthcare. This discrimination that is so deeply ingrained in American society has led to a deep mistrust in institutions by BIPOC individuals and can cause these individuals to be more likely to avoid seeking treatment, including visiting an audiologist [13].

Because OTCs are still relatively new, the research from this paper on the skin tone offerings for these devices is unique but warrants further reflection and expansion to other hearing-health-related devices. These findings may allow OTC manufacturers to improve the acceptability of their product offerings for BIPIC people early in the life cycle of the United States OTC market. Hearing aid colorways have also not been traditionally compared to the PERLA skin tone chart, but while this may be novel, the method is still used in many disciplines [31,34]. Additionally, these methods may be valuable in analyzing the availability of prescription hearing aids across the spectrum of human skin colors.

The OTC products that were examined were not put into the context of the company/device's market share value. This allows for a possible alternative explanation where the diverse brand options take up a larger percentage of the market, meaning that OTC devices would still allow for adequate colorway options for BIPOC individuals in most products available. While this context is important to consider, it does not negate the fact that there are still enough companies offering only lighter skin tone colors as device options that there is a clear skew available products for purchase. BIPOC people have less diversity in brand choices due to racial discrimination, and it just may be less evident in a high-level market analysis because of the market shares of particular devices.

4.3. Limitations

The primary limitation is the constraint of finding complete device codes with model colors clearly displayed. Out of 997 unique OTC models registered in the FDA database, only 83 unique OTC hearing aid models were able to be compared according to the study criteria due to incomplete product information in the FDA database. Further studies should incorporate a larger device base, possibly from OTC hearing aid markets in other countries. Future studies should also consider the market share of the individual devices/brands and how colorway offering may impact sales. This will aid in comprehending the intentionality behind the colorways as well as link back to a larger movement occurring in the marketing industry.

5. Conclusions

Over-the-counter hearing aids have great potential to improve equity in hearing healthcare for BIPOC individuals. They are cheaper, do not require a prescription from a healthcare professional, and can be a good starting point for people who have mild-to-moderate hearing loss. Based on this project, it has become clear that while these benefits may exist for people with relatively lighter skin, BIPOC people do not have the same opportunities to choose devices that best fit their skin tones. When discretion is a common desire for new hearing aid wearers, the lack of choice offered to BIPOC individuals by the current OTC market is further perpetuation of the racist history plaguing the United States. Future OTC offerings should be expanded to allow for more diverse colorways to afford BIPOC people the same range of product choices that white people are currently allowed.

Author Contributions: Conceptualization, methodology, software, formal analysis, data curation, and writing, S.A.K. Writing, S.J.F. All authors have read and agreed to the published version of the manuscript.

Funding: This research received no external funding.

Institutional Review Board Statement: Not applicable.

Informed Consent Statement: Not applicable.

Data Availability Statement: Data used in this study can be made available by contacting the authors.

Acknowledgments: The authors would like to thank Darnisha Starr Draughter and Junghwa Kim at the University of California, Irvine for their support in preparing this manuscript.

Conflicts of Interest: The authors declare no conflicts of interest.

References

1. World Health Organization. *World Report on Hearing*; World Health Organization: Geneva, Switzerland, 2021; Available online: https://www.who.int/publications/i/item/9789240020481 (accessed on 8 January 2024).
2. Department of Health and Human Services. Medical Devices; Ear, Nose, and Throat Devices; Establishing Over-the-Counter Hearing Aids; 2022; Code Number RIN 0910–AI21. Available online: https://www.federalregister.gov/documents/2022/08/17/2022-17230/medical-devices-ear-nose-and-throat-devices-establishing-over-the-counter-hearing-aids (accessed on 8 January 2024).
3. Jilla, A.M.; Johnson, C.E.; Huntington-Klein, N. Hearing aid affordability in the United States. *Disabil. Rehabil. Assist. Technol.* **2020**, *18*, 246–252. [CrossRef]
4. McNeal, M.H. Say what: The Affordable Care Act, Medicare, and hearing aids. *Harv. J. Legis.* **2016**, *53*, 621. [CrossRef]
5. President's Council of Advisors on Science and Technology. Aging America & Hearing Loss: Imperative of Improved Hearing Technologies. October 2015. Available online: https://obamawhitehouse.archives.gov/sites/default/files/microsites/ostp/PCAST/PCAST%20hearing%20letter%20report.pdf (accessed on 8 January 2024).
6. Nieman, C.L.; Suen, J.J.; Dean, L.T.; Chandran, A. Foundational Approaches to Advancing Hearing Health Equity: A Primer in Social Epidemiology. *Ear Hearth* **2022**, *43* (Suppl. S1), 5S. [CrossRef]
7. Monk, E.P. Colorism and Physical Health: Evidence from a National Survey. *J. Health Soc. Behav.* **2021**, *62*, 37–52. [CrossRef]
8. Mitchell, G.; Sampath, U.; Maan, A.; Balu, N. Factbox: What Changes Are Companies Making in Response to George Floyd Protests? *Reuters*, 20 June 2020. Available online: https://www.reuters.com/article/idUSKBN23R059/ (accessed on 25 January 2024).
9. Alcorn, C. Band-Aid Will Make Black and Brown Flesh-Toned Bandages. *CNN*, 12 June 2020. Available online: https://www.cnn.com/2020/06/12/business/black-band-aids/index.html (accessed on 25 January 2024).
10. Crayola. When Did You Introduce Crayola Multicultural and Colors of the World Products? Crayola. Available online: https://www.crayola.com/faq/another-topic/when-did-you-introduce-crayola-multicultural-products/ (accessed on 25 January 2024).
11. Da Silva, J.C.; de Araujo, C.M.; Lüders, D.; Santos, R.S.; de Lacerda, A.B.; José, M.R.; Guarinello, A.C. The Self-Stigma of Hearing Loss in Adults and Older Adults: A Systematic Review. *Ear Hearth* **2023**, *44*, 1301–1310. [CrossRef]
12. David, D.; Werner, P. Stigma regarding hearing loss and hearing aids: A scoping review. *Stigma Health* **2016**, *1*, 59. [CrossRef]
13. Jorgensen, L.E.; Barrett, R.E. Relating Factors and Trends in Hearing Device Adoption Rates to Opportunities for Hearing Health Care Providers. *Semin. Hearth* **2022**, *43*, 289–300. [CrossRef]
14. Sindi, A.; Hanbazazah, K.; Alamoudi, M.M.; Al-Harbi, A.; Aljuhani, M.; Zawawi, F. The Hearing Aid Effect in the 2020s: Where Do We Stand? *Cureus* **2023**, *15*, e38302. [CrossRef]
15. Mallick, M. Marketing Still Has a Colorism Problem. *Harvard Business Review*, 20 May 2021. Available online: https://hbr.org/2021/05/marketing-still-has-a-colorism-problem (accessed on 13 January 2024).
16. Alexander, N.; Costandius, E. The 'Human Colour' Crayon: Investigating the Attitudes and Perceptions of Learners regarding Race and Skin Colour. *Educ. Chang.* **2017**, *21*, 113–136. [CrossRef]
17. Marx, D.M.; Ko, S.J.; Friedman, R.A. The 'Obama Effect': How a salient role model reduces race-based performance differences. *J. Exp. Soc. Psychol.* **2009**, *45*, 953–956. [CrossRef]
18. Hunter, M. The Persistent Problem of Colorism: Skin Tone, Status, and Inequality. *Sociol. Compass* **2007**, *1*, 237–254. [CrossRef]
19. Nieman, C.L.; Marrone, N.; Szanton, S.L.; Thorpe, R.J.; Lin, F.R. Racial/Ethnic and Socioeconomic Disparities in Hearing Health Care among Older Americans. *J. Aging Health* **2016**, *28*, 68–94. [CrossRef]
20. Liu, X.; Rosa-Lugo, L.I.; Cosby, J.L.; Pritchett, C.V. Racial and Insurance Inequalities in Access to Early Pediatric Cochlear Implantation. *Otolaryngol. Neck Surg.* **2021**, *164*, 667–674. [CrossRef]
21. Cienkowski, K.M.; Pimentel, V. The hearing aid 'effect' revisited in young adults. *Br. J. Audiol.* **2001**, *35*, 289–295. [CrossRef]
22. McManus, H.; Salbod, S.; Berg, A.L. The Hearing Aid 'Effect' as a Function of Race and Gender. *Hearth J.* **2016**, *69*, 1214. [CrossRef]
23. Qian, Z.J.; Nuyen, B.A.; Kandathil, C.K.; Truong, M.T.; Tribble, M.S.; Most, S.P.; Chang, K.W. Social Perceptions of Pediatric Hearing Aids. *Laryngoscope* **2021**, *131*, E2387–E2392. [CrossRef]
24. Castiglione, A.; Benatti, A.; Velardita, C.; Favaro, D.; Padoan, E.; Severi, D.; Pagliaro, M.; Bovo, R.; Vallesi, A.; Gabelli, C.; et al. Aging, Cognitive Decline and Hearing Loss: Effects of Auditory Rehabilitation and Training with Hearing Aids and Cochlear Implants on Cognitive Function and Depression among Older Adults. *Audiol. Neurotol.* **2016**, *21* (Suppl. S1), 21–28. [CrossRef]
25. Babajanian, E.E.; Gurgel, R.K. Cognitive and behavioral effects of hearing loss. *Curr. Opin. Otolaryngol. Head Neck Surg.* **2022**, *30*, 339–343. [CrossRef]
26. Uchida, Y.; Sugiura, S.; Nishita, Y.; Saji, N.; Sone, M.; Ueda, H. Age-related hearing loss and cognitive decline—The potential mechanisms linking the two. *Auris Nasus Larynx* **2019**, *46*, 1–9. [CrossRef]
27. Simpson, A.N.; Matthews, L.J.; Cassarly, C.; Dubno, J.R. Time From Hearing Aid Candidacy to Hearing Aid Adoption: A Longitudinal Cohort Study. *Ear Hearth* **2019**, *40*, 468. [CrossRef]

28. Alsan, M.; Wanamaker, M. Tuskegee and the Health of Black Men*. *Q. J. Econ.* **2018**, *133*, 407–455. [CrossRef]
29. U.S. Food & Drug Administration. Establishment Registration & Device Listing. 2023. Available online: https://www.accessdata.fda.gov/scripts/cdrh/cfdocs/cfRL/TextSearch.cfm (accessed on 1 January 2024).
30. Bailey, A. Full List of OTC Hearing Aids. February 2023. Available online: https://www.hearingtracker.com/full-list-of-otc-hearing-aids (accessed on 1 January 2024).
31. Telles, E.E. *Pigmentocracies: Ethnicity, Race, and Color in Latin America*, 1st ed.; University of North Carolina Press: Chapel Hill, NC, USA, 2014.
32. Sharma, G.; Wu, W.; Dalal, E.N. The CIEDE2000 color-difference formula: Implementation notes, supplementary test data, and mathematical observations. *Color Res. Appl.* **2005**, *30*, 21–30. [CrossRef]
33. Yearby, R. Racial Disparities in Health Status and Access to Healthcare: The Continuation of Inequality in the United States Due to Structural Racism. *Am. J. Econ. Sociol.* **2018**, *77*, 1113–1152. [CrossRef]
34. Levitt, H. A Historical Perspective on Digital Hearing Aids: How Digital Technology Has Changed Modern Hearing Aids. *Trends Amplif.* **2007**, *11*, 7–24. [CrossRef]

audiology research

MDPI

Article

Preliminary Validation of the Children's Auditory Performance Scale (CHAPS) and the Auditory Processing Domain Questionnaire (APDQ) in Greek Cypriot Children

Konstantinos Drosos [1,*], Dionysios Tafiadis [2], Louiza Voniati [1], Alexandra Papanicolaou [3] and Chryssoula Thodi [1]

[1] School of Sciences, Speech and Language Therapy, European University Cyprus, 2404 Nicosia, Cyprus; l.voniati@euc.ac.cy (L.V.); c.thodi@euc.ac.cy (C.T.)
[2] Department of Speech and Language Therapy, University of Ioannina, GR-45500 Ioannina, Greece; tafiadis@uoi.gr
[3] Department of Hearing and Speech Sciences, University of Maryland College Park, College Park, MD 20740, USA; apapani3@umd.edu
* Correspondence: k.drosos@external.euc.ac.cy; Tel.: +357-22029900

Abstract: Background: Identification of auditory processing disorders is achieved using questionnaires along with linguistic, non-linguistic, and auditory processing tests. Notably, the questionnaires "Children's Auditory Performance Scale" (CHAPS) and "Auditory Processing Domain Questionnaire" (APDQ) are widely recognized and used. The current study investigated the psychometric properties of the CHAPS and APDQ in Greek Cypriot children. Methods: The CHAPS and APDQ questionnaires were completed by parents of 40 Greek Cypriot children, 16 typically developing (TD) children, and 24 children with a history of Speech Sound Disorders (SSDs). Results: There were significant differences between the two groups on both questionnaires. Cronbach's alpha was calculated at $\alpha = 0.922$ for the CHAPS total score and $\alpha = 0.926$ for the APDQ total score. The Receiver Operating Curve (ROC) analysis provided a cut-off point equal to -0.30 (AUC 0.849, $p < 0.001$) for CHAPS and a cut-off point equal to 90.00 (AUC 0.820, $p < 0.001$) for APDQ. Significant positive Spearman ρ correlations were observed between the CHAPS and APDQ ($\rho = 0.639$, $p = 0.001$). Conclusions: The CHAPS and APDQ can identify distinct auditory processing characteristics between in children with SSDs and TD children.

Keywords: auditory processing; discrimination; screening; CHAPS; APDQ; speech sound disorders

1. Introduction

Auditory processing disorder (APD) refers to a deficit in the neural processing of auditory information that can result in higher-order disorders related to learning, attention, memory, cognitive, communicative, or language-related skills [1,2]. APD affects an individual's ability to adequately acquire auditory skills (i.e., detection, discrimination, identification, and comprehension of speech), especially in complex noisy listening environments [1,3]. In children, the estimated prevalence is between 0.2% and 5% [4–6] noting a 2:1 male-to-female ratio of APD diagnosis. Several studies suggest high comorbidity between APD and developmental disorders such as developmental language disorder (DLD), dyslexia, learning disabilities (LDs), attention-deficit hyperactivity disorder (ADHD), autism spectrum disorders (ASD) [7–9], and Speech Sound Disorders (SSDs) [10]. Recognizing auditory processing impairments in children early on is crucial for implementing successful auditory interventions. This takes advantage of the brain's adaptability and allows for accurate differentiation of children with APD from those with related disorders [8]. It is essential to gather detailed reports on a child's listening difficulties in everyday settings to identify children who may be at risk for suspected APD. This can be achieved by administering screening questionnaires to caregivers and teachers [11,12]. The

American Academy of Audiology (AAA) [3] and the American Speech–Language–Hearing Association (ASHA) [1] recommend employing screening tools to pinpoint those who may be susceptible to APD. Questionnaires and behavioral checklists that have been mentioned in the international literature include the following: (1) the Children's Auditory Performance Scale (CHAPS); (2) the Screening Instrument for Targeting Educational Risk (SIFTER); (3) the Test of Auditory Processing Skills–Revised (TAPS-R); (4) the Children's Home Inventory of Listening Difficulties (CHILD); (5) Fisher's Auditory Problems Checklist (FAPC); (6) the Auditory Processing Domains Questionnaire (APDQ); (7) the Listening Inventory for Education (LIFE); (8) the Listening Inventory for Education–Revised (LIFE-R); (9) the Scale of Auditory Behaviors (SAB); (10) the Listening Inventory (TLI); and (11) the Evaluation of Children's Listening and Processing Skills (ECLIPS). Worldwide, researchers are continuously evaluating the use of APD screening tools and questionnaires based on relevance and clinical applicability [10–14]. Children with SSDs, as well as children with suspected APD, may have differences in auditory processing skills from TD children and children with APD diagnosis [8,10,15]. A crucial effort of this study was to reflect findings from the available literature on the population of children in Cyprus. Hence, we proceeded to administer the CHAPS and APDQ to record the auditory processing skills of Greek Cypriot children with typical development and children with SSDs. Therefore, this study examines the effectiveness of two established and commonly utilized questionnaires, the CHAPS and APDQ [12,16–18], in detecting and differentiating children with APD from TD children and children with SSDs. Additionally, this study aims to evaluate the suitability of these questionnaires as screening tools in Greek Cypriot children. The two questionnaires chosen for the present study are commonly accepted by the scientific community, are bibliographically recorded internationally in the existing knowledge of systematic reviews on the subject, and offer detailed results with relative subdomains covering audiological, linguistic, and non-linguistic fields [11,12].

2. Materials and Methods

2.1. Sample

The parents of 40 children between seven and ten years old filled out the CHAPS and APDQ questionnaires. Sixteen children who exhibited typical psychosocial and language development, of average age 8.40 years (7.85–8.70 years), formed the typically developing (TD) group. Twenty-four children diagnosed with Speech Sound Disorders (SSDs), of average age 8.1 years (7.90–8.40 years) formed the experimental group. All children were monolingual Greek Cypriot dialect speakers. Children in both groups had normal pure-tone thresholds, no history of middle ear disease, and no sensory, cognitive, psychomotor, communication, or learning disorders.

2.2. Translation Procedures of APDQ

The APDQ questionnaire was translated and adapted following the Cognitive Debriefing Method as outlined by Hall et al. [19]. Following communication with the original creators of the APDQ questionnaire, we proceeded to translate and adapt the questions to the Greek language. Initially, two native speakers of Greek proficient in English translated the questionnaire from English to Greek. A reconciliation version of the two translations was developed with the mediation of a third native Greek Speaker fluent in English. Following the initial stage, a proficient English Speaker back-translated the questionnaire to English, and the points showing discrepancies with the original were reworked in the translation to Greek. Following a consensus review of the two procedures, the form was finalized. The questionnaire was administered to three parents to ensure feasibility. Upon feedback from the pilot study, the team finalized the questionnaire.

2.3. Participant Recruitment and Assessment

The recruitment process and consent form were approved by the Cyprus National Bioethics Committee (EEBK/EP/2022/37). Invitations to participate in the study were extended to all parents of children undergoing therapy for SSDs at the Speech, Language, and Hearing Clinic of the European University Cyprus. The parents who agreed to allow their children to participate completed and signed the consent form. Parents provided information on their children's health history. TD children were recruited from public schools. The inclusion of children in public schools was approved by the Pedagogical Institute of the Ministry of Education, Sport, and Youth of the Republic of Cyprus KEEA-148053. A pure-tone audiogram was completed by an audiologist at the Speech, Language, and Hearing Clinic of the European University Cyprus.

Following audiometric testing, the children completed an auditory processing battery comprising the Gap Detection Test [20]; Gap-in-Noise Test [21]; Dichotic Hearing (words) [18]; Greek Speech in Bubble Test [22]; Duration and Pitch Pattern Sequence Tests [23]; Forward/Backward digit span [24]; and words presented in various signal-to-noise ratios. Children completed a battery of speech and language tests, consisting of the Action Picture Test (APT) [25] and the Metaphone test–full version (Test of Metaphonological Development and Reading Readiness in Phonological Awareness) [26]. The APT assesses the content and grammatical patterns in children's speech, effectively documenting the morphology in terms of grammar and syntax. The test considers grammatical structures and words used to convey information. The Metaphone test evaluates linguistic abilities related to rhyme, syllabic, and phonemic awareness. The Raven Colored Progressive Matrices Assessment (Raven) [27] was included in the protocol as an index of cognitive performance. The Raven is a non-verbal assessment of abstract and cognitive function, spatial reasoning, analogical reasoning, and problem-solving ability.

Parents of participating children filled out the CHAPS and APDQ questionnaires, which aimed to document the auditory processing profiles of the children and identify any distinguishing factors between the two groups.

The CHAPS questionnaire collects caregivers' and teachers' feedback on children's hearing difficulties at home and in academic settings [18,28]. The CHAPS includes thirty-six questions divided into six subscales: (1) perception in noise; (2) perception in quiet; (3) perception in ideal (one-on-one) situations; (4) perception with multiple inputs; (5) memory; and (6) attention. The first four subscales directly assess hearing-related difficulties, while the last two evaluate cognitive skills indirectly related to hearing. Responders are asked to rate the child's hearing difficulties relative to their peers using the following Likert scale: less difficulty (+1), same amount of difficulty (0), slightly more difficulty (−1), more difficulty (−2), considerably more difficulty (−3), significantly more difficulty (−4), and cannot function at all (−5). A raw score is calculated by adding the scores of individual question items; the overall result is divided by 7 to obtain an average overall score. Raw scores are available for each subscale; when divided by the number of questions, we obtain an overall score. The CHAPS questionnaire is utilized to screen and complement the diagnostic auditory processing evaluation. Silva et al. [29] published a systematic review. They investigated the accuracy of screening instruments for identifying APD and determined that the sensitivity of the CHAPS was higher than 70% among reviewed articles. In our research study, we used the Greek version of the CHAPS [18].

The APDQ was developed by O'Hara and Mealings in 2018 and revised in 2021 [16]. In the current iteration, the APDQ contains fifty questions divided into three sub-scales: (1) the Auditory Processing (AP) scale; (2) the Attention Control (ATT) scale; and (3) the Language (Lang) scale. One question overlaps between the AP and ATT scales, one question overlaps between the AP and Lang scales, and two questions are used to compare listening in quiet versus listening in noise. A behavior is attributed four points if it is performed regularly (>3/4 of the time), three points if it is performed often (1/2–3/4 of the time), one point if it is performed sometimes (1/4–1/2 of the time), and zero points if it is performed rarely (<1/4 of the time). Scale scores are calculated as the sum of item scores per scale divided by the number of items in each scale multiplied by four. Scale scores are reported as "percent of perfect score": scores above 75% are interpreted as greater skill competency, whereas scores below 25% are interpreted as reduced skill competency. Additionally, the APDQ includes an algorithmic indicator called Target AP, which is derived by subtracting the Auditory Processing domain score from the Attention domain score.

2.4. Statistical Analysis

Variables were evaluated for normality using the Kolmogorov–Smirnov and Shapiro–Wilk tests; descriptive variables reported included the Median (Mdn) and Interquartile range (IQR). The Mann–Whitney test was used to investigate differences between the two independent groups. A size effect analysis was performed with a partial eta squared coefficient for non-parametric values (n^2). The estimation of cut-off values for the CHAPS was computed through a Receiver Operating Characteristics (ROC) curve analysis. The optimal cut-off values were determined using the robust and effective Youden index. The Cronbach's alpha coefficient technique was used to evaluate the internal consistency of the Greek version of the two questionnaires.

To determine questionnaire sensitivity and specificity, we computed Spearman's rho between the total scores of the CHAPS, the APDQ, and the auditory processing scores.

The significance level was set at 0.05 for two-tailed comparisons. Statistical analyses were performed using IBM SPSS 28 statistical software [30].

3. Results

3.1. Demographic and Group Performance Findings

TD and children with SSDs had similar age and cognitive characteristics. Participants' demographics, language, and language performance are shown in Table 1. Bonferroni's adjustment for multiple comparisons was applied on the acceptable α level for the subdomain comparisons of the Action Pictures Test; for four comparisons, the acceptable level would be 0.05/4 = 0.0125. For the Metaphone test subdomain comparisons, the acceptable level would be 0.05/9 = 0.0056. Table 2 shows the auditory processing battery findings.

Table 1. Sample characteristics and language performance.

	TD Group (N = 16)	Experimental Group (N = 24)		
	Mdn (IQR)	**Mdn (IQR)**	p	n^2
Children's Age in Years	8.40 (7.85–8.70)	8.10 (7.90–8.40)	0.486	0.007
Raven Total Score	33.00 (31.50–33.50)	32.00 (31.00–33.00)	0.153	0.004
Action Picture Test Total Score	71.00 (62.50–76.00)	68.00 (60.00–71.00)	0.170	0.102
Action Picture Test: information	37.00 (32.00–38.50)	33.00 (31.00–36.00)	0.930	0.007
Action Picture Test: grammar	34.00 (30.50–36.50)	30.00 (28.00–32.00)	<0.005 *	0.150
Metaphone Total Score	180.00 (166.50–187.50)	169.00 (163.00–175.00)	0.220	0.099
Words from Same Syllable Score	13.00 (12.00–13.00)	13.00 (12.00–13.00)	0.936	0.002
Syllabication Score	8.00 (8.00–8.00)	8.00 (8.00–8.00)	0.830	0.006
First Syllable Identification Score	12.00 (12.00–12.00)	12.00 (12.00–12.00)	0.936	0.000
Final Syllable Localization Score	24.00 (23.00–26.00)	24.00 (22.00–26.00)	0.630	0.006
Word Finding Syllable Criterion Score	8.00 (7.00–8.00)	8.00 (8.00–8.00)	0.708	0.006
First Phoneme Identification Score	27.00 (24.50–28.50)	23.00 (22.00–26.00)	<0.005 *	0.216
Word Finding Phoneme Criterion Score	15.00 (13.50–17.00)	14.00 (12.00–15.00)	0.099	0.071
Word Repetition Score	37.00 (34.50–39.50)	34.00 (32.00–37.00)	<0.005 *	0.075

Abbreviations: TD group, typical developing children; Mdn, Medians; IQR, interquartile range; * p level at $p < 0.005$; n^2, partial eta squared.

Table 2. Auditory processing performance.

	TD Group (N = 16)	Experimental Group (N = 24)		
	Mdn (IQR)	Mdn (IQR)	*p*	n^2
Gap Detection 500 Hz	10.00 (10.00–10.00)	10.00 (10.00–10.00)	0.147	0.053
Gap Detection 1000 Hz	10.00 (10.00–10.00)	10.00 (10.00–10.00)	=0.005	0.095
Gap Detection 2000 Hz	10.00 (10.00–10.00)	10.00 (10.00–10.00)	0.809	0.001
Gap Detection 4000 Hz	10.00 (10.00–10.00)	10.00 (9.25–10.00)	0.127	0.059
Gap Detection in Noise 1	7.00 (7.00–7.00)	7.00 (7.00–7.00)	0.147	0.053
Gap Detection in Noise 5	6.00 (5.00–7.00)	5.00 (2.25–5.75)	<0.005	0.195
Speech in Bubble Right Ear	64.50 (58.25–66.00)	54.00 (39.75–62.00)	<0.005	0.143
SNR 7	70.00 (60.00–78.75)	60.00 (51.25–73.75)	0.165	0.049
SNR 5	67.50 (55.00–70.00)	60.00 (45.00–73.75)	0.284	0.029
SNR 3	65.00 (55.00–70.00)	55.00 (40.00–63.75)	=0.005	0.093
SNR 1	62.50 (55.00–70.00)	60.00 (50.00–65.00)	0.151	0.052
SNR Minus 1	50.00 (36.25–55.00)	40.00 (20.00–45.00)	<0.005	0.156
SNR 50%	2.40 (1.85–2.95)	3.00 (2.25–4.40)	=0.005	0.092
Dichotic Words—Right Ear 1st	21.00 (21.00–22.00)	19.50 (18.25–21.00)	<0.001	0.336
Dichotic Words Synchronized	21.00 (20.00–22.00)	18.00 (16.25–21.00)	=0.001	0.264
Duration Pattern Sequence	30.00 (29.50–30.00)	28.00 (26.25–29.00)	<0.001	0.323
Pitch Pattern 1000 to 2000 Hz	8.00 (7.25–8.00)	7.50 (7.00–8.00)	0.067	0.086
Pitch Pattern 4000 to 6000 Hz	8.00 (8.00–9.00)	7.00 (7.00–8.00)	=0.001	0.269
Forward Digit Span	8.00 (7.00–9.00)	7.00 (7.00–8.00)	0.200	0.042
Backward Digit Span	6.00 (5.00–7.00)	5.00 (4.25–6.00)	<0.005	0.108

Abbreviations: TD group, typical developing children; Mdn, Medians; IQR, interquartile range; SNR, signal-to-noise ratio; *p* level at $p < 0.005$; n^2, partial eta squared.

3.2. CHAPS Questionnaire and APDQ Findings

Table 3 shows the group performance and comparisons on the CHAPS questionnaire. The CHAPS questionnaire results indicate that the experimental group had significantly higher difficulty than the TD group [U = 1.500, $p < 0.001$] in all six CHAPS subdomains. Bonferroni's adjustment for multiple comparisons was applied on a level for the subdomain comparisons of the CHAPS test; for six comparisons the acceptable level would be 0.05/6 = 0.008. Table 4 shows the group performance and comparisons on the APDQ questionnaire There was a significant difference between the groups on the APDQ total score [U = 49.000, $p = 0.001$] and on the APDQ subdomains.

Table 3. Group performance and comparisons on the CHAPS questionnaire.

	Parents of Experimental Group Children (N = 24)	Parents of TD Children (N = 16)			
	Mdn (IQR)	Mdn (IQR)	Mann-Whitney U	*p*	n^2
CHAPS Total score	−0.50 (−0.70–−0.15)	0.20 (−0.20–0.80)	38.500	<0.001	0.455
CHAPS Noise subdomain	−1.30 (−1.65–−0.70)	0.30 (−0.30–0.70)	16.000	<0.001	0.682
CHAPS Quiet subdomain	−0.40 (−0.65–0.00)	0.40 (0.00–1.00)	49.000	<0.001	0.387
CHAPS Ideal subdomain	−0.30 (−0.70–0.70)	1.00 (0.00–1.00)	61.500	<0.005	0.314
CHAPS Multiple Inputs subdomain	−0.30 (−0.70–0.700)	0.70 (0.00–1.00)	33.500	<0.001	0.526

Table 3. *Cont.*

	Parents of Experimental Group Children (N = 24)	Parents of TD Children (N = 16)			
	Mdn (IQR)	**Mdn (IQR)**	**Mann-Whitney U**	***p***	**n²**
CHAPS Auditory Memory Sequencing subdomain	−0.50 (−0.85–−0.20)	0.00 (−0.50–1.00)	73.500	<0.005	0.235
CHAPS Auditory Attention Span subdomain	−0.10 (−0.90–0.50)	0.30 (−0.10–0.80)	68.000	<0.005	0.364

Abbreviations: CHAPS, Children's Auditory Performance Scale; Mdn, Medians; IQR, interquartile range; *p* level at $p < 0.005$; n^2, partial eta squared.

Table 4. Group performance and comparisons on the APDQ questionnaire.

	Parents of Experimental Group Children (N = 24)	Parents of TD Children (N = 16)			
	Mdn (IQR)	**Mdn (IQR)**	**Mann-Whitney U**	***p***	**n²**
APDQ Total Score	95.00 (81.50–107.00)	79.50 (68.75–85.00)	49.000	=0.001	0.253
APDQ Auditory Processing subdomain	60.00 (54.75–68.25)	50.50 (44.25–55.25)	35.000	<0.001	0.340
APDQ Attention Control subdomain	18.00 (14.75–22.00)	15.50 (12.50–17.00)	79.000	<0.005	0.109
APDQ Language subdomain	20.00 (18.00–24.00)	17.50 (16.25–19.75)	58.000	<0.005	0.202
APDQ Auditory Processing Target subdomain	−42.00 (50.00–39.00)	−36.00 (37.00–31.25)	29.000	<0.001	0.383

Abbreviations: APDQ, Auditory Processing Domains Questionnaire; Mdn, Medians; IQR, interquartile range; *p* level at $p < 0.005$; n^2, partial eta squared.

3.3. Receiver Operating Characteristics (ROC) Analysis for CHAPS and APDQ Questionnaires

3.3.1. ROC Analysis for CHAPS Questionnaire

The cut-off point of the CHAPS questionnaire total score was computed using ROC analysis. There was positive discrimination between children in the experimental group and TD children [AUC 0.849 (95% CI: 0.715–0.983), $p = 0.001$]. According to the Youden Index, the optimal cut-off point was −0.30 with a sensitivity of 0.800 and specificity of 0.765 for the CHAPS questionnaire total score (see Table 5; Figure 1).

Table 5. ROC data analysis of the *CHAPS* total score and its 6 domains.

Subdomains	Cut-Off	AUC (95% CI)	*p*
CHAPS Total Score	−0.30	0.849 (0.715–0.983)	=0.001
CHAPS Noise	−0.60	0.937 (0.858–1.000)	<0.001
CHAPS Quiet	−0.20	0.808 (0.657–0.959)	<0.005
CHAPS Ideal	−0.80	0.759 (0.591–0.926)	<0.005
CHAPS Multiple Inputs	0.10	0.869 (0.745–0.993)	<0.001
CHAPS Auditory Memory Sequencing	−0.10	0.712 (0.528–0.896)	<0.005
CHAPS Auditory Attention Span	0.30	0.733 (0.556–0.910)	<0.005

Abbreviations: CHAPS, Children's Auditory Performance Scale; AUC, area under curve; *p* level at $p < 0.005$.

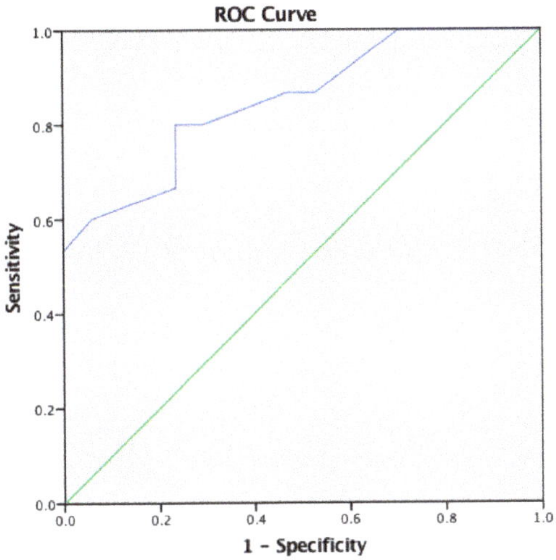

Figure 1. Receiver Operating Characteristics (ROC) curve for the CHAPS questionnaire total score—between parents of experimental group and parents of TD children.

Additionally, an ROC analysis revealed a positive discrimination for all CHAPS total score and CHAPS six subdomains as shown in Table 5 and Figures 1 and 2.

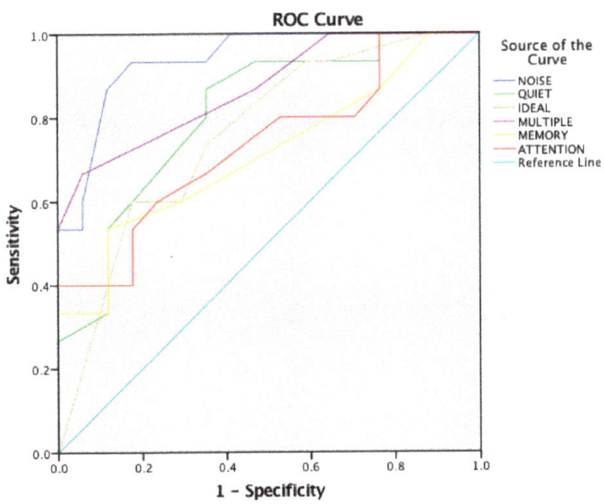

Figure 2. Receiver Operating Characteristics (ROC) curve for the six subdomains of CHAPS questionnaire—between parents of experimental group and parents group of TD children.

3.3.2. ROC Analysis for APDQ Questionnaire

The cut-off point of the APDQ questionnaire total score was computed using an ROC analysis. There was positive discrimination between children in the experimental group and TD children [AUC 0.820 (95% CI: 0.679–0.961), $p < 0.001$]. The optimal cut-off point was 90.00 with a sensitivity of 0.647 and 1-specificity of 0.750 according to the Youden Index for the APDQ questionnaire total score (see Table 6; Figure 3).

Table 6. ROC data analysis of the APDQ total score and its 4 domains.

	Cut-Off	AUC (95% CI)	*p*
APDQ Total Score	90.00	0.820 (0.679–0.961)	<0.001 *
APDQ Auditory Processing subdomain	53.00	0.871 (0.753–0.989)	<0.001 *
APDQ Attention Control subdomain	18.00	0.710 (0.532–0.887)	<0.005 *
APDQ Language subdomain	18.00	0.785 (0.632–0.938)	=0.005 *
Auditory Processing Target subdomain	38.00	0.871 (0.753–0.989)	<0.001 *

Abbreviations: APDQ, Auditory Processing Domains Questionnaire; AUC, area under curve; * p level at $p <$ 0.005.

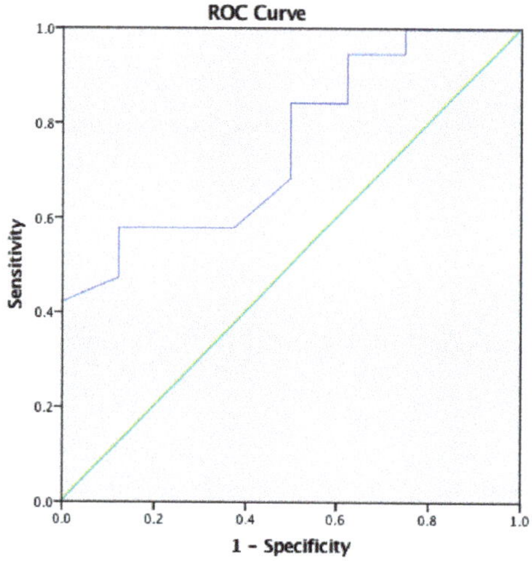

Figure 3. Receiver Operating Characteristics (ROC) curve for the APDQ questionnaire total score—between parents of experimental group and parents of TD children.

An ROC analysis revealed significant positive discrimination for the three APDQ subdomains as shown in Table 6 and Figure 4 and the APDQ Auditory Processing Target subdomain in Figure 5.

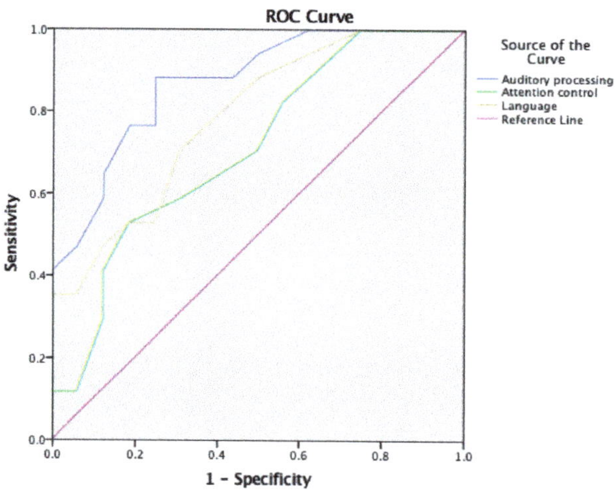

Figure 4. Receiver Operating Characteristics (ROC) curve of APDQ questionnaire—between parents of experimental group and parents of TD children for the APDQ Auditory Processing, Attention, and Language factors.

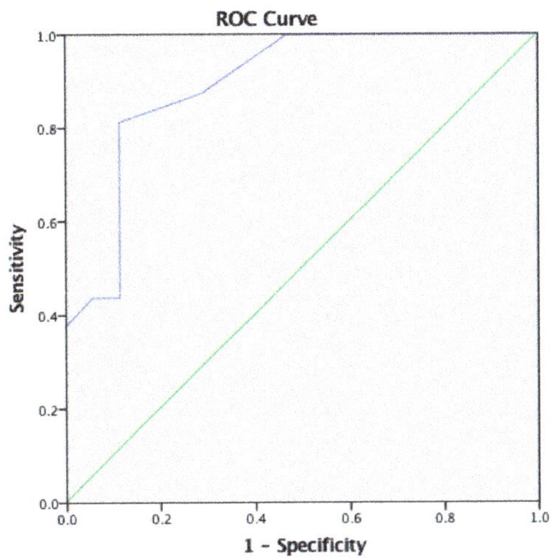

Figure 5. Receiver Operating Characteristics (ROC) curve of APDQ questionnaire—between parents of experimental group and parents of TD children for the APDQ Auditory Processing Target subdomain.

3.4. Reliability and Validity Measures for CHAPS and APDQ Questionnaires

The CHAPS total score internal consistency was excellent (Cronbach's alpha $\alpha = 0.922$). The item scale correlations of the CHAPS six items ranged from 0.896 to 0.930. Similarly, an excellent internal consistency was estimated for the APDQ total score (Cronbach's alpha $\alpha = 0.926$), with item scale correlations of APDQ 50 items ranging from 0.922 to 0.931.

The Spearman ρ correlations were computed between the Greek versions of the CHAPS Total Score and the APDQ for determining the sensitivity against an external validity criterion and the analysis returned a statistically significant positive result ($\rho = 0.639$, $p = 0.001$).

APD is a multifactorial process that requires audiological, linguistic, and non-linguistic as well as electrophysiological tests [12,22,29]. Correlations between CHAPS and APDQ questionnaire scores and auditory processing performance provide external validation for the capacity of the questionnaires to identify APD. The statistically significant correlations are presented in Table 7.

Table 7. Correlations between the CHAPS and APDQ test findings and auditory processing performance (only significant findings are included in the table).

Parameters	CHAPS	APDQ
CHAPS		$\rho = 0.639$ **
APDQ	$\rho = 0.639$ **	
DPS		$\rho = -0.522$ **
DICHOTIC WORDS RE first	$\rho = -0.354$ *	
SNR − 1		$\rho = -0.323$ *
SNR 7	$\rho = -0.392$ **	
Pitch pattern 1000 to 2000 Hz	$\rho = 0.256$ **	
Pitch pattern 4000 to 6000 Hz		$\rho = -0.316$ *

Abbreviations: CHAPS, Children's Auditory Performance Scale; APDQ, Auditory Processing Domains Questionnaire; DPS, Duration Pattern Sequence; RE, Right Ear, SNR, signal-to-noise ratio; ρ, Spearman's rank correlation coefficient; *: $p < 0.005$; **: $p < 0.001$.

4. Discussion

The current study investigated auditory processing characteristics among Greek Cypriot children aged 7–10 years (typically developing and with SSD), as reflected by the CHAPS and APDQ questionnaires. Findings highlight the capacity of the questionnaires to differentiate between the two populations in terms of auditory processing and explore correlations between questionnaire indices and auditory processing performance. A recent systematic review indicated that APD may be a major underlying factor in children with SSD, as lower scores on auditory processing tasks are often observed in children with varying SSD [10,29]. Kalnak and Nakena von Mentez [31] reported that children with phonological disorders have significant auditory processing and auditory sensitivity difficulties compared to children with typical development.

Our findings align with previous reports and underscore the utility of CHAPS and APDQ as effective tools for identifying listening difficulties. We concur with the recommendations that questionnaires can be used to identify children at risk for auditory processing disorders (APD) across diverse populations, as supported by the literature [10–12,15,18,31–33]. Furthermore, our findings add the SSD population to the clinical groups that might benefit from the identification of auditory processing through the CHAPS and APDQ questionnaires [11,12].

4.1. CHAPS Questionnaire

The CHAPS can distinguish between typical and clinical populations as it successfully differentiated children with suspected APD [34] from typically developing children of similar age to our study [35]. It was also effective in distinguishing children with listening difficulties from typically developing children in the older age range of 7–12 years [28]. Additionally, the CHAPS identified listening difficulties in children diagnosed with ADHD [35]. The CHAPS successfully discriminated typically developing Greek children from children diagnosed with APD at the age of 12 years [18]. Our results indicated that the CHAPS can be used to distinguish auditory processing characteristics between TD children and children with SSDs: children in our SSD group had lower scores in the total scores in all subdomains of the CHAPS. Our findings further corroborate previous reports [28,32,34,35].

Notably, ours is the first study to specifically investigate children with SSDs and compare their performance on the CHAPS and APDQ to the performance of typically developing children. Our findings indicate that the CHAPS can effectively differentiate children with listening difficulties or a lower auditory processing profile, placing them in a high-risk category for APD. The CHAPS may guide specialists to refer children for a comprehensive AP evaluation when these difficulties are identified. The use of CHAPS as a screening tool has been discussed in prior research reports [11,12,18,28,32,34–36].

4.1.1. CHAPS ROC Analysis

There is a paucity of reported cut-off points using the area under the curve (AUC) from ROC analysis. The two reports with cut-off points are Ahmmed and Ahmmed's [34] report on children with suspected APD, 6–11 years, and Sanchez and Lam [36], who report on children diagnosed with ADHD 7–10 years of age. Sanchez and Lam's study reported cut-off points with no statistical significance, rendering comparisons quite difficult [36]; however, the study is included in Table 8 to be exhaustive in our report.

Table 8. Reported ROC curves of CHAPS across clinical populations.

	Cut-Off Ahmmed and Ahmmed, 2016 [34]	*p*	Cut-Off Sanchez and Lam, 2007 [36]	*p*	Cut-Off in Current Paper	*p*
CHAPS total			0.61	=0.124	−0.30	=0.001
CHAPS Noise subdomain			0.60	=0.248	−0.60	<0.001
CHAPS Quiet subdomain			0.63	=0.182	−0.20	<0.005
CHAPS Ideal subdomain	0.684	=0.932	0.50	=0.481	−0.80	<0.005
CHAPS Multiple Inputs subdomain			0.66	=0.124	0.10	<0.001
CHAPS Auditory Memory Sequencing subdomain	0.632	=0.016	0.66	=0.138	−0.10	<0.005
CHAPS Auditory Attention Span subdomain	0.697	=0.043	NR	NR	0.30	<0.005

Abbreviations: CHAPS, Children's Auditory Performance Scale; NR, no report; p level at $p < 0.005$.

Ahmmed and Ahmmed [34] established specific cut-off points for children with suspected APD by determining whether the children's performance fell one standard deviation lower (SD), 1.5 SD lower, or 2 SD lower than the norm. They further evaluated the likelihood of an APD diagnosis based on the criteria outlined by the ASHA [1] and the AAA [3] guidelines. Cut-off values were not reported for the "Noise" subdomain, the "Quiet" subdomain, the "Multiple inputs" subdomain, and for the overall performance. Our cut-off points are quite different from Ahmmed and Ahmmed's [34] study, with slightly higher values overall; differences can be attributed to the clinical populations assessed and the method of cut-off point estimation. Their study parallels our findings in that both clinical populations had indications of listening difficulties as identified by CHAPS.

Sanchez and Lam's [36] results differ from ours as a whole and in the given subdomains: they included children with a diagnosis of ADHD and co-morbidity of learning difficulties. Children with ADHD may have a different auditory processing profile compared to children with typical development or children with comorbid learning difficulties.

Despite variations arising from different populations, age groups, cultural characteristics, and diagnoses, the specified cut-off points have consistently distinguished study populations from typically developing individuals. It is essential to consider these indicators alongside comprehensive assessments of linguistic and non-linguistic test results and auditory processing evaluations.

4.1.2. CHAPS Psychometric Properties

The CHAPS psychometric properties we report here concur with related international studies; most importantly, our findings agree with the Greek research by Iliadou and Bamiou [18] and others [17,28,34,36,37]. Similarly, the current study's intraclass classification coefficient Cronbach's alpha ($\alpha = 0.922$) was excellent. Our findings further documented that the CHAPS is a reliable and valid index questionnaire for screening and identifying auditory processing difficulties in the Cypriot Greek population.

4.2. APDQ Questionnaire

The APDQ has successfully differentiated clinical populations from typically developing children and effectively identified distinct auditory processing characteristics in children diagnosed with APD, ADHD, and learning disabilities [16]. Similarly, we found that the total scores and measurements in the four subdomains of the APDQ were poorer in children with SSDs compared to typically developing children. Our study has confirmed that the APDQ can effectively differentiate the auditory processing difficulties of children with SSDs from those of typically developing children. These findings underscore the clinical value of the APDQ.

4.2.1. APDQ ROC Analysis

To date, only Ahmadi et al. [38] have reported cut-off points for the APDQ. They indicated cut-off values of 76.20 for auditory processing, 80.92 for target auditory processing, 78.40 for language, and 61.25 for attention, based on the differentiation between children diagnosed with APD and children diagnosed with APD and learning difficulties. The authors did not detail the methodology they followed, nor did they estimate the overall cut-off point. The cut-off values they reported related to children diagnosed with APD and do not compare with a typically developing population. We have found significantly lower APDQ performance and cut-off levels from Ahmad et al. [38]; this finding can be attributed to the significantly younger age of our sample (children aged 7–10 years), whereas Ahmadi et al. evaluated children aged 7–17 years. Population variations notwithstanding, children with comorbid conditions would be expected to have poorer auditory processing performance [8,10,32]. Our exclusion criteria warranted the absence of neurodevelopmental disorders, thus excluding children with ADHD from our experimental group; the attention subdomain yielded the poorest scores in the Ahmadi et al. study. It is important to note that our study found that both the total score and individual APDQ subdomains effectively differentiate clinical populations [16,38].

4.2.2. APDQ Psychometric Properties

The APDQ psychometric properties reported here are in agreement with existing reports [16,38]. The Greek APDQ showed very good internal consistency comparable to that of the original English version and the Persian APDQ adaptation. Similarly, the current study's intraclass classification coefficient Cronbach's alpha ($\alpha = 0.926$) was excellent. Our findings further document that the APDQ is a reliable and valid screening questionnaire for auditory processing difficulties in Greek Cypriot children.

4.2.3. Correlation between CHAPS and APDQ with Auditory Processing Indices

Our findings indicate that children with SSDs perform lower than TD children on dichotic hearing tests, word discrimination in noise, and tests related to temporal processing, in agreement with the literature [10,39–44]. Shaikh, Baker, and Levya [40] reported significant correlations between CHAPS, DDT, and GIN. This underscores the potential value of screening tests to eliminate the necessity for further evaluation as well as the need to investigate the value of questionnaires as screening instruments for auditory processing difficulties in clinical populations. Furthermore, our study population aligns with the systematic review of Hearnshaw, Baker, and Munro [41], which indicated that most articles reported difficulties in speech perception tasks among preschool- and early-school-age children with SSDs. The persistence of these difficulties beyond the age of seven suggests a probable link to auditory processing issues, as highlighted in the systematic review by Drosos et al. [10] in children with SSDs. Therefore, it is crucial to identify distinguishing characteristics among populations and promptly refer individuals to an audiologist for accurate diagnosis, guidance for caregivers, and appropriate consultation with a rehabilitation specialist.

The current study contributes a valuable clinical perspective for the use of questionnaires to identify children with listening difficulties: we established that both the CHAPS and the APDQ have mostly moderate or strong correlations with Auditory Processing indices like duration and pitch patterns and reflect the listening difficulties in noise [22,41–44].

4.3. Limitations and Future Extensions

The relatively small sample size may present a limitation that lowers the applicability of our findings. Future research may involve a larger sample and inclusion of children with various comorbidities. A detailed follow-up of children referred for a comprehensive AP evaluation would strengthen the questionnaires' value as screening instruments to identify children with listening difficulties.

5. Conclusions

This study is a preliminary validation of the Greek version of the CHAPS and APDQ in Greek Cypriot-speaking children. The questionnaires showed good validity and reliability, and our findings verified the psychometric properties of the tests and their clinical applicability for children with SSDs.

Validity findings for the CHAPS and the APDQ were consistent with those reported for other languages. As current practice indicates that children with APD are initially assessed by special educators, educational psychologists, and/or speech pathologists before a full diagnostic AP assessment, reliable instruments to identify children at risk for APD can be of tremendous help to the interdisciplinary team. The CHAPS and APDQ can identify children at risk for APD and facilitate early detection. They may guide the non-audiology specialists of the interdisciplinary team to appropriate referrals for children suspected of APD and other comorbidities and provide a valuable counseling basis to their families and caregivers.

It should be emphasized that questionnaires should not be used in isolation for APD diagnosis nor replace diagnostic protocols that include linguistic and non-linguistic tests and specialized audiological tests. These questionnaires are useful in assessing listening difficulties in an academic environment, especially in children with learning difficulties and persisting SSDs. Language and phonological awareness difficulties often resolve after treatment, whereas the AP challenges may persist and affect overall academic performance [8,18,32].

Author Contributions: Conceptualization, K.D. and C.T.; methodology, K.D., C.T. and D.T.; validation, D.T., K.D. and C.T.; formal analysis, K.D., D.T. and C.T.; investigation, K.D., A.P. and L.V.; resources, K.D., L.V. and A.P.; data curation, K.D., A.P. and C.T.; writing—original draft preparation, K.D., D.T., L.V. and A.P.; writing—review and editing, L.V. and C.T.; visualization, K.D., L.V. and C.T.; supervision, C.T.; project administration, C.T. All authors have read and agreed to the published version of the manuscript.

Funding: This research received no external funding.

Institutional Review Board Statement: The study was conducted in accordance with the Declaration of Helsinki. This study has been approved by the National Bioethics Committee EEBK/EP/2022/37 on 8 July 2022 and the Pedagogical Institute of Ministry of Education, Sport, and Youth of the Republic of Cyprus KEEA-148053 on 9 November 2022.

Informed Consent Statement: Informed consent was obtained from the parents of all subjects involved in the study; oral consent from the children involved in the study was obtained before assessment.

Data Availability Statement: The data presented in this study are available on request from the corresponding author due to ethical and privacy reasons.

Conflicts of Interest: The authors declare no conflicts of interest.

References

1. American Speech-Language-Hearing Association. (Central) Auditory Processing Disorders—The Role of the Audiologist. Available online: https://www.asha.org/policy/ps2005-00114/ (accessed on 2 January 2024).
2. DeBonis, D.A. It is time to rethink central APD protocols for school-aged children. *Am. J. Audiol.* **2015**, *24*, 124–136. [CrossRef] [PubMed]
3. American Academy of Audiology. Clinical practice guidelines: Diagnosis, Treatment, and Management of Children and Adults with Central APD. Available online: https://www.audiology.org/practice-guideline/clinical-practice-guidelines-diagnosis-treatment-and-management-of-children-and-adults-with-central-auditory-processing-disorder/ (accessed on 2 January 2024).
4. Bamiou, D.E.; Musiek, F.E.; Luxon, L.M. Aetiology and clinical presentations of auditory processing disorders—A review. *Arch. Dis. Child.* **2001**, *85*, 361–365. [CrossRef] [PubMed]
5. Hind, S.E.; Haines-Bazrafshan, R.; Benton, C.L.; Brassington, W.; Towle, B.; Moore, D.R. Prevalence of clinical referrals having hearing thresholds within normal limits. *Int. J. Audiol.* **2011**, *50*, 708–716. [CrossRef] [PubMed]
6. Nagao, K.; Riegner, T.; Padilla, J.; Greenwood, L.A.; Loson, J.; Zavala, S.; Morlet, T. Prevalence of auditory processing disorder in school-aged children in the Mid-Atlantic region. *J. Am. Acad. Audiol.* **2016**, *27*, 691–700. [CrossRef] [PubMed]
7. WHO. The ICD-10 Classification of Mental and Behavioural Disorders: Clinical Descriptions and Diagnostic Guidelines. Available online: https://www.who.int/publications/i/item/9241544228 (accessed on 2 January 2024).
8. De Wit, E.; van Dijk, P.; Hanekamp, S.; Visser-Bochane, M.I.; Steenbergen, B.; van der Schans, C.P.; Luinge, M.R. Same or different: The overlap between children with auditory processing disorders and children with other developmental disorders: A systematic review. *Ear Hear.* **2018**, *39*, 1–19. [CrossRef] [PubMed]
9. Rosen, S. Auditory processing in dyslexia and specific language impairment: Is there a deficit? What is its nature? Does it explain anything? *J. Phon.* **2003**, *31*, 509–527. [CrossRef]
10. Drosos, K.; Papanicolaou, A.; Voniati, L.; Panayidou, K.; Thodi, C. Auditory Processing and Speech-Sound Disorders. *Brain Sci.* **2024**, *14*, 291. [CrossRef] [PubMed]
11. Volpatto, F.L.; Rechia, I.C.; Lessa, A.H.; Soldera, C.L.; Ferreira, M.I.; Machado, M.S. Questionnaires and checklists for central auditory processing screening used in Brazil: A systematic review. *Braz. J. Otorhinolaryngol.* **2019**, *85*, 99–110. [CrossRef] [PubMed]
12. Samara, M.; Thai-Van, H.; Ptok, M.; Glarou, E.; Veuillet, E.; Miller, S.; Reynard, P.; Grech, H.; Utoomprurkporn, N.; Sereti, A.; et al. A systematic review and metanalysis of questionnaires used for auditory processing screening and evaluation. *Front. Neurol.* **2023**, *14*, 1243170. [CrossRef]

13. Musiek, F.E.; Gollegly, K.M.; Lamb, L.E.; Lamb, P. Selected issues in screening for central auditory processing dysfunction. In *Seminars in Hearing*; Thieme Medical Publishers: New York, NY, USA, 1990; Volume 11, pp. 372–383. [CrossRef]
14. Barry, J.G.; Tomlin, D.; Moore, D.R.; Dillon, H. Use of questionnaire-based measures in the assessment of listening difficulties in school-aged children. *Ear Hear.* **2015**, *36*, e300–e313. [CrossRef]
15. De Wit, E.; Visser-Bochane, M.I.; Steenbergen, B.; van Dijk, P.; van der Schans, C.P.; Luinge, M.R. Characteristics of auditory processing disorders: A systematic review. *J. Speech Lang. Hear. Res.* **2016**, *59*, 384–413. [CrossRef] [PubMed]
16. O'Hara, B.; Mealings, K. Developing the auditory processing domains questionnaire (APDQ): A differential screening tool for auditory processing disorder. *Int. J. Audiol.* **2018**, *57*, 764–775. [CrossRef] [PubMed]
17. Smoski, W.; Brunt, M.A.; Tannahill, J.C. *Children's Auditory Performance Scale (CHAPS)*; Educational Audiology Association: Tampa, FL, USA, 1998.
18. Iliadou, V.; Bamiou, D.E. Psychometric evaluation of children with auditory processing disorder (APD): Comparison with normal-hearing and clinical non-APD groups. *J. Speech Lang. Hear. Res.* **2012**, *55*, 791–799. [CrossRef] [PubMed]
19. Hall, D.A.; Zaragoza Domingo, S.; Hamdache, L.Z.; Manchaiah, V.; Thammaiah, S.; Evans, C.; Wong, L.L. International Collegium of Rehabilitative Audiology and Tinnitus Research Network. *A good practice guide for translating and adapting hearing-related questionnaires for different languages and cultures. Int. J. Audiol.* **2018**, *57*, 161–175. [CrossRef] [PubMed]
20. Keith, R.W. *SCAN C: Test for Auditory Processing Disorders in Children*; Psychological Corporation: San Antonio, TX, USA, 2000.
21. Musiek, F.E.; Shinn, J.B.; Jirsa, R.; Bamiou, D.E.; Baran, J.A.; Zaida, E. GIN (Gaps-In-Noise) test performance in subjects with confirmed central auditory nervous system involvement. *Ear Hear.* **2005**, *26*, 608–618. [CrossRef] [PubMed]
22. Sidiras, C.; Iliadou, V.V.; Chermak, G.D.; Nimatoudis, I. Assessment of functional hearing in Greek-speaking children diagnosed with central auditory processing disorder. *J. Am. Acad. Audiol.* **2016**, *27*, 395–405. [CrossRef]
23. Musiek, F.E.; Baran, J.A.; Pinheiro, M.L. *Neuroaudiology: Case Studies*; Singular Publishing Group: San Diego, CA, USA, 1994.
24. Wechsler, D. *Wechsler Memory Scale-Revised*; Psychological Corporation: San Antonio, TX, USA, 1987.
25. Vogindroukas, I.; Protopapas, A.; Stavrakaki, S. *Action Pictures Test*; Glafki: Chania, Greece, 2011.
26. Giannetopoulou, A.; Kirpotin, L. *Metaphon Test*; Konstantaras: Athens, Greece, 2007.
27. Sideridis, G.; Antoniou, F.; Mouzaki, A.; Simos, P. *Raven's Coloured Progressive Matrices and Vocabulary*; Motivo: Athens, Greece, 2015.
28. Bieńkowska, K.; Gos, E.; Skarżyński, P.H. Psychometric properties of the Polish version of the Children's Auditory Performance Scale. *Med. Ogólna I Nauk. O Zdrowiu* **2020**, *26*, 261. [CrossRef]
29. Silva, T.D.; Nunes, A.D.; Farias, T.R.; Santos, A.B.; Taveira, K.V.; Balen, S.A. Accuracy of screening instruments in identifying central auditory processing disorders: An integrative literature review. *Rev. CEFAC* **2021**, *23*, e11720. [CrossRef]
30. *IBM SPSS Statistics for Windows*; Version 28.0; IBM Corp: Armonk, NY, USA, 2021.
31. Kalnak, N.; Nakeva von Mentzer, C. Listening and Processing Skills in Young School Children with a History of Developmental Phonological Disorder. *Healthcare* **2024**, *12*, 359. [CrossRef]
32. Sharma, M.; Purdy, S.C.; Kelly, A.S. Comorbidity of auditory processing, language, and reading disorders. *J. Speech Lang. Hear. Res.* **2009**, *52*, 706–722. [CrossRef]
33. Emanuel, D.C.; Ficca, K.N.; Korczak, P. Survey of the diagnosis and management of auditory processing disorder. *Am. J. Audiol.* **2011**, *20*, 48–60. [CrossRef] [PubMed]
34. Ahmmed, A.U.; Ahmmed, A.A. Setting appropriate pass or fail cut-off criteria for tests to reflect real life listening difficulties in children with suspected auditory processing disorder. *Int. J. Pediatr. Otorhinolaryngol.* **2016**, *84*, 166–173. [CrossRef]
35. Ghuzlan, G.; Mohsen, S.M. Validity and reliability of the Arabic version of children's auditory performance scale. *Audit. Vestib. Res.* **2022**, *31*, 158–164. [CrossRef]
36. Sanchez, L.; Lam, E. Evaluation of screening instruments for auditory processing disorder (APD) in a sample of referred children. *Aust. N. Z. J. Audiol.* **2007**, *29*, 26–39. Available online: https://search.informit.org/doi/10.3316/informit.904481097563048 (accessed on 4 February 2023).
37. Baydan, M.; Aslan, F.; Yılmaz, S.; Yalçınkaya, F. Children's auditory performance scale: Turkish validity and reliability. *Hacet. Univ. Fac. Health Sci. J.* **2020**, *7*, 32–40.
38. Ahmadi, Z.; Jarollahi, F.; Ahadi, M.; Hosseini, F.; Khamisabadi, S. Screening of auditory processing disorder in children with learning disabilities using the Persian version of the auditory processing domains questionnaire. *Audit. Vestib. Res.* **2020**, *29*, 156–164. [CrossRef]
39. Wilson, W.J. *Screening for Central Auditory Processing Disorder. Handbook of Central Auditory Processing Disorder*; Plural Publishing: San Diego, CA, USA, 2013.
40. Shaikh, M.A.; Baker, B.; Levy, A. Comparison of questionnaire-based and performance-based screening tools as predictors of auditory processing disorder. *Am. J. Audiol.* **2020**, *29*, 143–151. [CrossRef] [PubMed]
41. Hearnshaw, S.; Baker, E.; Munro, N. Speech perception skills of children with speech sound disorders: A systematic review and meta-analysis. *J. Speech Lang. Hear. Res.* **2019**, *62*, 3771–3789. [CrossRef] [PubMed]
42. Carvalho, N.G.; Ubiali, T.; Amaral, M.I.; Colella-Santos, M.F. Procedures for central auditory processing screening in schoolchildren. *Braz. J. Otorhinolaryngol.* **2019**, *85*, 319–328. [CrossRef]

43. Valente, D.L.; Plevinsky, H.M.; Franco, J.M.; Heinrichs-Graham, E.C.; Lewis, D.E. Experimental investigation of the effects of the acoustical conditions in a simulated classroom on speech recognition and learning in children. *J. Acoust. Soc. Am.* **2012**, *131*, 232–246. [CrossRef]
44. Jain, C.; Priya, M.B.; Joshi, K. Relationship between temporal processing and phonological awareness in children with speech sound disorders. *Clin. Linguist. Phon.* **2019**, *34*, 566–575. [CrossRef] [PubMed]

audiology research

Review

Congenital Cytomegalovirus-Related Hearing Loss

Nicoleta Gana [1], Iulia Huluță [1,2], Mihai-Ștefan Cătănescu [1], Livia-Mihaela Apostol [2], Florina Mihaela Nedelea [2,*], Romina-Marina Sima [1], Radu Botezatu [1,2], Anca Maria Panaitescu [1,2] and Nicolae Gică [1,2]

[1] Filantropia Clinical Hospital, 011171 Bucharest, Romania; gana_nicoleta@yahoo.com (N.G.); iuliahuluta16@gmail.com (I.H.); stefan.catanescu0920@stud.umfcd.ro (M.-Ș.C.); romina.sima@umfcd.ro (R.-M.S.); radu.botezatu@umfcd.ro (R.B.); anca.panaitescu@umfcd.ro (A.M.P.); gica.nicolae@umfcd.ro (N.G.)

[2] Gynecology Department, Faculty of Medicine, Carol Davila University of Medicine and Pharmacy, 020021 Bucharest, Romania; livia-mihaela.cosma@rez.umfcd.ro

* Correspondence: ina.nedelea@gmail.com

Abstract: Congenital hearing loss is a significant global health concern that affects millions of newborns and infants worldwide, posing substantial challenges for affected individuals, their families, and healthcare systems. This condition, present at birth, can stem from genetic factors, in utero exposures, infections, or complications during pregnancy or childbirth. The spectrum of congenital hearing loss ranges from mild to profound, impacting the development of speech, language, and cognitive skills, thereby influencing educational achievements, social integration, and future employment opportunities. Early detection and intervention strategies, such as newborn hearing screenings, genetic counseling, and the use of hearing aids or cochlear implants, are crucial for mitigating these impacts. This review article aims to explore the diagnostic approaches and management strategies for congenital cytomegalovirus-related hearing loss, emphasizing the importance of interdisciplinary care and the potential for technological advances to improve outcomes for affected individuals.

Keywords: hearing loss; CMV infection; congenital infections; screening

1. Introduction

Since the turn of the 21st century, newborn hearing screening programs have been implemented across North America, Europe, and most developed nations. These programs, which screen all newborns for hearing loss rather than just those considered at risk, have led to the identification of permanent bilateral hearing loss at a rate of approximately 1.33 per 1000 live births [1]. The incidence of severe to profound bilateral hearing loss in newborns remains steady at 1.1 per 1000, while an additional 1 to 2 per 1000 newborns exhibit mild to moderate bilateral hearing loss or unilateral hearing loss of varying degrees. Despite these consistent prevalence rates, the age at diagnosis has significantly decreased, thanks to effective screening initiatives [2].

The etiology of congenital hearing loss can be divided into genetic causes and acquired conditions [1]. Overall, 80% of congenital hearing loss is caused by genetic conditions. They classify as syndromic (10%) or non-syndromic (90%), the latter being autosomal recessive, autosomal dominant, or X-linked transmitted [3]. The acquired conditions refer to congenital infections such as CMV (cytomegalovirus), Zika virus, Rubella, and intrauterine exposure to toxins [1,4].

The general occurrence of hearing loss in congenital CMV infection (cCMV) is 12.6% [5–7]. cCMV ranks as the most prevalent congenital infection globally, with reported birth prevalence rates ranging from 0.64% to 0.7% [5–7]. Symptomatic children face a higher risk, with one in three experiencing hearing loss, compared with one in ten asymptomatic children [5–7]. When these findings are applied to the broader population, it suggests that out of every 10,000 children born annually, 5 will develop hearing loss due to cCMV [5–7].

Morton et al. approximated that cCMV is implicated in 21% of hearing loss cases at birth and contributes to 25% of childhood hearing loss by the age of 4 [8]. The exact mechanisms leading to sensorineural hearing loss from congenital CMV infection remain largely unknown [1]. Besides the direct damage caused by the virus, there is also evidence of immune system damage triggered by the host's immune reaction and the virus's pro-inflammatory chemokines [9,10]. The severity of the infection and the immune response from the mother, fetus, and placenta play a vital role in the health outcomes of the infection [9,10]. At birth, about 10% of newborns with CMV are symptomatic, with the highest risk of neonatal symptoms occurring when the mother is infected around the time of conception or during the first trimester [9,10].

2. Materials and Methods

Under the Preferred Reporting Items for Systematic Reviews and Meta-Analyses (PRISMA) criteria, a systematic search was conducted across scientific literature databases including PubMed, Science Direct, and Google Scholar to identify relevant studies published up to 2024 on congenital cytomegalovirus (CMV) and hearing loss (Figure 1). Only studies focusing on congenital CMV-related hearing impairment were included, while articles that did not meet the defined diagnosis criteria and addressed different causes of hearing loss were excluded.

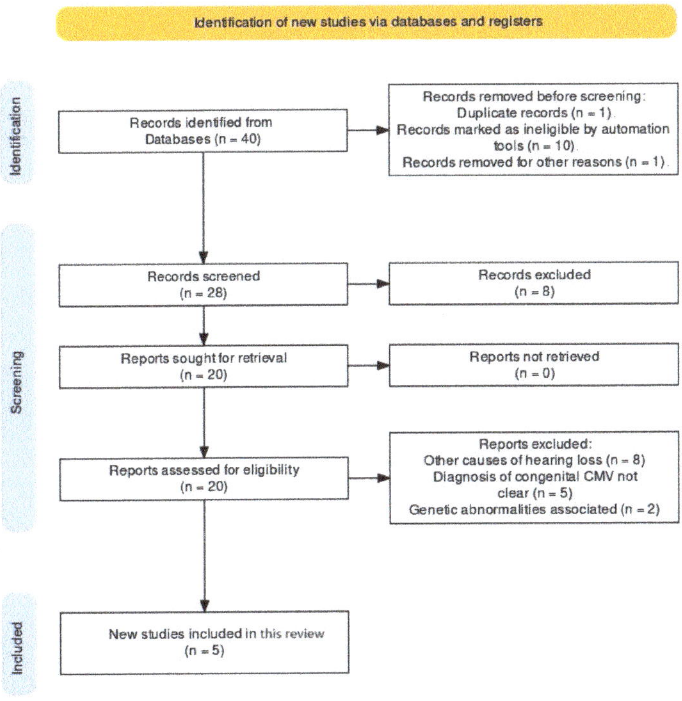

Figure 1. PRISMA flow diagram.

3. CMV Infection during Pregnancy

CMV, belonging to the human herpesvirus family, is the predominant viral reason for congenital infections. It stands as the primary non-genetic reason behind sensorineural hearing loss (SNHL) and is a significant source of neurological disorders [11]. Table 1 summarizes the findings of recent studies on the association between CMV infection during pregnancy and SNHL in neonates. Approximately 10–15% of newborns with congenital CMV exhibit symptoms at birth, with up to 25% of these children facing long-term health issues [12].

CMV infection during pregnancy can either be a primary infection or result from the reactivation of a previous infection or infection with another strain of the virus. The virus is transmitted to the fetus through the placenta, with the likelihood of transmission being higher during a primary infection in pregnancy than with a non-primary infection. The risk of congenital CMV infection is roughly 30–40% for infants whose mothers have a primary infection during pregnancy, compared with a 1–2% risk for infants following a non-primary maternal infection [7,13]. The risk of congenital infection also changes depending on when during the pregnancy the primary infection occurs, rising from about 30% in the first trimester to 47% in the third trimester [14–19]. Although viral transmission risk is lower early in pregnancy, the risk of diagnosing severe fetal infection prenatally is greater if the infection happens in the first rather than the third trimester. Consequently, the adverse outcomes for the fetus tend to be more serious, particularly with infections in the first trimester [14–19] (in Figure 2). Most women experiencing a primary CMV infection during pregnancy do not show symptoms, but a small number may exhibit symptoms similar to infectious mononucleosis, such as fever, fatigue, muscle pain, swollen lymph nodes, and, in rarer cases, hepatitis and pneumonia, with few experiencing lasting effects. Like other herpesviruses, CMV can stay dormant in the body, especially in the salivary glands, and can reactivate at any time, including during pregnancy [1,2].

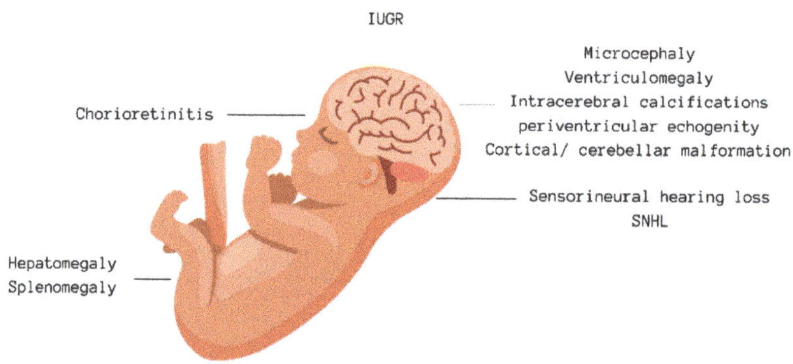

Figure 2. Fetal abnormalities potentially indicative of CMV infection [11,14–19].

Diagnosing maternal CMV infection involves identifying primary infection either by the emergence of CMV-specific IgG in previously seronegative women or through the detection of CMV IgM antibodies alongside low IgG avidity. However, it is challenging to rule out non-primary maternal infections using serological tests. Because of the absence of effective treatments during pregnancy and the failure to meet several criteria for an effective screening test, routine antenatal CMV screening is not commonly recommended [20]. Thus, serological testing for CMV is typically reserved for pregnant women presenting with flu-like symptoms, signs of glandular fever not attributed to Epstein–Barr virus, hepatitis symptoms with negative tests for hepatitis A, B, and C, or when routine ultrasounds suggest fetal abnormalities potentially indicative of CMV infection [20]. These include intracranial calcifications, ventriculomegaly, and microcephaly, which may signal neurological implications, while hepatomegaly and polyhydramnios may denote hepatic and amniotic fluid abnormalities, respectively. Additionally, intrauterine growth restriction (IUGR) and echogenic bowel patterns might suggest compromised fetal development and gastrointestinal issues linked with CMV. Detection of echogenic foci in the heart chambers and hyperechogenicity in the kidneys further aids in recognizing cardiac and renal complications associated with congenital CMV infection [11] A woman's immunity before conception does not ensure the protection of the fetus from infection [21].

Table 1. Prevalence of hearing impairment in children with CMV.

Study	Conclusion
Lanzieri et al., 2017 [22]	At age 18, SNHL prevalence was 25% among case patients and 8% among controls. The risk of delayed-onset SNHL was not significantly greater for case patients than for controls. For case patients, the risk of delayed-onset SNHL was significantly greater among those with unilateral congenital/early-onset hearing loss than those without. The prevalence of severe to profound bilateral SNHL among case patients was 2%.
Palma et al., 2019 [23]	Urinary CMV testing was carried out in 2966 children, representing 3.9% of total live births, between 2004 and 2014. CMV infection was confirmed in 339 children, and information on hearing loss was available in 250 (73.8%), of which 45/250 were cCMV, while 205/250 were acquired. A few children (n = 6/250-13%) with cCMV infection had confirmed hearing impairment. Among them, two were diagnosed after 2012 through the neonatal hearing screening program and were positive. The prevalence of symptomatic cCMV after the introduction of newborn hearing screening (2/10) was 20%, while the proportion of symptomatic cCMV with hearing loss before the screening was 11%. Among the 205 children (82%) with acquired CMV, 6 (2.9%) had moderate to severe hearing impairment. The remaining three cases were attributed to a delayed diagnosis of cCMV. All six cases with acquired CMV were born before the implementation of the newborn hearing screening.
Forner et al., 2014 [24]	The study aimed to analyze the kinetics of CMV viremia and viruria clearance in postnatal life after primary CMV intrauterine infection. All of the 33 newborns included were born full-term. Ten of thirty-tree infants (30%) developed postnatal sequelae during the first months or years of life. Eight children developed unilateral or bilateral hearing loss, where four infants developed severe bilateral hearing loss (average tone loss, 71–90 dB hearing level) four children presented moderate unilateral hearing loss (average tone loss, 41–70 dB hearing level). Two children developed psychomotor retardation, and one baby developed progressive right-side hemiparesis. The time of appearance of clinical abnormalities ranged from 3 months to 5 years of age. The remaining 23 infants (70%) presented no symptoms when the follow-up was concluded at 6 years of age.
Bradford et al., 2015 [25]	In the study, among 50 infants with serum samples, 37 tested positive for CMV DNA at enrollment, indicating viremia. These viremic infants were more prone to developing hearing loss at both the initial assessment and the 6-month follow-up. Additionally, they displayed other markers of active CMV disease, including elevated alanine aminotransferase levels, petechial rash, and organomegaly.
Picone et al., 2018 [15]	Following a retrospective analysis of 238 patients with maternal primary CMV infection identified during routine screening, the cohort underwent monitoring with serial ultrasound scans. The rate of intrauterine transmission was 24.9%, varying across different pregnancy periods. Maternal infections during the preconception or periconceptional period and the first trimester were associated with a significantly higher risk of ultrasound abnormalities compared with later periods. Among the infected newborns, three were symptomatic, all previously flagged during prenatal ultrasounds. Interestingly, no symptomatic fetal infections were observed when maternal infection occurred after the 14th week of gestation. Overall, 5.5% of clinically asymptomatic cases later developed hearing loss.

Lanzieri et al. defined sensorineural hearing loss as a hearing level of ≥25 dB for the ABR click or at any frequency for the corrected tone-burst or pure-tone air conduction results. This definition enabled the identification and categorization of sensorineural hearing loss in children with congenital cytomegalovirus infection. The audiometric configuration of hearing loss due to congenital CMV infection is not specific, and its severity varies. Children with congenital CMV infection may experience unilateral or bilateral hearing losses, ranging from unilateral high-frequency losses (4–8 kHz frequencies only) to profound bilateral losses. Progression and fluctuations in SNHL have been observed in these children as well. Additionally, there is a significantly higher risk of delayed-onset SNHL in children with unilateral congenital/early-onset hearing loss compared with those without it [22].

cCMV infection is primarily confirmed through PCR analysis by detecting CMV DNA in amniotic fluid, which is recommended to be conducted no sooner than 8 weeks following the estimated time of maternal infection and after 20 weeks of gestation. This timing is crucial as it aligns with established fetal urination, which affects the virus's appearance in amniotic fluid. The sensitivity of amniotic fluid PCR for diagnosing fetal infection is influenced by the timing of amniocentesis relative to the maternal infection and the gestational age at which the procedure is performed [11].

The diagnosis of newborn hearing loss. Two screening tests have been validated by international consensus conferences for several years including otoacoustic emissions (OAEs) and automated auditory brainstem response (AABR). Both tests are designed to be administered by non-specialized personnel and yield a binary outcome as pass or fail. Each test has its advantages and disadvantages [26].

Otoacoustic emissions (OAEs) are sounds emitted from the outer hair cells of the cochlea in response to a sound stimulus calibrated at 35 decibels (dB) for screening purposes and are collected in the external auditory canal. OAE tests assess the entire auditory pathway from the outer ear to the inner ear [26,27]. The test is conducted 24 h post-birth during the infant's natural sleep by placing a probe in the ear canal and recording from one ear to the other [26]. The rate of false positives, where OAEs are not detected despite no deafness, ranges from 3 to 8% on the first test and between 0.7 and 6% on a retest after 48 h; known causes include residual fluid in the outer or middle ear, movement, or excessive ambient noise [26,27]. Depending on the presence of risk factors, the rate of false negatives, where OAEs are detected in a deaf newborn, is between 0.009 and 0.2% [26]. This can occur in cases of auditory neuropathy due to damage to the inner hair cells of the cochlea (the actual sensory cells that transmit sound information to the auditory nerve fibers), auditory synaptopathy, or damage to the auditory pathways [26].

Automated auditory brainstem response (AABR) tests record the electrical activity of the auditory pathways up to the brainstem in response to a sound stimulus exploring frequencies between 2000 and 4000 Hz, with the device calibrated to deliver sounds at an intensity of 35 dB [26]. The test is performed on a naturally sleeping child, stimulating both ears simultaneously (with two disposable earphones attached to each ear) and recording the electrical activity with electrodes placed on the child's forehead and nape. The rate of false positives (no electrical activity recorded despite no deafness) is between 0.2 and 0.8% after a retest. False negatives (normal AABR despite deafness) are limited to hearing losses affecting frequencies of 1000 Hz or lower [26–29].

A crucial factor in choosing between these techniques is that only AABR can detect deafness due to damage to the inner hair cells, the auditory nerve, or the auditory pathways in the brainstem. For newborns at risk (e.g., in level 3 maternity units, neonatology, and intensive care departments), hearing loss due to auditory pathway damage is much more common (about 10% of detected hearing losses) than in the general new-born population (1% of hearing losses), with varied causes like hyperbilirubinemia, anoxia, and neurological conditions or syndromes. Therefore, AABR is the preferred method for screening at-risk newborns [26].

Screening is typically conducted during the maternity hospital stay; a practice adopted by nearly all countries to ensure comprehensive coverage [26]. A targeted CMV approach testing newborns who fail hearing screening is useful to identify most children with CMV-related sensorineural hearing loss as the impact of environmental and genetic factors on viral infection rates is still not fully understood [21]. Unfortunately, many newborns and children affected by cCMV infection do not exhibit hearing loss at birth and later go on to have delayed onset hearing loss [21].

A case-controlled retrospective study performed on 35 adult patients with moderate to profound sensorineural hearing loss showed that cervical vestibular evoked myogenic potentials (VEMPs) are useful in increasing the diagnosis of underlying causes of SNHL [30].

In the newborn period, the diagnosis of congenital CMV (cCMV) is often made by detecting high levels of the virus in the infant's saliva and urine. Finding viruses or viral DNA in these samples confirms cCMV infection. Testing urine or saliva within the first 2–3 weeks of life is crucial to differentiate cCMV from infections acquired at birth or through breastfeeding. While postnatal CMV infections can cause severe symptoms in very premature infants or those with significant immune deficiencies, they typically do not lead to long-term issues like sensorineural hearing loss (SNHL). Saliva testing for CMV using PCR technology is both highly accurate and reliable. To prevent contamination in breast milk, saliva samples should be collected at least an hour and a half after the last breastfeeding. Additionally, the integrity of PCR results is generally unaffected by the conditions under which samples are stored and transported [31,32].

Approximately 10% of infants infected with congenital CMV (cCMV) show symptoms at birth, including an enlarged liver and spleen, rashes such as petechiae or purpura, jaundice with elevated conjugated bilirubin levels, and/or a smaller head size (microcephaly). The consequences of cCMV infections vary widely; a significant number of symptomatic infants experience complications like sensorineural hearing loss (SNHL), cerebral palsy, delays in neurodevelopment, and vision loss [32]. Around half of these symptomatic newborns go on to develop SNHL, and among these, two-thirds exhibit neurological impairments. In contrast, 10–15% of infants who are asymptomatic but have SNHL will face permanent effects. For symptomatic infants, factors like intrauterine growth restriction and petechiae are linked to a higher risk of hearing loss, indicating a need for more research to pinpoint which children with asymptomatic cCMV are at risk for hearing loss.

SNHL associated with CMV can emerge later, progress over time, and vary in severity among children, regardless of whether they showed symptoms initially. About 50% of asymptomatic children with hearing loss have impairment in both ears. Because of the lack of visible symptoms at birth and the potential for SNHL to develop or worsen after birth, many infants with cCMV are not diagnosed through newborn hearing screenings [31]. Since it is challenging to predict which children, especially those who are asymptomatic, will develop SNHL, regular monitoring for hearing loss is advised for all children with cCMV every six months for the first 5–6 years. Early detection and timely intervention can significantly improve speech and language outcomes for children affected by CMV-related hearing loss. Both initial and subsequent CMV infections in the mother can lead to symptomatic cCMV infections and SNHL in the infant. While bilateral hearing loss, affecting speech development, occurs in nearly half of these infants, recent findings also highlight the negative impact of unilateral SNHL on a child's overall development [31].

4. Advanced Diagnostic Approaches for Congenital Cytomegalovirus Infection

CMV DNAemia. Forner et al. investigated viral loads in the blood at birth as prognostic indicators for asymptomatic newborns after primary CMV infection during pregnancy. Significant differences in viral loads were found between infants developing late-onset diseases and those remaining asymptomatic. A threshold (≥12,000 copies/mL) indicated a high risk of CMV-related sequelae. Another threshold (≥17,000 copies/mL) was defined for predicting sensorineural hearing loss. These thresholds can aid early identification of at-risk infants, allowing for careful monitoring with audiological and neurodevelopmental assessments [33].

Amniotic fluid peptide biomarkers. A study analyzing the peptidome in CMV-infected amniotic fluids identified a prognostic classifier of 34 peptides, outperforming current fetal biomarkers in predicting asymptomatic or symptomatic status at birth. Emphasizing the significance of viral replication intensity, this classifier was associated with a subset of highly up-regulated proteins within a neurological disease network. Hence, this peptidome classifier could find application in clinical settings during pregnancy to enhance prenatal counseling [34].

Dried blood spot screening. One study presented an improved method for detecting CMV DNA in dried blood spots (DBSs) using a novel single-tube nested protocol, outperforming single-round PCR. DBS samples, already collected for newborn screening, provide a feasible avenue for CMV screening in high throughput settings. The research demonstrated an overall sensitivity of 81%, emphasizing the importance of assay methodology in newborn screening for CMV. The findings suggest the potential inclusion of CMV screening in newborn programs, enabling early identification and intervention for infected infants [35].

Apparent diffusion coefficient values of white matter in magnetic resonance imaging of the neonatal brain. Vande Walle et al. investigated the correlation between white matter apparent diffusion coefficient (ADC) values and clinical outcomes in newborns with cCMV. Elevated ADC values were significantly associated with neonatal hearing loss, cognitive impairment, and motor impairment during follow-up, serving as a predictive tool with an area under the curve ranging from 0.73 to 0.89. The findings suggest that white matter signal alterations are part of the symptomatic spectrum of cCMV. While the study has limitations, including small sample sizes and short follow-up periods, it highlights the potential of white matter ADC as a promising tool for predicting clinical outcomes in newborns with cCMV infection. Further research with larger cohorts and extended follow-up is needed to refine predictive models and establish clear cutoff values for clinical applications [36].

5. Congenital CMV Infection Treatment

To date, the possibility of treating fetal CMV infections with antiviral medication has been explored, particularly with Valaciclovir, showing potential benefits. A study assessed the effectiveness of administering a high dosage of oral valacyclovir, 8 g daily, to pregnant women whose fetuses were symptomatic with cytomegalovirus infection, focusing on those at high risk for neurosensory and neurological issues. The study was structured as a multicentric, open-label, phase II trial with a single arm. The findings suggest that when given at a high dosage during pregnancy, valacyclovir can positively impact the health outcomes of fetuses showing moderate symptoms of infection [32].

However, the use of more potent anti-CMV medications during pregnancy remains controversial because of concerns about their safety. Drugs like (val)ganciclovir, cidofovir, and foscarnet are not approved for pregnant women because of potential maternal and fetal risks. In contrast, valacyclovir, though less potent against CMV in vitro, has been deemed safer based on its track record of not increasing birth defect risks in the children of many women who used it during pregnancy. These medications work by blocking the virus's DNA polymerase, thus preventing viral replication [36,37]. New drugs like Letermovir (LMV) and Maribavir (MBV) have been introduced as specific and effective anti-CMV options that operate through novel mechanisms, potentially reducing the side effects and toxicities associated with older drugs [38].

Congenital CMV infection is likely under-recognized because of a lack of adequate information on its prevention, the absence of universal guidelines for maternal and/or neonatal screening, and strategies for management and treatment. This situation hampers health policies aimed at mitigating the impact of this infection. Currently, CMV screening at birth is not universally implemented. Implementing a routine CMV screening for all newborns, including those without symptoms, could enhance their prospects. Universal screening has the potential to lower healthcare costs across the population. Additionally, early intervention could markedly improve the language development of these children, thus enhancing their social skills and learning abilities [9].

On the other hand, for newborns with cCMV infection, the two primary medications utilized are intravenous ganciclovir, administered at 6 mg/kg twice daily, and oral valganciclovir, which is a prodrug of ganciclovir. Upon oral intake, valganciclovir is quickly converted into ganciclovir. When valganciclovir is given at a dose of 16 mg/kg twice daily, the achieved plasma concentration is comparable to that of ganciclovir at a 6 mg/kg dosage [36]. Valganciclovir leads to a temporary reduction in the viral load, which reverts to its original level upon cessation of the treatment. Extended use of the drug could lead to the emergence of resistant viral strains. However, randomized controlled clinical trials have demonstrated that a 6-week course of treatment with ganciclovir and valganciclovir can be effective in newborns with symptomatic CMV infection affecting the central nervous system. This regimen has been associated with a decreased likelihood of severe hearing loss and improved neurological outcomes after one year [22,23].

A diagnosis of hearing loss early in a child's life can lead to early intervention during the critical time of speech development. The goal of intervention is to improve the development of language, social skills, and literacy for children who are deaf or hard of hearing. Newborn hearing should be assessed no later than 1 month after birth, preferably before discharge from the birth hospital. Newborns who do not pass the initial hearing assessment should be given a comprehensive audiological examination at no later than 3 months of age and should receive intervention before 6 months of age [20,21].

Regarding congenital sensorineural hearing loss treatment, the universal screening of congenital hearing loss is recommended, as an early diagnosis promotes an early intervention to reduce the irreversible damage to speech development [38]. The treatment of congenital hearing loss depends on the underlying cause. When the cause is not known, an MRI should be performed to assess the anatomy of the internal ear. The first medication administered is oral corticosteroids. If no improvement is noted in 10–14 days, clinicians use salvage intratympanic steroids [39]. Hearing aids are used in chronic conditions. Surgical management is represented by cochlear implants in patients where hearing aids are not useful [40].

The evidence highlights a concerning lack of awareness among women regarding congenital cytomegalovirus (cCMV) infection when compared with other less prevalent congenital conditions such as Down syndrome, toxoplasmosis, and human immunodeficiency virus (HIV) infection. Insufficient awareness of cCMV infection is not limited to pregnant women alone; a mere fraction of healthcare providers currently address this issue with their patients. Recognizing this substantial gap, urgent action is warranted to implement health campaigns and sustained medical education initiatives. These efforts aim to raise awareness and enhance the standard of antenatal counseling, ultimately reducing the risk of cCMV transmission.

On the other hand, timely identification is crucial for prompt intervention, including providing auditory aids and specialized speech–language therapy before the age of 6 months, as recommended by the Joint Committee on Infant Hearing. This proactive approach significantly improves outcomes, facilitating smoother integration into mainstream education for affected children. While conducting clinical trials in pregnant women poses challenges, prioritizing preclinical studies is essential to advance our understanding and management strategies for cCMV infection.

6. Conclusions

This review sheds light on the significant impact of congenital cytomegalovirus (CMV) infection on newborn hearing loss, emphasizing its global health implications. By delving into the epidemiology, causes, diagnostic methods, management approaches, and recent advancements, our understanding of CMV-related hearing impairment was deepened. This review underscores the crucial role of early detection and intervention, particularly through newborn hearing screening programs, in promptly addressing hearing deficits. Additionally, it highlights the diverse clinical presentations of congenital CMV infection, underscoring the need for interdisciplinary collaboration and ongoing research endeavors.

Author Contributions: Conceptualization, N.G. (Nicoleta Gana), N.G. (Nicolae Gică) and I.H., methodology, N.G. (Nicolae Gica) and R.-M.S., formal analysis, F.M.N.; data curation, M.-Ș.C. and A.M.P.; writing—original draft preparation, N.G. (Nicoleta Gana), I.H. and M.-Ș.C.; writing—review and editing, N.G. (Nicolae Gică) and R.B.; visualization, L.-M.A., I.H. and R.B. All authors have read and agreed to the published version of the manuscript.

Funding: This research received no external funding.

Institutional Review Board Statement: Not applicable.

Informed Consent Statement: Not applicable.

Data Availability Statement: No new data were created or analyzed in this study. Data sharing is not applicable to this article.

Conflicts of Interest: The authors declare no conflicts of interest.

References

1. Korver, A.M.; Smith, R.J.; Van Camp, G.; Schleiss, M.R.; Bitner-Glindzicz, M.A.; Lustig, L.R.; Usami, S.I.; Boudewyns, A.N. Congenital hearing loss. *Nat. Rev. Dis. Primers* **2017**, *3*, 16094. [CrossRef] [PubMed]
2. Lieu, J.E.C.; Kenna, M.; Anne, S.; Davidson, L. Hearing Loss in Children: A Review. *JAMA* **2020**, *324*, 2195–2205. [CrossRef] [PubMed]
3. Tanaka-Ouyang, L.; Marlin, S.; Nevoux, J. Les surdités d'origine génétique [Genetic hearing loss]. *Presse Med.* **2017**, *46*, 1089–1096. (In French) [CrossRef] [PubMed]
4. Wiwanitkit, V. Hearing loss in congenital Zika virus. *Braz. J. Otorhinolaryngol.* **2017**, *83*, 239. [CrossRef] [PubMed]
5. Goderis, J.; De Leenheer, E.; Smets, K.; Van Hoecke, H.; Keymeulen, A.; Dhooge, I. Hearing Loss and Congenital CMV Infection: A Systematic Review. *Pediatrics* **2014**, *134*, 972–982. [CrossRef] [PubMed]
6. Dollard, S.C.; Grosse, S.D.; Ross, D.S. New estimates of the prevalence of neurological and sensory sequelae and mortality associated with congenital cytomegalovirus infection. *Rev. Med. Virol.* **2007**, *17*, 355–363. [CrossRef] [PubMed]
7. Kenneson, A.; Cannon, M.J. Review and meta-analysis of the epidemiology of congenital cytomegalovirus (CMV) infection. *Rev. Med. Virol.* **2007**, *17*, 253–276. [CrossRef] [PubMed]
8. Morton, C.C.; Nance, W.E. Newborn hearing screening—A silent revolution. *N. Engl. J. Med.* **2006**, *354*, 2151–2164. [CrossRef] [PubMed]
9. Andronaco, D.W. Congenital Cytomegalovirus and Hearing Loss. *J. Obstet. Gynecol. Neonatal Nurs.* **2020**, *49*, 293–304. [CrossRef]
10. Enders, G.; Daiminger, A.; Bader, U.; Exler, S.; Enders, M. Intrauterine transmission and clinical outcome of 248 pregnancies with primary cytomegalovirus infection in relation to gestational age. *J. Clin. Virol.* **2011**, *52*, 244–246. [CrossRef]
11. Khalil, A.; Sotiriadis, A.; Chaoui, R.; da Silva Costa, F.; D'Antonio, F.; Heath, P.T.; Jones, C.; Malinger, G.; Odibo, A.; Prefumo, F.; et al. ISUOG Practice Guidelines: Role of ultrasound in congenital infection. *Ultrasound Obstet. Gynecol.* **2020**, *56*, 128–151. [CrossRef]
12. Townsend, C.L.; Forsgren, M.; Ahlfors, K.; Ivarsson, S.A.; Tookey, P.A.; Peckham, C.S. Long-term outcomes of congenital cytomegalovirus infection in Sweden and the United Kingdom. *Clin. Infect. Dis.* **2013**, *56*, 1232–1239. [CrossRef] [PubMed]
13. Boppana, S.B.; Rivera, L.B.; Fowler, K.B.; Mach, M.; Britt, W.J. Intrauterine transmission of cytomegalovirus to infants of women with preconceptional immunity. *N. Engl. J. Med.* **2001**, *344*, 1366–1371. [CrossRef] [PubMed]
14. Pesch, M.H.; Saunders, N.A.; Abdelnabi, S. Cytomegalovirus Infection in Pregnancy: Prevention, Presentation, Management and Neonatal Outcomes. *J. Midwifery Womens Health* **2021**, *66*, 397–402. [CrossRef] [PubMed]

15. Picone, O.; Vauloup-Fellous, C.; Cordier, A.G.; Guitton, S.; Senat, M.V.; Fuchs, F.; Ayoubi, J.M.; Grangeot Keros, L.; Benachi, A. A series of 238 cytomegalovirus primary infections during pregnancy: Description and outcome. *Prenat. Diagn.* **2013**, *33*, 751–758. [CrossRef]
16. Pass, R.F.; Fowler, K.B.; Boppana, S.B.; Britt, W.J.; Stagno, S. Congenital cytomegalovirus infection following first trimester maternal infection: Symptoms at birth and outcome. *J. Clin. Virol.* **2006**, *35*, 216–220. [CrossRef]
17. Liesnard, C.; Donner, C.; Brancart, F.; Gosselin, F.; Delforge, M.L.; Rodesch, F. Prenatal diagnosis of congenital cytomegalovirus infection: Prospective study of 237 pregnancies at risk. *Obstet. Gynecol.* **2000**, *95*, 881–888. [CrossRef]
18. Nicloux, M.; Peterman, L.; Parodi, M.; Magny, J.F. Outcome and management of newborns with congenital cytomegalovirus infection. *Arch. Pediatr.* **2020**, *27*, 160–165. [CrossRef]
19. Schleiss, M.R. Cytomegalovirus in the neonate: Immune correlates of infection and protection. *Clin. Dev. Immunol.* **2013**, *2013*, 501801. [CrossRef]
20. Ville, Y. Advocating for cytomegalovirus maternal serologic screening in the first trimester of pregnancy: If you do not know where you are going, you will wind up somewhere else. *Am. J. Obstet. Gynecol. MFM.* **2021**, *3*, 100356. [CrossRef]
21. Denoyelle, F.; Rouillon, I.; Alvin, F.; Parodi, M.; Couloigner, V.; Loundon, N.; Garabédian, N. Le dépistage néonatal de la surdité [Neonatal hearing screening]. *Med. Sci.* **2021**, *37*, 519–527. (In French)
22. Lanzieri, T.M.; Chung, W.; Flores, M.; Blum, P.; Caviness, A.C.; Bialek, S.R.; Congenital Cytomegalovirus Group. Hearing loss in children with asymptomatic congenital cytomegalovirus infection. *Pediatrics* **2017**, *139*, e20162610. [CrossRef] [PubMed]
23. Palma, S.; Roversi, M.F.; Bettini, M.; Mazzoni, S.; Pietrosemoli, P.; Lucaccioni, L.; Berardi, A.; Genovese, E. Hearing loss in children with congenital cytomegalovirus infection: An 11-year retrospective study based on laboratory database of a tertiary paediatric hospital. *Acta Otorhinolaryngol. Ital.* **2019**, *39*, 40–45. [CrossRef]
24. Forner, G.; Abate, D.; Mengoli, C.; Palù, G.; Gussetti, N. High Cytomegalovirus (CMV) DNAemia Predicts CMV Sequelae in Asymptomatic Congenitally Infected Newborns Born to Women with Primary Infection During Pregnancy. *J. Infect. Dis.* **2015**, *212*, 67–71. [CrossRef]
25. Bradford, R.D.; Cloud, G.; Lakeman, A.D.; Boppana, S.; Kimberlin, D.W.; Jacobs, R.; Demmler, G.; Sanchez, P.; Britt, W.; Soong, S.; et al. Detection of cytomegalovirus (CMV) DNA by polymerase chain reaction is associated with hearing loss in newborns with symptomatic congenital CMV infection involving the central nervous system. *J. Infect. Dis.* **2005**, *191*, 227–233. [CrossRef]
26. Clemens, C.J.; Davis, S.A. Minimizing false-positives in universal newborn hearing screening: A simple solution. *Pediatrics* **2001**, *107*, E29. [CrossRef]
27. Caluraud, S.; Marcolla-Bouchetemblé, A.; de Barros, A.; Moreau-Lenoir, F.; de Sevin, E.; Rerolle, S.; Charrière, E.; Lecler-Scarcella, V.; Billet, F.; Obstoy, M.-F.; et al. Newborn hearing screening: Analysis and outcomes after 100,000 births in Upper-Normandy French region. *Int. J. Pediatr. Otorhinolaryngol.* **2015**, *79*, 829–833. [CrossRef] [PubMed]
28. Joint Committee of Infant Hearing (JCIH). Year, 2007 position statement: Principles and guidelines for early hearing detection and intervention programs. *Pediatrics* **2007**, *120*, 898–921. [CrossRef] [PubMed]
29. Singh, S.; Maheshwari, A.; Boppana, S. CMV-induced Hearing Loss. *Newborn* **2023**, *2*, 249–262.
30. Ciodaro, F.; Freni, F.; Alberti, G.; Forelli, M.; Gazia, F.; Bruno, R.; Sherdell, E.P.; Galletti, B.; Galletti, F. Application of Cervical Vestibular-Evoked Myogenic Potentials in Adults with Moderate to Profound Sensorineural Hearing Loss: A Preliminary Study. *Int. Arch. Otorhinolaryngol.* **2020**, *24*, e5–e10. [CrossRef]
31. Dollard, S.C.; Schleiss, M.R.; Grosse, S.D. Public health and laboratory considerations regarding newborn screening for congenital cytomegalovirus. *J. Inherit. Metab. Dis.* **2010**, *33*, 249–254. [CrossRef] [PubMed]
32. Leruez-Ville, M.; Ghout, I.; Bussières, L.; Stirnemann, J.; Magny, J.F.; Couderc, S.; Salomon, L.J.; Guilleminot, T.; Aegerter, P.; Benoist, G.; et al. In utero treatment of congenital cytomegalovirus infection with valacyclovir in a multicenter, open-label, phase II study. *Am. J. Obstet. Gynecol.* **2016**, *215*, 462.e1–462.e10. [CrossRef] [PubMed]
33. Desveaux, C.; Klein, J.; Leruez-Ville, M.; Ramirez-Torres, A.; Lacroix, C.; Breuil, B.; Froment, C.; Bascands, J.-L.; Schanstra, J.P.; Ville, Y. Identification of Symptomatic Fetuses Infected with Cytomegalovirus Using Amniotic Fluid Peptide Biomarkers. *PLoS Pathog.* **2016**, *12*, e1005395. [CrossRef]
34. Vande Walle, C.; Keymeulen, A.; Oostra, A.; Schiettecatte, E.; Dhooge, I.; Smets, K.; Herregods, N. Apparent diffusion coefficient values of the white matter in magnetic resonance imaging of the neonatal brain may help predict outcome in congenital cytomegalovirus infection. *Pediatr. Radiol.* **2024**, *54*, 337–346. [CrossRef] [PubMed]
35. Kim, J.H.; Robles, V.; Weimer, K.E.D.; Gehtland, L.M.; Kucera, K.S. Improved Dried Blood Spot PCR Assay for Universal Congenital Cytomegalovirus Screening in Newborns. *Microbiol. Spectr.* **2023**, *11*, e0404122. [CrossRef]
36. Kimberlin, D.W.; Acosta, E.P.; Sánchez, P.J.; Sood, S.; Agrawal, V.; Homans, J.; Jacobs, R.F.; Lang, D.; Romero, J.R.; Griffin, J.; et al. Pharmacokinetic and pharmacodynamic assessment of oral valganciclovir in the treatment of symptomatic congenital cytomegalovirus disease. *J. Infect. Dis.* **2008**, *197*, 836–845. [CrossRef]
37. Oliver, S.E.; Cloud, G.A.; Sánchez, P.J.; Demmler, G.J.; Dankner, W.; Shelton, M.; Jacobs, R.F.; Vaudry, W.; Pass, R.F.; Soong, S.J.; et al. Neurodevelopmental outcomes following ganciclovir therapy in symptomatic congenital cytomegalovirus infections involving the central nervous system. *J. Clin. Virol.* **2009**, *46*, S22–S26. [CrossRef]
38. Faure Bardon, V.; Peytavin, G.; Lê, M.P.; Guilleminot, T.; Elefant, E.; Stirnemann, J.; Leruez-Ville, M.; Ville, Y. Placental transfer of Letermovir & Maribavir in the ex vivo human cotyledon perfusion model. New perspectives for in utero treatment of congenital cytomegalovirus infection. *PLoS ONE* **2020**, *15*, e0232140.

39. Tanna, R.J.; Lin, J.W.; De Jesus, O. Sensorineural Hearing Loss. [Updated 23 August 2023]. In *StatPearls [Internet]*; StatPearls Publishing: Treasure Island, FL, USA, 2024.
40. Gazia, F.; Abita, P.; Alberti, G.; Loteta, S.; Longo, P.; Caminiti, F.; GarGano, R. NICU Infants & SNHL: Experience of a western Sicily tertiary care centre. *Acta Med. Mediterr.* **2019**, *35*, 1001.

audiology research

Review

Strategies to Mitigate Cisplatin-Induced Ototoxicity: A Literature Review of Protective Agents, Mechanisms, and Clinical Gaps

Alexandru Orasan [1], Mihaela-Cristina Negru [1,*], Anda Ioana Morgovan [1], Razvan Claudiu Fleser [2], Daniela Sandu [3], Adrian Mihail Sitaru [4], Alexandru-Catalin Motofelea [5] and Nicolae Constantin Balica [1]

1 ENT Department, "Victor Babes" University of Medicine and Pharmacy, Eftimie Murgu Square No. 2, 300041 Timisoara, Romania; alexandru.orasan@umft.ro (A.O.); anda.morgovan@umft.ro (A.I.M.); balica@umft.ro (N.C.B.)
2 Otorhinolaryngology Department, "Iuliu Hatieganu" University of Medicine and Pharmacy, 400347 Cluj-Napoca, Romania; fleser_razvan_claudiu@elearn.umfcluj.ro
3 OncoHelp Cancer Centre, Radiation Oncology Department, "Victor Babes" University of Medicine and Pharmacy, Str. Rusu Sireanu nr. 34 Timisoara, 300041 Timisoara, Romania; daniela.sandu@umft.ro
4 Department of Pediatric Surgery, "Louis Turcanu" Emergency Clinical Hospital for Children, Iosif Nemoianu Street 2, 300011 Timisoara, Romania; adrian.sitaru@umft.ro
5 Center for Molecular Research in Nephrology and Vascular Disease, Faculty of Medicine, "Victor Babeș" University of Medicine and Pharmacy, 300041 Timișoara, Romania; alexandru.motofelea@umft.ro
* Correspondence: mihaelaprodea@umft.ro

Abstract: Background: Cisplatin, a widely used chemotherapeutic agent, is associated with significant ototoxicity, leading to progressive and irreversible sensorineural hearing loss in up to 93% of patients. Cisplatin generates reactive oxygen species (ROS) in the cochlea, activating apoptotic and necroptotic pathways that result in hair cell death. Inflammatory processes and nitrative stress also contribute to cochlear damage. Methods: This literature review was conducted to explore the mechanisms underlying cisplatin-induced ototoxicity and evaluate protective strategies, including both current and emerging approaches. A structured search was performed in multiple scientific databases, including PubMed and ScienceDirect, for articles published up to November 2024. Results: Current otoprotective strategies include systemic interventions such as antioxidants, anti-inflammatory agents, and apoptosis inhibitors, as well as localized delivery methods like intratympanic injection and nanoparticle-based systems. However, these approaches have limitations, including potential interference with cisplatin's antitumor efficacy and systemic side effects. Emerging strategies focus on genetic and biomarker-based risk stratification, novel otoprotective agents targeting alternative pathways, and combination therapies. Repurposed drugs like pravastatin also show promise in reducing cisplatin-induced ototoxicity. Conclusions: Despite these advancements, significant research gaps remain in translating preclinical findings to clinical applications and developing selective otoprotective agents that do not compromise cisplatin's efficacy. This review examines the mechanisms of cisplatin-induced ototoxicity, current otoprotective strategies, and emerging approaches to mitigate this adverse effect.

Keywords: cisplatin; ototoxicity; chemotherapy; antioxidants; nanoparticles; apoptosis

1. Introduction

Cisplatin, a platinum-based chemotherapeutic agent, is widely used in treating various solid tumors due to its potent anticancer activity. It is particularly effective against testicular, ovarian, head and neck, bladder, lung, and cervical cancers, as well as melanoma and lymphomas [1,2]. The rate of head and neck cancer (HNC) is expected to increase by 30% by 2030, highlighting the growing need for effective treatments and comprehensive diagnostic approaches. However, there are many similarities between the symptomatology of benign and malignant diagnoses, underscoring the importance of a protocolized examination since the absence of adenopathy does not exclude a malignant diagnosis, which can affect prognosis [3]. Cisplatin's remarkable contribution to cancer treatment is most evident in testicular cancer, where it has significantly improved response and survival rates. Prior to cisplatin's introduction, testicular tumors had response rates of approximately 50%, but cisplatin-based therapy now cures the majority of patients with advanced stage disease [4]. Interestingly, while cisplatin has clearly improved response rates for testicular, ovarian, and small cell lung tumors, its impact on overall survival has been marginal in most cases [5]. This limitation is often attributed to the development of drug resistance in tumor cells. Its use is associated with significant side effects, particularly ototoxicity—progressive and irreversible sensorineural hearing loss [6,7]. Up to 93% of patients receiving cisplatin chemotherapy may develop hearing impairment, which can severely impact quality of life in cancer survivors [6,8]. Interestingly, the severity of cisplatin-induced ototoxicity is related to factors like age and cumulative dose, with younger patients and higher total doses leading to more severe hearing loss [9]. While cisplatin affects hearing, Mosalaei et al. found no statistically significant effect on the sense of smell at doses causing hearing impairment, highlighting the specificity of its ototoxic effects [10]. Despite its ototoxic potential, cisplatin remains a crucial component of cancer treatment due to its high efficacy. Currently, there is no approved treatment or prevention for cisplatin-induced ototoxicity in adult patients [6,11]. In the pediatric population, sodium thiosulfate (Pedmark) received approval in September 2022 in the USA for reducing the risk of ototoxicity associated with cisplatin in patients aged 1 month and older with localized, non-metastatic solid tumors [12].

A systematic review has identified sodium thiosulfate as the most promising intervention for preventing cisplatin-induced ototoxicity in adult cancer patients. However, current interventions have shown only mild benefits [13].

This presents a significant challenge in balancing the benefits of cisplatin therapy against its potential long-term effects on hearing, especially in pediatric patients where the impact on quality of life can be particularly profound [9,11]. Cisplatin remains a cornerstone in cancer chemotherapy, particularly for solid tumors. Its widespread use is due to its proven efficacy in improving response rates and, in some cases, survival rates. However, the challenges of drug resistance and side effects have led to ongoing research into combination therapies, novel drug delivery systems, and the development of other platinum-based and non-platinum metal complexes to enhance its therapeutic potential and mitigate its limitations [14,15]. The aim of this review is to provide a comprehensive evaluation of cisplatin-induced ototoxicity, focusing on its molecular mechanisms, existing protective strategies, and emerging therapeutic approaches. A key research gap lies in the translation of promising preclinical interventions into clinically viable therapies that selectively prevent ototoxicity without compromising cisplatin's antitumor efficacy. This gap is further compounded by the limited understanding of inter-individual variability in ototoxicity risk, driven by genetic, demographic, and treatment-related factors. By addressing these challenges, this review seeks to propose targeted, evidence-based strategies to mitigate cisplatin-induced ototoxicity while preserving its chemotherapeutic effectiveness.

2. Material and Methods

This literature review was conducted to explore the mechanisms underlying cisplatin-induced ototoxicity and evaluate protective strategies, including current and emerging approaches. A structured search was performed in multiple scientific databases, including PubMed and ScienceDirect, for articles published up to November 2024. The search utilized terms such as "cisplatin", "ototoxicity", "hearing loss", "otoprotective agents", and "oxidative stress". Boolean operators and Medical Subject Heading (MeSH) terms were employed to refine the results and ensure relevance. In addition to database searches, reference lists of key articles were manually reviewed to identify additional relevant studies.

The selection of articles followed a structured inclusion and exclusion process. Studies were included if they addressed the mechanisms of cisplatin-induced ototoxicity or evaluated otoprotective interventions. Eligible articles encompassed reviews, clinical studies, and preclinical research that provided mechanistic insights or discussed interventions aimed at mitigating cisplatin-induced hearing loss. Articles not focused on cisplatin-related ototoxicity or lacking substantial data on mechanisms or protective strategies were excluded. Only articles published in English or with accessible English translations were considered for this review.

The study selection process involved an initial screening of titles and abstracts to assess their relevance. Full-text reviews were then conducted to confirm the eligibility of the selected articles. Two independent reviewers performed the screening and selection, resolving discrepancies through consensus or, if necessary, by involving a third reviewer.

Key information included study design, mechanisms of cisplatin-induced ototoxicity, protective strategies, and their outcomes. Mechanistic data were categorized into oxidative stress, apoptosis, and emerging pathways, while otoprotective interventions were grouped into systemic and localized approaches. Outcomes were analyzed with a focus on their effectiveness in preventing ototoxicity and their potential impact on cisplatin's chemotherapeutic efficacy.

The synthesis of findings was conducted narratively. Mechanisms of cisplatin-induced ototoxicity were outlined, highlighting oxidative stress and other cellular pathways. Protective strategies were evaluated, emphasizing their strengths, limitations, and clinical applicability. Emerging therapeutic approaches were also discussed, with attention to the translation of preclinical findings to clinical settings. Throughout the review, research gaps and areas requiring further investigation were identified, providing a foundation for future studies.

3. Results

Mechanisms of Cisplatin-Induced Ototoxicity

Reactive oxygen species (ROS) play a significant role in cochlear cell damage and apoptosis, contributing to various forms of hearing loss. ROS are highly reactive molecules that can oxidize proteins, lipids, and DNA, potentially leading to cell death through apoptosis or necrosis [16]. In the cochlea, which is particularly vulnerable to oxidative stress, ROS generation is common in many conditions. This can result in cell death, making it a critical area of study for hearing loss prevention and treatment [17]. The cochlea is particularly vulnerable to oxidative stress, which can be induced by various factors such as noise exposure, ototoxic drugs, and aging. These stressors can trigger the production of ROS, leading to cochlear cell damage and ultimately hearing loss [18]. Interestingly, while ROS are generally considered harmful, they also serve as essential intracellular second messengers for certain cytokines and growth factors, highlighting their complex role in cellular processes [16]. To combat the detrimental effects of ROS, the cochlea employs various protective mechanisms. One such mechanism involves corticotropin-releasing factor

(CRF) signaling, which has been shown to protect against aminoglycoside-induced ROS production and activation of cell death pathways [17]. Additionally, antioxidant systems play a crucial role in neutralizing ROS, although their effectiveness may be limited during periods of high ROS production [19]. Understanding these protective mechanisms and the intricate balance between ROS production and elimination is essential for developing strategies to prevent and treat hearing loss caused by oxidative stress in the cochlea.

Cisplatin exposure activates both apoptotic and necroptotic pathways in the cochlea, leading to hair-cell death and hearing loss. Cisplatin generates reactive oxygen species (ROS) in the inner ear, which can trigger cell death pathways [20]. These ROS activate the c-Jun N-terminal kinase (JNK) and p38 mitogen-activated protein kinase (MAPK) pathways, ultimately inducing hair cell apoptosis [20]. Interestingly, while ex vivo studies suggest that only apoptosis contributes to cisplatin ototoxicity, in vivo research indicates that both apoptosis and necroptosis are involved in cisplatin-induced cochlear damage [21]. Necroptosis, a programmed form of necrosis, involves receptor-interacting protein kinase (RIPK) 1 and RIPK3 [21]. This finding contradicts the traditional view that necrosis in cisplatin ototoxicity is solely a passive process. Recent studies have also identified additional cell death pathways activated by cisplatin in the cochlea, including ferroptosis [22]. The involvement of multiple cell death pathways highlights the complexity of cisplatin ototoxicity and suggests that targeting a single pathway may not be sufficient for complete otoprotection. Understanding these diverse mechanisms provides new avenues for developing therapeutic strategies to prevent or mitigate cisplatin-induced hearing loss, such as the use of antioxidants, caspase inhibitors, and necroptosis inhibitors [21,22].

Recent research has highlighted the involvement of emerging pathways in cisplatin-induced ototoxicity, including autophagy and nitrative stress. Autophagy, traditionally considered a survival mechanism, has been shown to play a dual role in cisplatin ototoxicity. Early upregulation of autophagy via the class III PI3K pathway exerts cytoprotective effects, while later increases in autophagy through mTOR pathway suppression can induce cell death [23]. This suggests that modulating the autophagic pathway could be a potential strategy against cisplatin-induced hearing loss. Nitrative stress, particularly induced by S-nitrosylation of cochlear proteins, has been implicated in cisplatin ototoxicity. Studies have shown that cisplatin treatment leads to increased S-nitrosylation of at least three cochlear proteins in the organ of Corti, stria vascularis, and spiral ganglions, which are known targets of cisplatin toxicity.

Although direct evidence identifying specific S-nitrosylated proteins remains limited, available proteomic and immunohistochemical data suggest that nitrative modifications, including S-nitrosylation, contribute to cochlear dysfunction. For example, LIM Domain Only 4 (LMO4) is notably downregulated in response to cisplatin treatment, with its decreased expression correlating with increased ototoxicity severity [24]. Additionally, the localization of nitrotyrosine-bearing proteins within outer hair cells indicates that nitrative stress—potentially encompassing S-nitrosylation—compromises protein function in the cochlea [25]. Furthermore, the observed downregulation of Ras-related proteins, such as Rab-2A and Rab-6A, in cisplatin-treated cochlear tissues supports the hypothesis that nitrative modifications disrupt intracellular signaling pathways critical for hair cell survival [26]. Collectively, these findings underscore the likely role of S-nitrosylation as one component of the nitrative stress response that exacerbates oxidative damage and promotes apoptotic cascades in cisplatin-induced ototoxicity. Further targeted research is required to directly identify and characterize S-nitrosylated cochlear proteins, which could ultimately lead to novel therapeutic strategies aimed at mitigating cisplatin-induced hearing loss [27].

Importantly, the inhibition of peroxynitrite formation by Trolox attenuated both S-nitrosylation and hearing loss, suggesting a crucial role for this modification in mediating cisplatin's ototoxic effects [28]. Parthanatos, a PARP-1-dependent form of programmed cell death, has been linked to oxidative stress-induced cell death in various tissues [29,30]. While not directly studied in the context of cisplatin ototoxicity, the involvement of oxidative stress and PARP-1 activation in cisplatin-induced hearing loss suggests that parthanatos may play a role in this process. Further research is needed to elucidate the specific contribution of parthanatos to cisplatin ototoxicity and its potential as a therapeutic target. These emerging pathways provide new insights into the complex mechanisms underlying cisplatin-induced hearing loss. Understanding the interplay between autophagy, nitrative stress, and potentially parthanatos could lead to the development of novel protective strategies against cisplatin ototoxicity, ultimately improving the quality of life for cancer patients undergoing chemotherapy. Table 1 highlights the main mechanisms through which cisplatin induces ototoxicity.

Table 1. Summary of mechanisms of cisplatin-induced ototoxicity, pathways, key studies, and therapeutic implications.

Mechanism	Pathway/Details	Key Studies	Therapeutic Implications
Oxidative Stress	ROS generation causing lipid, protein, and DNA damage; activation of apoptotic pathways.	[16–18]	Antioxidants like NAC and vitamin E could neutralize ROS.
Apoptosis	Activation of JNK and p38 MAPK pathways, leading to hair cell apoptosis.	[20]	Caspase inhibitors and agents targeting JNK/MAPK pathways.
Necroptosis	Involves RIPK1 and RIPK3; a programmed necrosis contradicting earlier views of passive necrosis.	[21]	Necroptosis inhibitors targeting RIPK1 and RIPK3 pathways.
Ferroptosis	Iron-dependent lipid peroxidation; recently linked to cochlear cell death in cisplatin ototoxicity.	[22]	Potential use of ferroptosis inhibitors in preclinical research.
Autophagy	Dual role: cytoprotective effects early, but later induction of cell death via mTOR suppression.	[23]	Agents modulating autophagy pathways may reduce cell death.
Nitrative Stress	S-nitrosylation of cochlear proteins; peroxynitrite formation linked to cellular damage.	[28]	Inhibitors of nitrative stress, such as Trolox, show potential.
Parthanatos	PARP-1-dependent cell death; linked to oxidative stress and cochlear cell damage.	[22,23]	Targeting PARP-1 pathways could mitigate ototoxic effects.

4. Current Otoprotective Strategies

4.1. Systemic Interventions

Antioxidants have shown promise in mitigating cisplatin-induced nephrotoxicity, which affects approximately one-third of patients receiving this treatment [31]. Oxidative stress is a significant mechanism in cisplatin nephrotoxicity, stimulating apoptosis, inflammation, mitochondrial damage, and endoplasmic reticulum stress. The administration of antioxidants could be a suitable approach for preventing these adverse effects [31]. Studies have demonstrated that radical scavengers like α-tocopherol and N-N′-diphenyl-p-phenylenediamine can decrease blood urea nitrogen induced by cisplatin, suggesting that the toxic effects of cisplatin may be related to free radical-induced damage [32]. Additionally, trans-3,3′,5,5′-tetrahydroxy-4′-methoxystilbene and resveratrol have shown significant inhibition of protein carbonylation, reduction of thiol group oxidation, and decreased lipid peroxidation in blood platelets treated with platinum compounds [33]. However, it is important to note that while antioxidants may help reduce cisplatin-induced toxicity, there are concerns about potential interference with cisplatin's antitumor effect. The anticancer properties of platinum compounds are primarily attributed to their ability to form covalent adducts on DNA [34,35]. Antioxidants could potentially interfere with this mechanism, potentially reducing the drug's efficacy. Therefore, further research is needed to determine the optimal balance between reducing toxicity and maintaining antitumor activity when combining antioxidants with cisplatin treatment. In conclusion, while antioxidants show promise in mitigating cisplatin-induced toxicity, careful consideration must be given to their potential impact on the drug's antitumor efficacy.

Apoptosis inhibitors have shown promising results in reducing cochlear cell death and protecting against hearing loss in various studies. Tabuchi et al. showed that X-linked inhibitor of apoptosis protein (XIAP) decrease caspase-3 activation and hair cell loss during gentamicin ototoxicity, acting as part of a protective response [36]. XIAP inhibitors increased gentamicin-induced hair cell loss, indicating XIAP's protective role. Antioxidants like L-N-Acetylcysteine (L-NAC) have demonstrated effectiveness in reducing radiation-induced apoptosis in cochlear cells by decreasing reactive oxygen species (ROS) generation [37]. L-NAC increased cell viability and diminished apoptosis after irradiation. Apaf-1 inhibitors have shown potential in preventing cell and tissue damage in animal models of apoptotic damage by decreasing cytochrome c release and apoptosome-mediated activation of procaspase-9 [38]. This suggests Apaf-1 inhibition may have therapeutic potential for apoptosis-related diseases. Oral administration of antioxidant vitamins A, C, E, and magnesium (ACEMg) improved auditory function and increased survival of sensory outer hair cells after noise-induced hearing loss in rats [39]. ACEMg modulated the expression of antioxidant enzymes, diminished pro-apoptotic proteins, and increased anti-apoptotic Bcl-2 levels. In summary, various apoptosis inhibitors, including XIAP, antioxidants, and Apaf-1 inhibitors, have demonstrated efficacy in reducing cochlear cell death through different mechanisms. These findings highlight the potential of targeting apoptotic pathways for hearing protection and treatment of hearing loss.

Studies have demonstrated that inhibition of NF-κB activation or suppression of inflammatory mediators can attenuate hearing loss, highlighting the significance of inflammatory pathways in cisplatin-induced ototoxicity [40]. The NF-κB signaling cascade plays a central role in inflammation by regulating the release of pro-inflammatory mediators, including inducible nitric oxide synthase (iNOS) and tumor necrosis factor-alpha (TNF-α), which both contribute to cochlear damage and hearing loss [40]. Various compounds have shown potential in mitigating this inflammatory response by inhibiting NF-κB activation and reducing the production of pro-inflammatory cytokines. Notably, rhein, alantolactone, celastrol, and parthenolide have been identified as effective inhibitors of NF-κB signaling, thereby exerting otoprotective effects [41–44].

While targeting NF-κB activation appears to be a promising strategy, its role in immune homeostasis must be carefully considered. Some studies suggest that NF-κB plays a protective role in certain tissues by maintaining immune equilibrium and preventing excessive inflammatory damage [45]. This dual function highlights the complexity of inflammatory pathways and underscores the need for targeted approaches in treating cisplatin-induced hearing loss.

Cisplatin-induced activation of NF-κB and the subsequent release of inflammatory mediators such as TNF-α, interleukin-6 (IL-6), and cyclooxygenase-2 (COX-2) contribute to both cochlear cell death and nephrotoxicity [46]. Hyperin, a flavonoid compound, has been shown to reduce cisplatin-induced acute kidney injury by inhibiting NF-κB activation and suppressing inflammatory cytokines such as TNF-α, IL-1β, and IL-6 (Chao et al., 2016). Similarly, polysulfide and hydrogen sulfide donors have demonstrated protective effects against cisplatin nephrotoxicity by inhibiting NF-κB phosphorylation and preventing the degradation of IκBα, ultimately reducing the expression of pro-inflammatory factors [47].

These findings reinforce the notion that targeting NF-κB could be a viable therapeutic strategy to mitigate cisplatin-induced toxicity.

Interestingly, the relationship between NF-κB activation and cell death appears to be context-dependent. In hepatic cells, for instance, pretreatment with TNF-α or IL-1β has been found to activate NF-κB and prevent apoptosis under specific conditions [48]. This paradox suggests that while NF-κB inhibition may be beneficial in attenuating inflammatory damage in the cochlea, its broader physiological functions should be carefully evaluated.

Overall, the suppression of NF-κB activation and inflammatory mediators presents a compelling strategy for mitigating cisplatin-induced ototoxicity. Several compounds, including flavonoids and sulfur-containing molecules, have demonstrated efficacy in reducing inflammation-driven cochlear damage. Future research should focus on refining targeted anti-inflammatory therapies that selectively block pathological NF-κB activation while preserving its essential physiological functions.

4.2. Localized Delivery Strategies

4.2.1. Intratympanic Delivery:

Intratympanic (IT) drug delivery has emerged as a promising approach for treating inner ear disorders while minimizing systemic exposure and potential interference with cisplatin's antitumor effects [49,50]. This method allows for high drug concentrations in the inner ear while maintaining low systemic levels, thus reducing the risk of side effects and drug interactions [49]. Several studies have demonstrated the efficacy of IT administration for otoprotection against cisplatin-induced hearing loss. For instance, IT injection of N-acetylcysteine (NAC) resulted in very restricted systemic uptake while achieving substantially higher intracochlear drug levels compared to systemic administration [49]. Similarly, IT dexamethasone showed modest otoprotection against cisplatin ototoxicity without interfering with its chemotherapeutic effects [51]. However, there are some contradictions and challenges associated with IT delivery. While a 2% NAC concentration provided significant otoprotection, a 4% concentration resulted in reduced hearing capacity, highlighting the importance of optimal dosing [52]. Additionally, high-concentration NAC caused considerable inflammatory reactions, suggesting that not all formulations are suitable for IT administration [53]. In conclusion, IT drug delivery shows great potential for minimizing systemic exposure while maintaining cisplatin efficacy. It offers a targeted approach to otoprotection, allowing for high local drug concentrations with limited systemic effects. However, careful consideration must be given to drug formulations, concentrations, and delivery methods to optimize efficacy and safety. Further research is needed to refine IT delivery techniques and expand its applications in treating inner ear disorders [54].

4.2.2. Nanoparticles and Hydrogels

Novel drug delivery systems for targeted release to the cochlea have shown significant promise in improving treatment efficacy for inner ear disorders. Nanoparticle-based approaches represent a major advancement, offering enhanced biocompatibility, stability, and cell/tissue uptake compared to traditional methods [55]. These nanocarriers can be designed for controlled and sustained release of therapeutic agents directly to specific cell types within the cochlea, maximizing therapeutic effects while minimizing systemic side effects [56]. Interestingly, microfluidics-based systems are emerging as a cutting-edge technology for cochlear drug delivery. These wearable or implantable microsystems provide improved control over pharmacokinetics and enable longer-term delivery, with potential applications in hair cell regeneration [57]. Additionally, cochlear implant-mediated drug delivery represents an innovative approach, combining electrical stimulation with localized drug administration [58]. Targeted drug delivery to the cochlea is rapidly evolving, with promising developments in nanoparticle-based systems, microfluidic technologies, and implant-mediated approaches. Novel biomaterials like chitosan-glycerophosphate hydrogels have also demonstrated sustained local drug release to the inner ear [59]. As research progresses, these advanced delivery systems have the potential to significantly improve treatment outcomes for a range of inner ear disorders, from ototoxicity to sensorineural hearing loss [60,61].

5. Emerging and Experimental Approaches

5.1. Genetic and Biomarker-Based Risk Stratification

Genetic predisposition, age, renal function, and comorbidities significantly influence the risk of ototoxicity in patients undergoing cisplatin treatment. Genetic association studies have identified several candidate genes that may contribute to cisplatin-induced ototoxicity. For instance, polymorphisms in genes such as *ACYP2*, *WFS1*, and *SLC16A5* have been linked to a higher risk of hearing loss following cisplatin therapy [62,63].

Beyond genetic markers, biomarkers play a crucial role in predicting patient susceptibility to ototoxicity and developing personalized otoprotection strategies. Genetic association studies have identified several candidate genes that may contribute to cisplatin-induced ototoxicity. The thiopurine methyltransferase (TPMT) gene is considered critical for susceptibility to cisplatin-induced hearing loss, as highlighted in a pharmacogenetic guideline [64]. Other genes of interest include ABCC3, OTOS, SLC22A2, NFE2L2, SLC16A5, LRP2, GSTP1, SOD2, WFS1, and ACYP2 [64]. Additionally, the APOE gene has been associated with biological age measures, which may indirectly influence ototoxicity susceptibility [65]. Interestingly, there are contradictions in the current research. While some studies have found promising genetic markers, others report low evidence due to small cohort sizes and contradictory replication studies [66]. The A1555G mitochondrial DNA mutation has shown a strong association with aminoglycoside ototoxicity, but evidence for other genetic variants remains limited [66]. Biomarkers for personalized otoprotection are an active area of research, with genetic markers showing potential for predicting patient susceptibility to ototoxicity. However, further studies with larger cohorts and consistent replication are needed to validate these findings. Future research should focus on developing a unified set of clinical, treatment, and genetic risk factors to create flexible models for forecasting post-treatment audiograms and improving patient care [67] (Table 2).

Table 2. Genetic polymorphisms associated with cisplatin-induced ototoxicity.

Gene	Polymorphism	Associated Risk	Study Findings	References
ACYP2	rs1872328	Increased risk of hearing loss	Polymorphism linked to higher susceptibility to cisplatin-induced hearing loss in pediatric patients	[62]
WFS1	rs62283056	Increased risk of hearing loss	Dose-dependent effect; individuals with the minor allele exhibit greater hearing loss at higher cumulative cisplatin doses; replicated in a cohort of 18,620 patients	[68]
SLC16A5	rs4788863	Protection against hearing loss	Identified as protective against cisplatin-induced ototoxic effects in two independent cohorts. Functional validation revealed that SLC16A5 silencing altered cellular responses to cisplatin, suggesting its role in ototoxic mechanisms. Previous studies highlight potential otoprotective strategies using SLC16A5 inhibitors like cimetidine.	[63]
TPMT	rs12201199	Increased risk of hearing loss	Genetic variant associated with cisplatin-induced hearing loss in children. Found in two cohorts ($p = 0.00022$); functional validation suggested significant susceptibility.	[69]
COMT	rs9332377	Increased risk of hearing loss	Genetic variant linked to higher susceptibility to cisplatin ototoxicity in pediatric patients; association replicated ($p = 0.00018$).	[70]

5.2. Novel Otoprotective Agents

Epigenetic modifications and non-apoptotic pathways are promising targets for cancer therapy and other diseases. Agents targeting DNA methylation and histone modifications have shown considerable potential in clinical studies for treating various cancers [71]. These epigenetic alterations significantly influence gene expression, cellular proliferation, differentiation, and apoptosis, making them attractive targets for therapeutic intervention. Epigenetic modifications, including histone modifications and DNA methylation, play crucial roles in regulating gene expression and can potentially modulate the expression of antioxidant defense genes in cochlear cells exposed to cisplatin. DNA methylation and histone modifications are known to influence gene expression in response to various environmental stresses, including oxidative stress [72]. Cisplatin, a chemotherapeutic agent, can induce oxidative stress in cells, potentially triggering epigenetic changes. Epigenetic modifications play a significant role in regulating genes involved in oxidative stress response, particularly SOD2 (superoxide dismutase) and GPX1 (glutathione peroxidase). In human multiple myeloma cells, the SOD2 gene encoding manganese superoxide dismutase (MnSOD) is epigenetically silenced through promoter hypermethylation. Treatment with the DNA methyltransferase inhibitor Zebularine reverses this methylation, increasing SOD2 gene expression and enzyme levels [73]. Similarly, in pulmonary artery endothelial cells, histone deacetylase (HDAC) inhibitors such as scriptaid and trichostatin A induce the expression of extracellular superoxide dismutase (EC-SOD) up to 10-fold. This induction is associated with increased histone H3 (Lys27) acetylation and H3 (Lys4) trimethylation at the gene promoter [74]. Interestingly, the regulation of oxidative stress-related genes can differ between antioxidant and pro-oxidant genes. While HDAC inhibitors increase EC-SOD expression, they simultaneously decrease the expression of the pro-oxidant gene NADPH oxidase 4 by more than 95% in pulmonary artery endothelial cells [74]. This differential regulation results in a significant reduction of cellular reactive oxygen species levels. Similarly, sound conditioning, a pretreatment using low-level non-damaging sound, has been found to protect against subsequent acoustic trauma by suppressing apoptotic pathways. This approach upregulates bcl-2, an inducible neuroprotective gene, and prevents the release of cytochrome c from mitochondria, thereby preserving hair cell function and hearing [75]. Consequently, it is an interesting alternative to traditional approaches for preventing noise-induced hearing loss. Targeting non-apoptotic pathways through epigenetic modifications or sound conditioning offers promising avenues for treating various diseases. Epigenetic drugs, such as DNA methyltransferase inhibitors and histone deacetylase inhibitors, have shown efficacy in clinical trials for cancer treatment [76,77]. Additionally, epigenetic alterations play a significant role in influencing apoptotic pathways in various cell types, including cochlear cells. While the provided context does not specifically address cochlear cells, we can draw insights from the general mechanisms of epigenetic regulation of apoptosis. Epigenetic modifications, such as DNA methylation, histone modifications, and non-coding RNAs, can significantly impact the expression of apoptosis-related genes, including BCL2 and TP53 [78]. These modifications can either promote or suppress cancer development by influencing various programmed cell death processes, particularly autophagy and apoptosis. In the context of BCL2, an anti-apoptotic gene, epigenetic alterations can lead to its overexpression, which has been associated with chemotherapy resistance in various human cancers (Kang & Reynolds, 2009) [79]. For instance, histone deacetylase inhibitors (HDACis) like vorinostat and romidepsin have been shown to selectively kill transformed cells by inducing a tumor-cell-selective pro-apoptotic gene expression signature, including the downregulation of the pro-survival gene BCL2A1 [80]. Regarding TP53, although not explicitly mentioned in the provided context, it is known to be a crucial pro-apoptotic gene. Epigenetic modifications can potentially influence its expression and activity, thereby affecting the balance between pro- and anti-apoptotic factors in cells. Table 3 shows the main agents and their effects.

Table 3. Overview of epigenetic modifications, sound conditioning, and combination therapies with their therapeutic potential and key studies.

Approach	Description	Key Studies	Therapeutic Potential
Epigenetic Modifications	Targets DNA methylation and histone modifications to influence gene expression and apoptosis.	[71,76,77]	Epigenetic drugs show efficacy in cancer treatment by modulating cellular processes.
Sound Conditioning	Uses low-level non-damaging sound to upregulate neuroprotective genes (e.g., bcl-2) and prevent cytochrome c release.	[75]	Promising alternative for preventing noise-induced and other types of hearing loss.
Combination Therapies	Targets multiple pathways simultaneously to enhance therapeutic efficacy and overcome single-drug limitations.	[81,82]	Addresses limitations of single-drug therapies; applicable in cancer, cardiac arrest, and HIV/AIDS.
Nanotechnology-based Carriers	Employs nanocarriers for controlled drug release, tumor sensitization, and improved drug distribution.	[81,82]	Improves bioavailability and targeted drug delivery with minimized side effects.
Multi-drug Cocktails	Combines multiple drugs to address complex diseases; used in HIV/AIDS, cardiac arrest, and Alzheimer's.	[83,84]	Provides life-saving benefits and addresses multiple disease mechanisms; requires optimization.

Combination therapies have emerged as a promising approach for treating complex diseases by targeting multiple pathways simultaneously. This strategy aims to overcome the limitations of single-drug treatments and enhance therapeutic efficacy. Nanotechnology-based carriers have shown potential for sequential combination therapy, allowing for the controlled release of multiple drugs to target tumor cells [81]. These nanoformulations can sensitize tumor cells through cascaded drug delivery or can remodel the tumor microenvironment to enhance drug distribution. Similarly, in cardiac arrest treatment, a multi-drug cocktail targeting multiple pathways of ischemia-reperfusion injury has demonstrated improved neurologically survival rates in animal studies [82]. This approach addresses the complex metabolic disturbances following cardiac arrest, which single-drug therapies have failed to effectively target. Interestingly, the concept of polypharmacology has been successfully applied in HIV/AIDS treatment, with combined antiretroviral therapy (cART) providing life-saving benefits [83]. However, the development of new drugs remains crucial due to emerging resistant strains and poor adherence to cART. In the context of Alzheimer's disease, a multitargeted anti-aging approach using drug cocktails has been proposed to address the complex age-related mechanisms involved in the disease progression [84]. The development of multi-drug cocktails offers a promising strategy for comprehensive protection against complex diseases. However, optimizing these combinations remains challenging. Advanced techniques such as microfluidic systems for precise drug dispensing [85] and information-theoretic active learning approaches [86] may help streamline the process of identifying effective drug combinations. Further research and clinical validation are needed to fully realize the potential of these multi-targeted therapies.

5.3. Statin–Cisplatin Interactions and Their Implications for Ototoxicity-Reducing Therapies in Cancer Treatment

Cisplatin exerts its ototoxic effects primarily by inducing reactive oxygen species (ROS) generation, leading to oxidative damage in cochlear hair cells and spiral ganglion neurons. Excess ROS triggers mitochondrial dysfunction, activating intrinsic apoptotic pathways that result in progressive hearing loss [27,87]. Statins, particularly pravastatin and atorvastatin, have demonstrated antioxidant properties, enhancing the activity of key antioxidant enzymes such as superoxide dismutase (SOD) and glutathione peroxidase (GPX), which help scavenge ROS and reduce oxidative damage [88].

In addition to oxidative stress, inflammation plays a critical role in CIO. Cisplatin activates the NF-κB signaling pathway, leading to the upregulation of pro-inflammatory cytokines such as TNF-α, IL-6, and COX-2, which exacerbate cochlear damage [89,90]. Statins have been shown to suppress NF-κB activity, reducing inflammation-mediated hair cell degeneration. Pravastatin, in particular, has demonstrated downregulation of inflammatory cytokines in models of cardiovascular and renal injury, suggesting a potential protective role in the cochlea [90].

Mitochondrial dysfunction and apoptosis further contribute to CIO, with p53 upregulation playing a key role in promoting cisplatin-induced programmed cell death. Studies have shown that pravastatin can suppress p53 expression, thereby inhibiting mitochondrial-dependent apoptosis and preserving cell viability in cisplatin-treated tissues [91]. Given that mitochondrial dysfunction is a major contributor to hearing loss, pravastatin's ability to modulate apoptotic pathways may offer substantial otoprotective benefits.

Finally, cochlear ischemia due to endothelial dysfunction is another key contributor to CIO. Cisplatin impairs endothelial nitric oxide synthase (eNOS) activity, reducing cochlear blood flow and exacerbating ischemic damage. Pravastatin and atorvastatin have been shown to enhance nitric oxide bioavailability, improving microvascular perfusion and oxygen delivery, which may help maintain cochlear function during cisplatin therapy [92].

Several studies have investigated the efficacy of statins in mitigating CIO. Lovastatin has been found to protect against cisplatin-induced hearing loss in adult mice, with greater protection observed in females compared to males, suggesting that sex-based differences may influence statin efficacy (Fernandez et al., 2020) [8]. Atorvastatin users experienced a significantly lower incidence of hearing loss (9.7%) compared to non-statin users (29.4%) during cisplatin treatment, further supporting statins' potential role in otoprotection [93].

Despite these promising findings, clinical studies on statins as otoprotective agents remain inconclusive. Some trials have reported no significant differences in hearing loss rates between statin users and non-users, highlighting variability in efficacy (McCullough et al., 2022) [90]. The inconsistency in findings underscores the need for extensive clinical trials to validate these results and optimize dosing regimens to ensure maximum benefit without interfering with cisplatin's chemotherapeutic activity [92].

One major concern regarding otoprotective agents is the potential for interference with cisplatin's antitumor effects. Unlike many antioxidant therapies, statins have demonstrated anticancer properties, including inhibition of tumor growth, induction of apoptosis, and suppression of metastasis [94].

6. Clinical Implications

Biomarker-based risk assessment holds promise for tailoring protective interventions against cisplatin-induced ototoxicity (CIO). Genetic variants contributing to CIO have been identified through genome-wide association studies, highlighting the polygenic nature of this adverse drug reaction [95]. This genetic information can be leveraged to develop polygenic scores (PGSs) for predicting CIO risk, potentially enabling more targeted prevention efforts. A study demonstrated the development of a biologically informed PGS for CIO (PGSCIO) using large-scale hearing loss genome-wide association study data combined with single-cell RNA sequencing data from cisplatin-treated murine inner ears. This PGSCIO showed superior performance in predicting CIO risk compared to a general hearing loss PGS, suggesting its potential for identifying high-risk individuals [95]. Such biomarker-based risk assessments could guide the implementation of personalized protective strategies. Interestingly, while personalized medicine approaches show promise, current interventions for preventing CIO in adult cancer patients have shown only mild benefits. Sodium thiosulfate appears to be the most promising preventive strategy, but there is still a need for more rigorous, high-quality research to evaluate potential symptoms and innovative treatment modalities [13]. The integration of genetic risk assessment with other clinical factors could lead to more effective, tailored interventions. For instance, considering that one in five adult cancer patients treated with cisplatin develops symptomatic high-frequency hearing loss [96], combining genetic risk scores with clinical risk factors could help identify those most likely to benefit from protective interventions. In conclusion, biomarker-based risk assessment, particularly using polygenic scores, offers a promising approach for tailoring protective interventions against cisplatin-induced ototoxicity. By identifying high-risk individuals, clinicians could implement targeted prevention strategies, potentially including pharmacological interventions like sodium thiosulfate or other emerging therapies. However, further research is needed to translate these genetic insights into clinically actionable interventions and to evaluate their effectiveness in preventing or mitigating cisplatin-induced ototoxicity. A team-based approach involving oncologists, audiologists, and nurses is crucial for effectively managing ototoxicity in cancer patients: Oncologists play a central role in ototoxicity management as the primary source of information for patients about the potential ototoxic effects of chemotherapy [97]. They are responsible for considering treatment modifications if alternative options are available to reduce ototoxicity risks [98]. However, studies have found that oncologists' awareness and practices regarding ototoxicity monitoring vary widely, with some routinely referring patients for audiological evaluation while others rely on patient self-referral [98,99]. Audiologists are essential team members for implementing ototoxicity monitoring programs and providing specialized hearing assessments [97,100]. Their involvement allows for the early identification of hearing loss and timely intervention. However, the role of audiologists is not always fully realized within oncology teams, and there is often a lack of established protocols for ototoxicity monitoring in hospitals [97,101]. Nurses, especially oncology nurses, play a critical role in patient care and education. However, studies have found varying levels of awareness about ototoxicity among nursing staff, highlighting the need for improved education and training [97,99]. Interestingly, some studies advocate for an expanded multidisciplinary approach, including pharmacists in the ototoxicity monitoring team. [100,102] This interdisciplinary collaboration can lead to more effective service delivery and patient management. In conclusion, while a team-based approach is recognized as crucial for managing ototoxicity [103], implementation remains challenging. There is a need for improved awareness, established protocols, and better integration of audiological services within cancer care teams to enhance ototoxicity monitoring and management [99,104]. Future strategies should focus on fostering collaboration among team members and standardizing ototoxicity monitoring practices across healthcare facilities.

Healthcare providers play a crucial role in managing ototoxicity and implementing protective strategies. Training in this area is essential for several reasons: Firstly, effective ototoxicity management requires a multidisciplinary approach involving audiologists, clinical pharmacists, and physicians [103,105]. Healthcare providers need to be aware of the potential effects of ototoxic medications and be able to identify patients at increased risk of developing ototoxicity [105]. This knowledge is critical for implementing appropriate administration and monitoring protocols to prevent auditory impairment. Interestingly, despite widespread recommendations for early and effective ototoxicity monitoring and management, there is limited evidence of implementation in healthcare services across the UK [106]. About 72% of surveyed centers reported the absence of ototoxicity management protocols, highlighting a significant gap in provider education and practice guidelines [106]. To address these educational needs, healthcare providers should be trained in several key areas. These include understanding ototoxic medications and their effects, implementing pharmacological and audiological monitoring strategies, and utilizing otoprotective substances where appropriate [103,105]. Additionally, providers should be educated on the importance of proactive ototoxicity management strategies, which aim to minimize exposure, avoid symptom onset, provide ongoing monitoring, and manage auditory and vestibular changes as patients' clinical needs evolve [107]. By improving education and awareness in these areas, healthcare providers can better contribute to preserving patients' hearing and vestibular function while effectively treating life-threatening conditions [103].

7. Conclusions

Even if cisplatin shows good anti-cancer response, one important disadvantage is ototoxicity. Ototoxicity can appear due to oxidative stress induced by cisplatin. It is necessary to develop different technologies and techniques that can have an anti-cancer effect, but also show a protective effect against ROS. Antioxidants and anti-inflammatory substances showed promising results for anti-cancer effects and ROS protection, but further research is necessary to establish the combination and dosage for the best results. Apoptosis inhibitors such as XIAP, L-NAC, and Apaf-1 inhibitors have shown promise in reducing cochlear cell death and protecting against hearing loss caused by toxic agents like gentamicin and cisplatin. These findings show the therapeutic potential of targeting apoptotic pathways to prevent hearing loss, especially in ototoxicity treatment. Interesting findings show that epigenetic modifications and non-apoptotic pathways present new avenues for treating various diseases, including cancer and hearing loss. Approaches like sound conditioning and epigenetic drugs have shown potential in preventing hearing loss and modulating gene expression. These novel therapies offer new possibilities for targeting complex disease mechanisms. Also, pravastatin's potential goes beyond its decreasing cholesterol effects, with evidence suggesting benefits in reducing cardiovascular risks and protecting against nephrotoxicity. Its antioxidant properties and impact on cellular stress responses, particularly through modulation of the p53 pathway, make it a promising candidate for diverse therapeutic applications. Further studies are needed to fully explore its potential across various clinical scenarios.

Author Contributions: Conceptualization, A.O. and M.-C.N.; methodology, A.I.M.; software, R.C.F.; validation, D.S., A.M.S. and A.-C.M.; formal analysis, M.-C.N.; investigation, A.I.M.; resources, A.O.; data curation, A.-C.M.; writing—original draft preparation, M.-C.N.; writing—review and editing, M.-C.N. and N.C.B.; visualization, D.S.; supervision, A.O.; project administration, M.-C.N.; funding acquisition, R.C.F. All authors have read and agreed to the published version of the manuscript.

Funding: We would like to acknowledge Victor Babes University of Medicine and Pharmacy, Timișoara, for their support in covering the costs of publication for this research paper.

Institutional Review Board Statement: Not applicable.

Informed Consent Statement: Not applicable.

Conflicts of Interest: The authors declare no conflicts of interest.

References

1. Ghosh, S. Cisplatin: The First Metal Based Anticancer Drug. *Bioorg Chem.* **2019**, *88*, 102925. [CrossRef] [PubMed]
2. Jadon, A.S.; Bhadauriya, P.; Sharma, M. An Integrative Review of Cisplatin: The First Metal Anti-Tumor Drug. *J. Drug Deliv. Ther.* **2019**, *9*, 673–677. [CrossRef]

3. Kis, A.M.; Watz, C.G.; Motofelea, A.C.; Chiriac, S.; Poenaru, M.; Dehelean, C.A.; Borza, C.; Ionita, I. Challenges of Pharyngeal Cancer Screening in Lower-Income Countries during Economic and Social Transitions: A Population-Based Analysis. *Eur. J. Investig. Health Psychol. Educ.* **2023**, *13*, 2226–2237. [CrossRef]
4. Roberts, D.; O'Dwyer, P.J.; Johnson, S.W. Platinum Complexes for the Treatment of Cancer. In *Cancer Management in Man: Chemotherapy, Biological Therapy, Hyperthermia and Supporting Measures*; Minev, B., Ed.; Cancer Growth and Progression; Springer: Dordrecht, The Netherlands, 2011; Volume 13, pp. 145–164. [CrossRef]
5. Canon, J.-L.; Humblet, Y.; Symann, M. Resistance to Cisplatin: How to Deal with the Problem? *Eur. J. Cancer Clin. Oncol.* **1990**, *26*, 1–3. [CrossRef]
6. Waissbluth, S.; Daniel, S.J. Cisplatin-Induced Ototoxicity: Transporters Playing a Role in Cisplatin Toxicity. *Hear. Res.* **2013**, *299*, 37–45. [CrossRef]
7. Benkafadar, N.; Menardo, J.; Bourien, J.; Nouvian, R.; François, F.; Decaudin, D.; Maiorano, D.; Puel, J.-L.; Wang, J. Reversible P53 Inhibition Prevents Cisplatin Ototoxicity without Blocking Chemotherapeutic Efficacy. *EMBO Mol. Med.* **2017**, *9*, 7–26. [CrossRef] [PubMed]
8. Brock, P.; Rajput, K.; Edwards, L.; Meijer, A.; Simpkin, P.; Hoetink, A.; Kruger, M.; Sullivan, M.; van den Heuvel-Eibrink, M. Cisplatin Ototoxicity in Children. IntechOpen. 2021. Available online: https://www.intechopen.com/chapters/75723 (accessed on 4 November 2024).
9. Brock, P.R.; Bellman, S.C.; Yeomans, E.C.; Pinkerton, C.R.; Pritchard, J. Cisplatin Ototoxicity in Children: A Practical Grading System. *Med. Pediatr. Oncol.* **1991**, *19*, 295–300. [CrossRef] [PubMed]
10. Mosallai, A.; Heydari, M.H.; Khademi, B.; Omidvari, S.; Ahmadloo, N.; Mohammadian Panah, M. Effects of Cisplatin on Olfactory Function in Cancer Patients Receiving Cisplatin-Based Chemotherapy. *Iran. J. Otorhinolaryngol.* **2008**, *20*, 7–12.
11. Peleva, E.; Emami, N.; Alzahrani, M.; Bezdjian, A.; Gurberg, J.; Carret, A.S.; Daniel, S.J. Incidence of Platinum-Induced Ototoxicity in Pediatric Patients in Quebec. *Pediatr. Blood Cancer* **2014**, *61*, 2012–2017. [CrossRef]
12. Dhillon, S. Sodium Thiosulfate: Pediatric First Approval. *Paediatr. Drugs* **2023**, *25*, 239–244. [CrossRef] [PubMed]
13. Correa-Morales, J.E.; Giraldo-Moreno, S.; Mantilla-Manosalva, N.; Cuellar-Valencia, L.; Borja-Montes, O.F.; Bedoya-Muñoz, L.J.; Iriarte-Aristizábal, M.F.; Quintero-Muñoz, E.; Zuluaga-Liberato, A.M. Prevention and Treatment of Cisplatin-Induced Ototoxicity in Adults: A Systematic Review. *Clin. Otolaryngol.* **2024**, *49*, 1–15. [CrossRef]
14. Chen, D.; Milacic, V.; Frezza, M.; Dou, Q.P. Metal Complexes, Their Cellular Targets and Potential for Cancer Therapy. *Curr. Pharm. Des.* **2009**, *15*, 777–791. [CrossRef] [PubMed]
15. Alkahtani, S.; Alarifi, S.; Albasher, G.; Al-Zharani, M.; Aljarba, N.H.; Almarzoug, M.H.; Alhoshani, N.M.; Al-Johani, N.S.; Alothaid, H.; Alkahtane, A.A. Poly Lactic-Co-Glycolic Acid- (PLGA-) Loaded Nanoformulation of Cisplatin as a Therapeutic Approach for Breast Cancers. *Oxid. Med. Cell. Longev.* **2021**, *2021*, 5834418. [CrossRef]
16. Kang, S.W. Role of Reactive Oxygen Species in Cell Death Pathways. *Hanyang Med. Rev.* **2013**, *33*, 77–82. [CrossRef]
17. Basappa, J.; Turcan, S.; Vetter, D.E. Corticotropin-Releasing Factor-2 Activation Prevents Gentamicin-Induced Oxidative Stress in Cells Derived from the Inner Ear. *J. Neurosci. Res.* **2010**, *88*, 2976–2990. [CrossRef] [PubMed]
18. Kamogashira, T.; Fujimoto, C.; Yamasoba, T. Reactive Oxygen Species, Apoptosis, and Mitochondrial Dysfunction in Hearing Loss. *Biomed. Res. Int.* **2015**, *2015*, 617207. [CrossRef] [PubMed]
19. Mohan, H.; Vandna; Soni, S.; Syed, S. Targeting Reactive Oxygen Species (ROS) for Cancer Therapy. In *Handbook of Oxidative Stress in Cancer: Therapeutic Aspects*; Chakraborti, S., Ed.; Springer: Singapore, 2022; pp. 1–16. [CrossRef]
20. Tabuchi, K.; Nishimura, B.; Nakamagoe, M.; Hayashi, K.; Nakayama, M.; Hara, A. Ototoxicity: Mechanisms of Cochlear Impairment and Its Prevention. *Curr. Med. Chem.* **2011**, *18*, 4866–4871. [CrossRef]
21. Ruhl, D.; Du, T.T.; Wagner, E.L.; Choi, J.H.; Li, S.; Reed, R.; Kim, K.; Freeman, M.; Hashisaki, G.; Lukens, J.R.; et al. Necroptosis and Apoptosis Contribute to Cisplatin and Aminoglycoside Ototoxicity. *J. Neurosci.* **2019**, *39*, 2951–2964. [CrossRef] [PubMed]
22. Ramkumar, V.; Mukherjea, D.; Dhukhwa, A.; Rybak, L.P. Oxidative Stress and Inflammation Caused by Cisplatin Ototoxicity. *Antioxidants* **2021**, *10*, 1919. [CrossRef]
23. Youn, C.K.; Kim, J.; Park, J.-H.; Do, N.Y.; Cho, S.I. Role of Autophagy in Cisplatin-Induced Ototoxicity. *Int. J. Pediatr. Otorhinolaryngol.* **2015**, *79*, 1814–1819. [CrossRef]
24. Jamesdaniel, S.; Rathinam, R.; Neumann, W.L. Targeting Nitrative Stress for Attenuating Cisplatin-Induced Downregulation of Cochlear LIM Domain Only 4 and Ototoxicity. *Redox. Biol.* **2016**, *10*, 257–265. [CrossRef] [PubMed]
25. Jamesdaniel, S.; Ding, D.; Kermany, M.H.; Davidson, B.A.; Knight, P.R.; Salvi, R.; Coling, D.E. Proteomic Analysis of the Balance between Survival and Cell Death Responses in Cisplatin-Mediated Ototoxicity. *J. Proteome Res.* **2008**, *7*, 3516–3524. [CrossRef]
26. Waissbluth, S.; Garnier, D.; Akinpelu, O.V.; Salehi, P.; Daniel, S.J. The Impact of Erdosteine on Cisplatin-Induced Ototoxicity: A Proteomics Approach. *Eur. Arch. Otorhinolaryngol.* **2017**, *274*, 1365–1374. [CrossRef]
27. Tan, W.J.T.; Vlajkovic, S.M. Molecular Characteristics of Cisplatin-Induced Ototoxicity and Therapeutic Interventions. *Int. J. Mol. Sci.* **2023**, *24*, 16545. [CrossRef]

28. Jamesdaniel, S.; Manohar, S.; Hinduja, S. Is S-Nitrosylation of Cochlear Proteins a Critical Factor in Cisplatin-Induced Ototoxicity? *Antioxid. Redox Signal.* **2012**, *17*, 929–933. [CrossRef] [PubMed]
29. Jiang, H.-Y.; Yang, Y.; Zhang, Y.-Y.; Xie, Z.; Zhao, X.-Y.; Sun, Y.; Kong, W.-J. The Dual Role of Poly(ADP-Ribose) Polymerase-1 in Modulating Parthanatos and Autophagy under Oxidative Stress in Rat Cochlear Marginal Cells of the Stria Vascularis. *Redox. Biol.* **2018**, *14*, 361–370. [CrossRef]
30. Zhang, J.; Hu, X.; Geng, Y.; Xiang, L.; Wu, Y.; Li, Y.; Yang, L.; Zhou, K. Exploring the Role of Parthanatos in CNS Injury: Molecular Insights and Therapeutic Approaches. *J. Adv. Res.* **2024**, *in press*. [CrossRef]
31. Tolouian, R.; Tolouian, A.; Dastan, F.; Farhangi, V.; Peymani, P.; Saeifar, S.; Montes, O.F.B.; Mohmoodnia, L.; Khosravifarsani, M.; Sadighpour, T. Antioxidants and Cisplatin Nephrotoxicity; an Updated Review on Current Knowledge. *J. Nephropharmacol.* **2022**, *12*, e10556. [CrossRef]
32. Sugihara, K.; Gemba, M. Modification of Cisplatin Toxicity by Antioxidants. *Jpn. J. Pharmacol.* **1986**, *40*, 353–355. [CrossRef] [PubMed]
33. Olas, B.; Wachowicz, B.; Majsterek, I.; Blasiak, J.; Stochmal, A.; Oleszek, W. Antioxidant Properties of trans-3,3′,5,5′-Tetrahydroxy-4′-Methoxystilbene Against Modification of a Variety of Biomolecules in Human Blood Cells Treated with Platinum Compounds. *Nutrients* **2006**, *22*, 1202–1209. [CrossRef]
34. Bose, R.N. Biomolecular Targets for Platinum Antitumor Drugs. *Mini Rev. Med. Chem.* **2002**, *2*, 103–111. [CrossRef] [PubMed]
35. Brabec, V. DNA Modifications by Antitumor Platinum and Ruthenium Compounds: Their Recognition and Repair. *Prog. Nucleic Acid Res. Mol. Biol.* **2002**, *71*, 1–68. [CrossRef] [PubMed]
36. Tabuchi, K.; Pak, K.; Chavez, E.; Ryan, A.F. Role of Inhibitor of Apoptosis Protein in Gentamicin-Induced Cochlear Hair Cell Damage. *Neuroscience* **2007**, *149*, 213–222. [CrossRef] [PubMed]
37. Low, W.K.; Sun, L.; Tan, M.G.; Chua, A.W.; Wang, D.Y. L-N-Acetylcysteine Protects Against Radiation-Induced Apoptosis in a Cochlear Cell Line. *Acta Otolaryngol.* **2008**, *128*, 440–445. [CrossRef]
38. Orzáez, M.; Sancho, M.; Marchán, S.; Mondragón, L.; Montava, R.; Valero, J.G.; Landeta, O.; Basañez, G.; Carbajo, R.J.; Pineda-Lucena, A.; et al. Apaf-1 Inhibitors Protect from Unwanted Cell Death in In Vivo Models of Kidney Ischemia and Chemotherapy Induced Ototoxicity. *PLoS ONE* **2014**, *9*, e110979. [CrossRef]
39. Alvarado, J.C.; Fuentes-Santamaría, V.; Melgar-Rojas, P.; Gabaldón-Ull, M.C.; Cabanes-Sanchis, J.J.; Juiz, J.M. Oral Antioxidant Vitamins and Magnesium Limit Noise-Induced Hearing Loss by Promoting Sensory Hair Cell Survival: Role of Antioxidant Enzymes and Apoptosis Genes. *Antioxidants* **2020**, *9*, 1177. [CrossRef] [PubMed]
40. Wen, Q.; Zhang, F.; Zhang, C.; Li, H.; Xu, Q.; Ye, P.; Chen, D.; Miao, J.; Mei, L.; Liu, X.; et al. Rhein Attenuates Lipopolysaccharide-Primed Inflammation through NF-κB Inhibition in RAW264.7 Cells: Targeting the PPAR-γ Signal Pathway. *Can. J. Physiol. Pharmacol.* **2019**, *98*, 357–365. [CrossRef] [PubMed]
41. Ren, Y.; Luo, X.; Sun, A.; Dou, W.; Wang, Z.; Han, M.; Yue, B.; Zhang, J.; Yu, Z.; Ren, G. Activation of PXR by Alantolactone Ameliorates DSS-Induced Experimental Colitis via Suppressing NF-\u03baB Signaling Pathway. *Sci. Rep.* **2019**, *9*, 16636. [CrossRef] [PubMed]
42. An, S.Y.; Park, J.; Kim, H.; Choi, S.Y.; Youn, G.S. Celastrol Suppresses Expression of Adhesion Molecules and Chemokines by Inhibiting JNK-STAT1/NF-κB Activation in Poly(I:C)-Stimulated Astrocytes. *BMB Rep.* **2017**, *50*, 25–30. [CrossRef] [PubMed]
43. Ju, S.M.; Park, J.; Cho, Y.S.; Youn, G.S.; Choi, S.Y. Celastrol Ameliorates Cytokine Toxicity and Pro-Inflammatory Immune Responses by Suppressing NF-κB Activation in RINm5F Beta Cells. *BMB Rep.* **2015**, *48*, 172–177. [CrossRef]
44. Nam, Y.J.; Lee, M.S.; Lee, D.H.; Lee, C.S. Sesquiterpene Lactone Parthenolide Attenuates Production of Inflammatory Mediators by Suppressing the Toll-like Receptor-4-Mediated Activation of the Akt, mTOR, and NF-κB Pathways. *Naunyn-Schmiedeberg Arch. Pharmacol.* **2015**, *388*, 921–930. [CrossRef] [PubMed]
45. Wullaert, A.; Pasparakis, M.; Bonnet, M.C. NF-κB in the Regulation of Epithelial Homeostasis and Inflammation. *Cell Res.* **2010**, *21*, 146–158. [CrossRef]
46. Chao, C.-S.; Tsai, C.-S.; Chang, Y.-P.; Chen, J.-M.; Chin, H.-K.; Yang, S.-C. Hyperin Inhibits Nuclear Factor Kappa B and Activates Nuclear Factor E2-Related Factor-2 Signaling Pathways in Cisplatin-Induced Acute Kidney Injury in Mice. *Int. Immunopharmacol.* **2016**, *40*, 517–523. [CrossRef] [PubMed]
47. Sun, H.-J.; Leng, B.; Bian, J.-S.; Wu, Z.-Y. Polysulfide and Hydrogen Sulfide Ameliorate Cisplatin-Induced Nephrotoxicity and Renal Inflammation through Persulfidating STAT3 and IKKβ. *Int. J. Mol. Sci.* **2020**, *21*, 7805. [CrossRef]
48. Nagaki, M.; Naiki, T.; Brenner, D.A.; Osawa, Y.; Imose, M.; Hayashi, H.; Banno, Y.; Nakashima, S.; Moriwaki, H. Tumor Necrosis Factor α Prevents Tumor Necrosis Factor Receptor—Mediated Mouse Hepatocyte Apoptosis, but Not Fas-Mediated Apoptosis: Role of Nuclear Factor-κB. *Hepatology* **2000**, *32*, 1272–1279. [CrossRef]
49. Gausterer, J.C.; Saidov, N.; Ahmadi, N.; Zhu, C.; Wirth, M.; Reznicek, G.; Arnoldner, C.; Gabor, F.; Honeder, C. Intratympanic Application of Poloxamer 407 Hydrogels Results in Sustained N-Acetylcysteine Delivery to the Inner Ear. *Eur. J. Pharm. Biopharm.* **2020**, *150*, 143–155. [CrossRef] [PubMed]

50. Videhult Pierre, P.; Fransson, A.; Kisiel, M.A.; Damberg, P.; Nikkhou Aski, S.; Andersson, M.; Hällgren, L.; Laurell, G. Middle Ear Administration of a Particulate Chitosan Gel in an in Vivo Model of Cisplatin Ototoxicity. *Front. Cell. Neurosci.* **2019**, *13*, 268. [CrossRef] [PubMed]
51. Murphy, D.; Daniel, S.J. Intratympanic Dexamethasone to Prevent Cisplatin Ototoxicity: A Guinea Pig Model. *Otolaryngol. Head Neck Surg.* **2011**, *145*, 452–457. [CrossRef]
52. Chen, B.C.; Lin, L.J.; Lin, Y.C.; Lee, C.F.; Hsu, W.C. Optimal N-Acetylcysteine Concentration for Intratympanic Injection to Prevent Cisplatin-Induced Ototoxicity in Guinea Pigs. *Acta Oto-Laryngol.* **2022**, *142*, 127–131. [CrossRef] [PubMed]
53. Nader, M.-E.; Théorêt, Y.; Saliba, I. The Role of Intratympanic Lactate Injection in the Prevention of Cisplatin-Induced Ototoxicity. *Laryngoscope* **2010**, *120*, 1208–1213. [CrossRef] [PubMed]
54. Yang, H.C.; Cho, H.H. Intratympanic Drug Injection for Inner Ear Disease. *Korean J. Otorhinolaryngol.-Head Neck Surg.* **2014**, *57*, 364–372. [CrossRef]
55. Valente, F.; Astolfi, L.; Simoni, E.; Danti, S.; Franceschini, V.; Chicca, M.; Martini, A. Nanoparticle Drug Delivery Systems for Inner Ear Therapy: An Overview. *J. Drug Deliv. Sci. Technol.* **2017**, *39*, 28–35. [CrossRef]
56. Nagaraja, S.H.; Nataraj, C.; Jang, Y.; Nair, A.; Attimarad, M.; Al-Dhubiab, B.; Meravanige, G.; Asdaq, S.; Anwer, M.K.; Gopalachar, J.; et al. An Overview of Nanoparticle Drug Delivery for Ototoxin and Noise Mediated Hearing Loss Treatment. *Indian. J. Pharm. Educ.* **2022**, *56*, S581–S598. [CrossRef]
57. Ayoob, A.M.; Borenstein, J.T. The Role of Intracochlear Drug Delivery Devices in the Management of Inner Ear Disease. *Expert Opin. Drug Deliv.* **2015**, *12*, 465–479. [CrossRef] [PubMed]
58. Richardson, R.T.; Wise, A.K.; Andrew, J.K.; O'Leary, S.J. Novel Drug Delivery Systems for Inner Ear Protection and Regeneration after Hearing Loss. *Expert. Opin. Drug Deliv.* **2008**, *5*, 1059–1076. [CrossRef] [PubMed]
59. Paulson, D.P.; Abuzeid, W.; Jiang, H.; Oe, T.; O'Malley, B.W.; Li, D. A Novel Controlled Local Drug Delivery System for Inner Ear Disease. *Laryngoscope* **2008**, *118*, 706–711. [CrossRef]
60. Delaney, D.S.; Liew, L.J.; Lye, J.; Atlas, M.D.; Wong, E.Y.M. Overcoming Barriers: A Review on Innovations in Drug Delivery to the Middle and Inner Ear. *Front. Pharmacol.* **2023**, *14*, 1207141. [CrossRef]
61. Swan, E.E.; Mescher, M.J.; Sewell, W.F.; Tao, S.L.; Borenstein, J.T. Inner Ear Drug Delivery for Auditory Applications. *Adv. Drug Deliv. Rev.* **2008**, *60*, 1583–1599. [CrossRef] [PubMed]
62. Xu, H.; Robinson, G.W.; Huang, J.; Lim, J.Y.-S.; Zhang, H.; Bass, J.K.; Broniscer, A.; Chintagumpala, M.; Bartels, U.; Gururangan, S.; et al. Common Variants in ACYP2 Influence Susceptibility to Cisplatin-Induced Hearing Loss. *Nat. Genet.* **2015**, *47*, 263–266. [CrossRef] [PubMed]
63. Drögemöller, B.I.; Monzon, J.G.; Bhavsar, A.P.; Borrie, A.E.; Brooks, B.; Wright, G.E.B.; Liu, G.; Renouf, D.J.; Kollmannsberger, C.K.; Bedard, P.L.; et al. Association Between SLC16A5 Genetic Variation and Cisplatin-Induced Ototoxic Effects in Adult Patients with Testicular Cancer. *JAMA Oncol.* **2017**, *3*, 1558–1562. [CrossRef] [PubMed]
64. Langer, T.; Clemens, E.; Broer, L.; Maier, L.; Uitterlinden, A.G.; de Vries, A.C.H.; van Grotel, M.; Pluijm, S.F.M.; Binder, H.; Mayer, B.; et al. Usefulness of Current Candidate Genetic Markers to Identify Childhood Cancer Patients at Risk for Platinum-Induced Ototoxicity: Results of the European PanCareLIFE Cohort Study. *Eur. J. Cancer* **2020**, *138*, 212–224. [CrossRef] [PubMed]
65. Kuo, C.-L.; Pilling, L.C.; Liu, Z.; Levine, M.E. Genetic Predisposition to Accelerated Biological Ages Predicted by Biochemical Markers. *Innov. Aging* **2019**, *3*, S947–S948. [CrossRef]
66. Lanvers-Kaminsky, C.; Ciarimboli, G. Pharmacogenetics of Drug-Induced Ototoxicity Caused by Aminoglycosides and Cisplatin. *Pharmacogenomics* **2017**, *18*, 1683–1695. [CrossRef] [PubMed]
67. DeBacker, J.R.; McMillan, G.P.; Martchenke, N.; Lacey, C.M.; Stuehm, H.R.; Hungerford, M.E.; Konrad-Martin, D. Ototoxicity Prognostic Models in Adult and Pediatric Cancer Patients: A Rapid Review. *J. Cancer Surviv.* **2023**, *17*, 82–100. [CrossRef] [PubMed]
68. Wheeler, H.E.; Gamazon, E.R.; Frisina, R.D.; Perez-Cervantes, C.; El Charif, O.; Mapes, B.; Fossa, S.D.; Feldman, D.R.; Hamilton, R.J.; Vaughn, D.J.; et al. Variants in WFS1 and Other Mendelian Deafness Genes Are Associated with Cisplatin-Associated Ototoxicity. *Clin. Cancer Res.* **2017**, *23*, 3325–3333. [CrossRef] [PubMed]
69. Ross, C.J.D.; Katzov-Eckert, H.; Dubé, M.-P.; Brooks, B.; Rassekh, S.R.; Barhdadi, A.; Feroz-Zada, Y.; Visscher, H.; Brown, A.M.K.; Rieder, M.J.; et al. Genetic Variants in TPMT and COMT Are Associated with Hearing Loss in Children Receiving Cisplatin Chemotherapy. *Nat. Genet.* **2009**, *41*, 1345–1349. [CrossRef]
70. de Souza Tesch, R.; Ladeira Bonato, L.; Quinelato, V.; Ladeira Casado, P.; Rezende Vieira, A.; Granjeiro, J.M.; Góes, C. Evaluation of Genetic Risk Related to Catechol-O-Methyltransferase (COMT) and B2-Adrenergic Receptor (ADRB2) Activity in Different Diagnostic Subgroups of Temporomandibular Disorder in Brazilian Patients. *Int. J. Oral. Maxillofac. Surg.* **2020**, *49*, 237–243. [CrossRef] [PubMed]
71. Kalebic, T. Epigenetic Changes: Potential Therapeutic Targets. *Ann. N. Y. Acad. Sci.* **2003**, *983*, 278–285. [CrossRef] [PubMed]
72. RM, S.K.; Hao, F.; Cheng, H.; Zhang, X.; Wang, Y.; He, S.; Sun, L. Redox Components: Key Regulators of Epigenetic Modifications in Plants. *Int. J. Mol. Sci.* **2020**, *21*, 1419. [CrossRef] [PubMed]

73. Hodge, D.R.; Peng, B.; Pompeia, C.; Thomas, S.B.; Cho, E.; Clausen, P.A.; Marquez, V.E.; Farrar, W.L. Epigenetic Silencing of Manganese Superoxide Dismutase (SOD-2) in KAS 6/1 Human Multiple Myeloma Cells Increases Cell Proliferation. *Cancer Biol. Ther.* **2005**, *4*, 585–592. [CrossRef]
74. Zelko, I.N.; Folz, R.J. Regulation of Oxidative Stress in Pulmonary Artery Endothelium. Modulation of Extracellular Superoxide Dismutase and NOX4 Expression Using Histone Deacetylase Class I Inhibitors. *Am. J. Respir. Cell Mol. Biol.* **2015**, *53*, 513–524. [CrossRef] [PubMed]
75. Niu, X.; Shao, R.; Canlon, B. Suppression of Apoptosis Occurs in the Cochlea by Sound Conditioning. *NeuroReport* **2003**, *14*, 1025. [CrossRef]
76. Issa, J. Epigenetic Therapy. *Cancer Res.* **2009**, *69*, ES4-3. [CrossRef]
77. Wang, Y.; Xie, Q.; Tan, H.; Liao, M.; Zhu, S.; Zheng, L.-L.; Huang, H.; Liu, B. Targeting Cancer Epigenetic Pathways with Small-Molecule Compounds: Therapeutic Efficacy and Combination Therapies. *Pharmacol. Res.* **2021**, *173*, 105702. [CrossRef]
78. Damiescu, R.; Efferth, T.; Dawood, M. Dysregulation of Different Modes of Programmed Cell Death by Epigenetic Modifications and Their Role in Cancer. *Cancer Lett.* **2024**, *584*, 216623. [CrossRef]
79. Kang, M.H.; Reynolds, C.P. Bcl-2 Inhibitors: Targeting Mitochondrial Apoptotic Pathways in Cancer Therapy. *Clin. Cancer Res.* **2009**, *15*, 1126–1132. [CrossRef] [PubMed]
80. Bolden, J.E.; Johnstone, R.W.; Cluse, L.; Martin, B.P.; Shi, W.; Jankowski, K.; Mackenzie, K.L.; Kan, C.-Y.; Smyth, G.K. HDAC Inhibitors Induce Tumor-Cell-Selective pro-Apoptotic Transcriptional Responses. *Cell Death Dis.* **2013**, *4*, e519. [CrossRef]
81. Shim, G.; Kim, M.-G.; Kim, D.; Park, J.Y.; Oh, Y.-K. Nanoformulation-Based Sequential Combination Cancer Therapy. *Adv. Drug Deliv. Rev.* **2017**, *115*, 57–81. [CrossRef]
82. Choudhary, R.C.; Shoaib, M.; Hayashida, K.; Yin, T.; Miyara, S.J.; d'Abramo, C.; Heuser, W.G.; Shinozaki, K.; Kim, N.; Takegawa, R.; et al. Multi-Drug Cocktail Therapy Improves Survival and Neurological Function after Asphyxial Cardiac Arrest in Rodents. *Cells* **2023**, *12*, 1548. [CrossRef] [PubMed]
83. Bianco, M.D.C.A.D.; Leite, D.I.; Branco, F.S.C.; Boechat, N.; Uliassi, E.; Bolognesi, M.L.; Bastos, M.M. The Use of Zidovudine Pharmacophore in Multi-Target-Directed Ligands for AIDS Therapy. *Molecules* **2022**, *27*, 8502. [CrossRef]
84. Ladiges, W.C. Time for an Alzheimer's Disease Cocktail. *Aging Pathobiol. Ther.* **2020**, *2*, 14–15. [CrossRef]
85. Huang, W.-Y.; Liu, C.-A.; Fan, R.-S.; Lin, Z.-D.; Wang, K.; Lee, G.-B. Automatic Optimization of Drug Cocktails on an Integrated Microfluidic System. *Biomicrofluidics* **2017**, *11*, 034109. [CrossRef]
86. Park, M.; Nassar, M.; Evans, B.L.; Vikalo, H. Adaptive Experimental Design for Drug Combinations. In Proceedings of the 2012 IEEE Statistical Signal Processing Workshop (SSP), Ann Arbor, MI, USA, 5–8 August 2012; pp. 712–715. [CrossRef]
87. Dai, D.; Chen, C.; Lu, C.; Guo, Y.; Li, Q.; Sun, C. Apoptosis, Autophagy, Ferroptosis, and Pyroptosis in Cisplatin-Induced Ototoxicity and Protective Agents. *Front. Pharmacol.* **2024**, *15*, 1430469. [CrossRef] [PubMed]
88. Hu, S.W.; Han, L.; Shu, Y. A Potential Therapeutic Approach for Cisplatin-Induced Hearing Loss. *Mol. Ther. Nucleic Acids* **2024**, *35*, 102207. [CrossRef] [PubMed]
89. Li, Y.; Zhang, T.; Song, Q.; Gao, D.; Li, Y.; Jie, H.; Huang, P.; Zheng, G.; Yang, J.; He, J. Cisplatin Ototoxicity Mechanism and Antagonistic Intervention Strategy: A Scope Review. *Front. Cell Neurosci.* **2023**, *17*, 1197051. [CrossRef] [PubMed]
90. Kaur, T.; Mukherjea, D.; Sheehan, K.; Jajoo, S.; Rybak, L.P.; Ramkumar, V. Short Interfering RNA against STAT1 Attenuates Cisplatin-Induced Ototoxicity in the Rat by Suppressing Inflammation. *Cell Death Dis.* **2011**, *2*, e180. [CrossRef]
91. Fujieda, M.; Morita, T.; Naruse, K.; Hayashi, Y.; Ishihara, M.; Yokoyama, T.; Toma, T.; Ohta, K.; Wakiguchi, H. Effect of Pravastatin on Cisplatin-Induced Nephrotoxicity in Rats. *Hum. Exp. Toxicol.* **2011**, *30*, 603–615. [CrossRef]
92. Schmitt, N.C.; Fernandez, K.; Newlands, S.; Allen, P.; Kaufman, A.; McMillan, G.P.; Switchenko, J.M.; Stokes, W.A.; Mehra, R.; Mandawat, A.; et al. Randomized, Placebo-Controlled Trial of Atorvastatin to Prevent Hearing Loss in Patients with Head and Neck Squamous Cell Carcinoma Receiving Cisplatin Based Chemoradiation (CRT). *JCO* **2024**, *42*, TPS12153. [CrossRef]
93. Fernandez, K.A.; Allen, P.; Campbell, M.; Page, B.; Townes, T.; Li, C.-M.; Cheng, H.; Garrett, J.; Mulquin, M.; Clements, A.; et al. Atorvastatin Is Associated with Reduced Cisplatin-Induced Hearing Loss. *J. Clin. Investig.* **2021**, *131*, 142616. [CrossRef] [PubMed]
94. Fernandez, K.; Spielbauer, K.K.; Rusheen, A.; Wang, L.; Baker, T.G.; Eyles, S.; Cunningham, L.L. Lovastatin Protects against Cisplatin-Induced Hearing Loss in Mice. *Hear. Res.* **2020**, *389*, 107905. [CrossRef] [PubMed]
95. Miao, D.N.R.; Wilke, M.A.; Pham, J.; Ladha, F.; Singh, M.; Arsenio, J.; Yang, W.; Yang, J.J.; Drögemöller, B.I. Leveraging Large-Scale Datasets and Single Cell Omics Data to Develop a Polygenic Score for Cisplatin-Induced Ototoxicity. *Hum. Genom.* **2024**, *18*, 112. [CrossRef]
96. Voruz, F.; Vuilleumier, A.; Migliorini, D.; Nacher-Soler, G.; Rousset, F.; De Maesschalck, T.; Senn, P. Cisplatin-Induced Ototoxicity in 401 Consecutive Geneva Cancer Patients. *Res. Sq.* **2022**. [CrossRef]
97. Govender, C.D.; Pillay, M.; Paken, J.; Sewram, V. Perspectives and Practices of Ototoxicity Monitoring. *S. Afr. J. Commun. Disord.* **2020**, *67*, 1–10. [CrossRef]

98. Garinis, A.C.; Cornell, A.; Allada, G.; Fennelly, K.P.; Maggiore, R.J.; Konrad-Martin, D. Ototoxicity Monitoring Through the Eyes of the Treating Physician: Perspectives from Pulmonology and Medical Oncology. *Int. J. Audiol.* **2018**, *57*, S42–S47. [CrossRef] [PubMed]
99. Nagdee, N.; de Andrade, V.M. Strengthening Cancer Care through the Inclusion of Audiological Services. *S. Afr. Health Rev.* **2024**, *26*, 152–161. [CrossRef]
100. Schellack, N.; Wium, A.M.; Ehlert, K.; van Aswegen, Y.; Gous, A. Establishing a Pharmacotherapy Induced Ototoxicity Programme within a Service-Learning Approach. *S. Afr. J. Commun. Disord.* **2015**, *62*, 7. [CrossRef] [PubMed]
101. De Andrade, V.; Khoza-Shangase, K.; Hajat, F. Perceptions of Oncologists at Two State Hospitals in Gauteng Regarding the Ototoxic Effects of Cancer Chemotherapy: A Pilot Study. *Afr. J. Pharm. Pharmacol.* **2009**, *3*, 307–318.
102. Rhainds, M.; Bussières, M.; L'Espérance, S.; Nourissat, A.; Coulombe, M. 137 Audiologic Monitoring of Cisplatin Ototoxicity in Cancer Treatment of Adults: A Balance between Overdiagnosis and Patient Safety? *BMJ Evid.-Based Med.* **2018**, *23*, A64. [CrossRef]
103. Ramma, L.; Schellack, N.; Heinze, B. Prevention of Treatment-Induced Ototoxicity: An Update for Clinicians. *S. Afr. Med. J.* **2019**, *109*, 145–149. [CrossRef]
104. Khoza-Shangase, K.; Masondo, N. In Pursuit of Preventive Audiology in South Africa: Scoping the Context for Ototoxicity Assessment and Management. *J. Pharm. Bioallied Sci.* **2021**, *13*, 46. [CrossRef]
105. Natalie, S.; Alida, N. An Overview of Pharmacotherapy-Induced Ototoxicity. *S. Afr. Fam. Pract.* **2013**, *55*, 357–365. [CrossRef]
106. Maru, D.; Malky, G.-A. Current Practice of Ototoxicity Management across the United Kingdom (UK). *Int. J. Audiol.* **2018**, *57*, S29–S41. [CrossRef] [PubMed]
107. Fernandez, K.A.; Garinis, A.; Knight, K.; Konrad-Martin, D.; Morata, T.; Poling, G.L.; Reavis, K.M.; Sanchez, V.A.; Dreisbach, L. What's New in Ototoxicity Management? *Perspect. ASHA Spec. Interest Groups* **2024**, *9*, 113–123. [CrossRef]

audiology research

MDPI

Article

Assessing the Effectiveness of Different Hyperbaric Oxygen Treatment Methods in Patients with Sudden Sensorineural Hearing Loss

Paweł Rozbicki [1,*], Jacek Usowski [1], Sandra Krzywdzińska [1], Dariusz Jurkiewicz [1] and Jacek Siewiera [2]

[1] Department of Otolaryngology with Division of Cranio-Maxillo-Facial Surgery, Military Institute of Medicine—National Research Institute, 04-141 Warsaw, Poland

[2] Department of Hyperbaric Medicine, Military Institute of Medicine—National Research Institute, 04-141 Warsaw, Poland

* Correspondence: prozbicki@wim.mil.pl; Tel.: +48-261-816-471

Abstract: Introduction: Hyperbaric oxygen therapy (HBOT) is one of the treatment methods in patients with sudden sensorineural hearing loss (SSNHL). It is recommended as an elective treatment in patients undergoing steroid therapy. According to current scientific reports, HBOT should be implemented within two weeks after the first symptoms. However, as far as the profile of HBOT is concerned, there are no straightforward recommendations. Methods: The data obtained from the medical records of 218 patients undergoing HBOT for SSNHL at the Military Institute of Medicine—National Research Institute were analyzed statistically for the impact of the duration and the delay in implementing HBOT on the end results of pure-tone audiometry (PTA). Results: A statistically significant hearing improvement in patients undergoing more than 15 cycles of HBOT was detected at all frequencies except for 1500 Hz; in the group reporting for treatment with a delay of more than 10 days, hearing improvement was statistically unsignificant at frequencies of 1500, 3000, and 4000 Hz. Conclusions: The statistical analysis showed that the urgent onset of HBOT could be a significant factor in the therapy of SSNHL.

Keywords: hyperbaric oxygen therapy; sudden sensorineural hearing loss; sudden deafness; audiology

1. Introduction

Hyperbaric oxygen therapy (HBOT) is a treatment method using molecular oxygen in a pressurized environment. Common indications for the therapy are decompression sickness, non-healing of wounds during radiotherapy or diabetes, carbon monoxide poisoning, and brain abscesses [1]. Sudden sensorineural hearing loss (SSNHL) is a disease in which HBOT is applied. This condition causes a significant decline in the performance of hearing organs, which motivates urgent medical consultations at the Emergency Department. In the United States of America, it occurs in 5–27 individuals per 100,000 people annually, and there are approximately 66,000 new cases annually [2–4]. Despite numerous studies, the etiology of SSNHL remains unknown. The presumptive underlying causes of SSNHL are autoimmune reactions, traumatic events, metabolic disorders, and vascular abnormalities [5–8]. Except for the aforementioned reasons, recent studies propose mechanisms including genetic and epigenetic interrelationships, also considering line-1 global DNA methylation, iron homeostasis genes, ferroptosis, and cellular stressors such as iron excess and dysfunctional mitochondrial superoxide dismutase activity [9]. Inadequate treatment or late diagnosis of SSNHL increases the risk of poor recovery. Potential outcomes, such as permanent hearing deficit and tinnitus, significantly decrease the quality of life [10]. Pure-tone audiometry (PTA) remains an essential diagnostic tool for identifying SSNHL, as it involves an analysis of both ways in which the acoustic impulses are conducted. PTA is performed in soundproof rooms with the use of regularly certified devices. A typical setup consists of headphones for air conduction (AC) and bonephones placed on mastoid processes for bone conduction (BC). During the study, clear sounds at specified frequencies are played, with the volume increasing by 5 dB HL until the patient confirms they can hear a tone. This increase occurs by pressing a special button which entails recording of the auditory stimulus threshold on a particular level. Typically, in PTA, the sound in AC is marked for the following frequencies: 125, 250, 500, 1000, 1500, 2000, 4000, 6000, and 8000 Hz. Indications for 6000 and 8000 Hz are not used in BC due to an intensified muffling of these sounds by cranial bones. This enables differentiating sensorineural, conductional, and mixed hearing losses. Sensorineural hypoacusis involves lowering both the air and bone audiometric curves.

Sensorineural hypoacusis implies damage to the acoustic organ above the conducting apparatus, that is, the organ of Corti and auditory pathway neurons along the cochlear nerve, cochlear nuclei, lateral lemniscus, medial geniculate body, and other central nervous system structures reaching the auditory cortex. A detailed distinction of the etiologies of various types of sensorineural hypoacusis was made during audiological studies, such as brainstem auditory evoked potential measurements, otoacoustic emission, verbal audiometry, and electrocochleography. The diagnostic criterion of SSNHL is an increase in the hearing threshold stimulus to >30 dB HL over at least three audiometric frequencies, developing over no longer than 72 h [11]. In compliance with the recommendations of the Academy of Otolaryngology–Head and Neck Surgery (AAO-HNS)'s Clinical Practice Guidelines: Sudden Hearing Loss, the primary treatment methods of SSNHL are oral, intravenous, or intratympanic steroid therapies (STs). Each method has advantages and disadvantages, so a choice of a given method should be made case by case. The AAO-HNS recommends a standard dose of systemic ST of 1 mg/kg of body mass for prednisone, with a maximum dose of 60 mg. Nonetheless, a detailed schedule of systemic ST application in SSNHL remains debatable and is the subject of scientific research. The AAO-HNS, in its Clinical Practice Guidelines: Sudden Hearing Loss, recommends HBOT within 14 days after the first symptoms as an elective treatment. HBOT might be used to improve outcomes in patients with SSNHL in conjunction with steroids or as salvage therapy [12,13]. Other relevant medical societies and associations also recommend HBOT [14–16]. HBOT can be distinguished into initial treatment or salvage treatment. Treatment combined with steroid therapy within two weeks of symptom onset is known as initial treatment. Salvage treatment means HBOT combined with steroid therapy implemented within one month after the onset of SSNHL. This involves exposing the patient to 100% oxygen at a pressure of 1.5–2 ATA; the purposes of an increased supply of oxygen to the cochlea are a positive impact on the patient's immunity and hemodynamics, a reduction in hypoxia and edema, and potentiation of normal host responses to infection and ischemia [17]. The healing impact of HBOT may be related to increased red blood cells, hematocrit, hemoglobin concentration, and superoxide dismutase [18]. Moreover, HBOT preserves the microcirculation by reducing venular leukocyte adherence and inhibiting progressive adjacent arteriolar vasoconstriction [17]. Currently, no guidelines point to a particular HBOT protocol in patients with SSNHL, but a greater interest in this area has recently been observed [19]. The cited study demonstrated a dependence of pressure applied in the hyperbaric chamber on hearing improvement. It appears that patients applied with a pressure of 2.5 ATA had better treatment results than those treated with 1.5 ATA. In the examined group, there were no statistically significant differences in the decrease in hearing threshold stimulus with respect to the total time of compression (1 vs. 2 h). A selective influence of pressure values on hearing threshold stimulus was, however, demonstrated by Krajcovicova et al. [20]. Application of 2.0 ATA improved treatment results in the speech frequency spectrum. Compressions of 2.5 ATA proved more effective at lower frequencies. Further study showed that a pressure of 2.0 ATA is ineffective in the treatment of hearing loss encompassing octave bands of 1–2 kHz. Brief instructions available in the present-day scientific literature are not backed by research on the recommended number of cycles of hyperbaric oxygen therapy. For instance, LeGros et al. [21] mention 10–20 days of therapy. HBOT protocols applied until now result from experiences at research centers and the protocols applied in other diseases treated with HBOT. The development of recommendations requires a statistical analysis of treatment results in patients suffering from SSNHL subjected to different protocols, constituting this manuscript's foundation. A significant proportion of patients with SSNHL do not fully recover despite proven idiopathic disease remissions. The risk of permanent hearing deficits and an impairment stemming from them is a reason behind scientific research on therapy optimization. Such research aims to maximize the percentage of full recovery in patients and to reduce adverse reactions to the performed interventions. This study aimed to evaluate the influence of different HBOT profiles on hearing improvement in patients with SSNHL.

2. Materials and Methods

The medical records of patients admitted to the Department of Hyperbaric Medicine, Military Institute of Medicine—National Research Institute, and the Department of Otolaryngology with Division of Cranio-Maxillo-Facial Surgery, Military Institute of Medicine—National Research Institute due to SSNHL between January 2018 and December 2019 were analyzed retrospectively. The number of patients treated by the Institute during the indicated period determined the scale of the study. The eligibility criteria for the research included diagnosed SSNHL and completeness of medical records, including details on whether the patient had PTA before and after HBOT. A diagnostic criterion of SSNHL, according to the guidelines of the AAO-HNS, is an increase in the hearing threshold stimulus to >30 dB HL over at least three audiometric frequencies, developing over no longer than 72 h.

Exclusion criteria were as follows: age < 18 years, age > 85 years, HBOT initiated 30 days after the first symptoms of SSNHL, coexistent cerebrospinal inflammation, neuropsychiatric disorders, Ménière's disease, hereditary hearing disorders, inner ear malformations, facial nerve neuromas, acoustic neuromas (or other tumors of the inner auditory canal, cerebellopontine angle), bilateral SSNHL, subsequent episode of SSNHL, and air-bone gaps on PTA.

PTA results were the key variables considered for the SSNHL diagnosis. The tests were conducted using an Interacoustics AC40 audiometer for the following frequencies [Hz] for air conduction (AC) (125, 250, 500, 1000, 1500, 2000, 3000, 4000, 6000, 8000) and bone conduction (BC) (125, 250, 500, 1000, 1500, 2000, 3000, 4000). To prevent the non-test ear from influencing the results, the study used tone masking. A statistical analysis was conducted only for BC, given the nature of SSNHL. Since PTA is subjective, its result as the only variable was potentially biased. Patients with diagnosed SSNHL were treated with ST schemes. Details on the pharmacotherapy used can be found in our team's previous work [22]. Patients underwent HBOT with the following protocol: compression to 2.5 ATA, total compression/decompression time: 10 min (0.025 m/s), oxygenation 3 × 20 min with 100% as a breathing factor, and oxygen breaks 2 × 5 min performed routinely to prevent toxic effect on the lungs. A medical staff member (a nurse, a doctor, or a paramedic) was present in the chamber during HBOT. The HBOT cycles were conducted daily, once a day. Compression during hyperbaric therapy was performed with a BAROXHBO device. Most patients underwent 15 cycles (1 cycle being equivalent to 1 day) of HBOT, given the previous experience of the institute. The patients were divided into subgroups for statistical analysis according to the delay in implementing HBOT (<5 days, 5–10 days, >10 days) and the number of cycles/duration of HBOT (<15 cycles, 15 cycles, >15 cycles). After the start of HBOT, patients underwent a monitoring hearing test. The data concerning the above-mentioned variables were extracted from the medical records of patients treated in the Department of Hyperbaric Medicine and Department of Otolaryngology with the Division of Cranio-Maxillo-Facial Surgery, Military Institute of Medicine—National Research Institute.

Statistical Analysis

The results were tabulated. First, the mean hearing threshold in patients before and after treatment was summarized for the entire study group. Using the visual method and the Kolmogorov–Smirnov test, a normal distribution was found in the studied variables. Next, using a paired Student's *t*-test, the significance of differences between the means before and after the treatment was verified.

Subsequently, the relationship between the delay in hyperbaric therapy and the end results of treatment was analyzed. After confirming a normal distribution in the subgroups, statistical analysis was performed using a paired Student's *t*-test. The first step was to compare the significance of differences in the mean hearing threshold in PTA before and after the treatment across the subgroups.

The final step of the statistical analysis was to compare the statistical significance of hearing improvement according to the number of hyperbaric chamber cycles. After confirming the normal distribution of the variables, the data were analyzed using a paired Student's *t*-test.

3. Results

The statistical analysis included 218 patients (mean age: 48.8 ± 14.5 years; 117 males, 101 females). Patients not meeting the study criteria were excluded from the study and the analysis. Each patient was observed for at least two months after admission to the Military Institute of Medicine—National Research Institute. No patient was disqualified due to HBOT contraindications. Patients administered <15 cycles of HBOT terminated treatment for personal reasons that were not related to the treatment itself.

The studied patients demonstrated a typical distribution for age structure and hearing depth in the Kolmogorov–Smirnov test. The average patient delay in reporting to the Department of Hyperbaric Medicine—Military Institute of Medicine—National Research Institute after the onset of SSNHL symptoms was 8.2 (±6.6) days. The average hearing threshold stimulus in the study group before the treatment was 54.6 (±31.3) dB HL and it was 39.6 (±32.2) dB HL after the treatment.

A significant lowering of hearing threshold was observed in BC, which directly indicates a recovery from SSNHL. The results are presented in Table 1.

Table 1. BC before and after combined treatment with ST and HBOT.

Frequency [Hz]	Before [dB]	After [dB]	Difference	*p*
250	41.22	26.03	15.19	<0.001
500	48.05	28.68	19.37	<0.001
1000	49.05	30.52	18.52	<0.001
1500	69.40	32.72	36.68	<0.001
2000	52.49	34.86	17.63	<0.001
3000	56.76	38.11	18.65	<0.001
4000	54.03	38.67	15.35	<0.001

Then, the respective results of hyperbaric treatment were analyzed. In the first step, patients treated with HBOT were divided into subgroups according to the delay in therapy initiation: <5 days (75 patients), 5–10 days (95 patients), and >10 days (48 patients). In the next step, the group was divided according to the number of applied compressions: <15 cycles (23 persons), 15 cycles (176 persons), and >15 cycles (19 persons). A normal distribution in variables resulting from the PTA study was confirmed for all the groups. This enabled a parametric analysis during further evaluation of the groups. The results of the Student's *t*-test with respect to the delay in HBOT are shown in Table 2.

Table 2. Delay in HBOT and improvement in hearing at different frequencies.

Frequency [Hz]	<5 Days (p-Value; Difference [dB])	5–10 Days (p-Value; Difference [dB])	>10 Days (p-Value; Difference [dB])
250	$p < 0.001$; 17.6	$p < 0.001$; 14.5	$p < 0.05$; 11.4
500	$p < 0.001$; 21.6	$p < 0.001$; 17.9	$p < 0.001$; 18.2
1000	$p < 0.001$; 21.3	$p < 0.001$; 17.7	$p < 0.05$; 13.5
1500	$p < 0.001$; 24.2	$p < 0.001$; 21.8	$p > 0.05$; 8.2
2000	$p < 0.001$; 19.8	$p < 0.001$; 16.2	$p < 0.05$; 12.1
3000	$p < 0.001$; 18.2	$p < 0.001$; 15.9	$p > 0.05$; 10.2
4000	$p < 0.001$; 15.9	$p < 0.001$; 13.7	$p > 0.05$; 10.9

The analysis presented here shows statistically significant improvements across all frequencies in the patient groups studied except for 1500, 3000 Hz, and 4000 Hz in the group who reported for treatment with a delay of more than 10 days.

Next, the groups were divided by therapy duration (number of cycles) and analyzed using a Student's t-test (Table 3).

Table 3. Cycle count in HBOT and improvement in hearing at different frequencies.

Frequency [Hz]	<15 Cycles (p-Value; Difference [dB])	15 Cycles (p-Value; Difference [dB])	>15 Cycles (p-Value; Difference [dB])
250	$p < 0.001$; 14.3	$p < 0.001$; 14.9	$p < 0.05$; 24.4
500	$p < 0.001$; 18.8	$p < 0.001$; 19.4	$p < 0.05$; 28.1
1000	$p < 0.001$; 17.7	$p < 0.001$; 18.2	$p < 0.01$; 24.7
1500	$p < 0.001$; 19.6	$p < 0.001$; 20.7	$p > 0.05$; 33.6
2000	$p < 0.001$; 16.0	$p < 0.001$; 15.7	$p < 0.05$; 25.3
3000	$p < 0.001$; 15.0	$p < 0.001$; 14.9	$p < 0.05$; 26.0
4000	$p < 0.001$; 12.6	$p < 0.001$; 11.8	$p < 0.01$; 29.7

A statistically significant hearing improvement was demonstrated for patients treated with 15 cycles or less across all frequencies analyzed. In patients treated with more than 15 cycles, hearing improvement was statistically significant across all frequencies except for 1500 Hz.

4. Discussion

The statistical analysis results complied with the purpose of the study, which was to confirm the impact of the HBOT profile on treatment outcomes. In the groups compared, delaying HBOT more than 10 days from the time of the first SSNHL symptoms was associated with a reduced treatment efficacy at 1500, 3000, and 4000 Hz. This is in line with current scientific evidence [12,20,23–25]. Cavaliere et al. demonstrated a complex relationship between the choice of therapeutical strategy for SSNHL and hearing improvement [26]. The cited report compared the HBOT results with and without simultaneous application of ST. The treatment was particularly effective 14 days after the first symptoms. Moreover, the use of ST with HBOT resulted in less satisfying therapy results in patients admitted for treatment up to seven days after the first symptoms of SSNHL. There is a need for further research in this field, focusing on the relationship between oxidative stress [18] occurring at the early stage of SSNHL and the choice of treatment protocol. The comparison of HBOT delays indicated that in patients admitted to hospital after 10 days, the hearing improvement was statistically significant for a frequency of 250, 500, 1000, and 2000 Hz. This means that hearing improvements in the examined group of patients were not statistically significant at higher frequencies in the speech spectrum. Tae-Min Rhee's team [27] conducted a meta-analysis encompassing 16 unrandomized tests and three RCTs, which showed the statistically significant benefits of HBOT lasting longer than 1200 min. Their findings are in agreement with our study. HBOT requires regular visits to a medical facility at a fixed time. These facilities may be located a certain distance from the patient's residence, causing difficulties related to commuting and accommodation. For this reason, one may expect differences in the availability of HBOT for patients with SSNHL depending on the country, and the distribution of hyperbaric medicine centers in the region inhabited by patients may impact the treatment outcomes. One potential solution to such problems would be the development of new HBOT facilities. However, this may prove problematic, particularly in countries with low spending on healthcare. Patients may have also resigned from the therapy due to a lack of motivation for regular visits to their medical facility. A patient undergoing therapy should, thus, always be informed by an attending physician on the chances and risks of the therapy. The communication between a doctor and a patient should be considered a key determinant of end-treatment results. In their meta-analysis encompassing 106 correlational studies and 21 experimental interventions, Zolnierek et al. demonstrated that the communication skills of medical staff strongly correlate with patients following their guidelines. The recommendations offered by staff members trained in soft skills were followed 1.62 times more often than by doctors who did not possess such skills [28].

Our study results also revealed a decreased significance of hearing improvements in patients treated with more than 15 cycles of HBOT. This could be induced by the negative impact of oxidate stress caused by hyperbaric oxygen or the smaller number of enrolled patients in this group. These relations should be solved in further studies.

The experience of the center and the retrospective character of this study directly led to the uneven distribution of patients in groups divided by the number of treatment cycles in a hyperbaric chamber. Differences in the number of patients in the study groups did not cause deviations from the normal distribution in the groups, which enabled their comparison using parametric statistical tests. The limitation of this study was the lack of a control group of patients who did not undergo HBOT. This was associated with clinical practice in our institute, based on evidence-based medicine describing the positive influence of HBOT on SSNHL [12–15].

Studies opposing the recommendations of the AAO-HNS's Clinical Practice Guideline: Sudden Hearing Loss [11] report no significant differences in end treatment results between groups treated exclusively with ST as opposed to groups treated with ST and HBOT [29]. In the cited study, there are the following differences in the HBOT protocols: intervals between compressions—5 min vs. 10 min—and minor differences in the decompression time—10 min vs. 6–12 min. In comparison with Skarżyński et al., the hearing improvement in our study was 15.3 dB HL vs. 14.1 dB HL. It can be expected that these dependencies will not achieve statistical significance. A difference in subjective hearing may also be clinically irrelevant. Nevertheless, a statistical calculation of raw data from both teams would need to be conducted to exclude the influence of a specific HBOT profile.

A metanalysis conducted by Eryigit et al. [30] of 16 articles published between 2002 and 2018 proved the relationship between the depth of hearing impairments and the final outcomes of HBOT treatment in SSNHL. In the cited study, no significant difference was demonstrated between the HBOT and control groups. On the contrary, in patients with severe and profound SSNHL, the hearing improvement was statistically significant. In the group of patients enrolled in our study, a significant number of patients presented moderate hearing impairments that could reduce the salience of the results. Studying the relationship between the severity of SSNHL and the influence of HBOT on final outcomes requires further prospective studies in diverse HBOT protocols.

Opposing to study conducted by Eryigit [30], Choi et al. stated there were no differences in hearing improvement between the HBOT and control group of patients with severe to profound SSNHL [31]. However, the differences of hearing improvement rate were observed in group of patients with diabetes mellitus. The cited study was performed on a group of patients undergoing an HBOT protocol including ventilation for 90 min per session with 2,4 ATA pressure. The number of sessions administered for patients was described as over 14 sessions. This means that the hyperbaric session properties were comparable to our study. On the other hand, the delay to HBOT was higher in our group than for the subjects enrolled by Choi et al. This could be a reason why hearing gains are higher in Choi's study in comparison to our 53.3 dB HL (53.4% difference prior to initial PTA) and 39.1 dB HL (39.6% difference prior to initial PTA) vs. 15,0 dB (27.5% difference prior to initial PTA). This corresponds with results of our study, where the hearing improvement was more significant in the group of patients with minor delays to HBOT administration.

Dynamically developing prosthetics are often essential in the treatment of hypoacusis, especially considering the poor prognosis for full recovery in many cases of SSNHL. Promising results of surveys on improvements in quality of life and quality of hearing were observed in a multicenter prospective examination of life quality in patients with surgically implanted cochlear implants (the Health Utility Index increased by 33%, SSQ improvement in the quality of comprehending speech of 180%, spatial hearing increased by 135%, quality of hearing increased by 98%) [32]. The priority remains to achieve the best possible results in improving hearing, despite the development of medical technologies that improve hypoacusis. Current scientific reports lack research that would standardize an HBOT profile used in the treatment of SSNHL regarding the number of compressions and the duration of a single compression cycle. The results of our study encourage further research across a wider population to establish an optimal therapy scheme, which may lead to an improvement in the SSNHL treatment outcomes.

5. Conclusions

In the group of patients who received HBOT after 10 days, there was no statistically significant improvement in the hearing threshold in high-frequency PTA. Thus, it seems beneficial to start HBOT for SSNHL within the first 10 days of illness. The statistical significance of hearing improvements decreased in the group of patients treated with more than 15 cycles of HBOT. Further prospective studies with standardized and randomized therapeutic protocols are required.

Author Contributions: Conceptualization, P.R., J.U., S.K., D.J. and J.S.; methodology P.R., J.U., D.J. and J.S.; validation J.U., D.J. and J.S.; investigation, P.R., J.U., S.K. and D.J.; resources, P.R., J.U. and D.J.; data curation, P.R. and J.U.; writing—original draft preparation, P.R., S.K. and J.U., writing—review and editing, D.J. and J.S.; supervision D.J. and J.S.; project administration, P.R. All authors have read and agreed to the published version of the manuscript.

Funding: This research received no external funding.

Institutional Review Board Statement: Ethical review and approval were waived due to the study's retrospective nature.

Informed Consent Statement: Patient consent was waived due to anonymized medical data and the retrospective type of study.

Data Availability Statement: Medical data are available at the Military Institute of Medicine—National Research Institute.

Acknowledgments: Our research team would like to thank the staff of the Audiology Outpatient Unit and Department of Hyperbaric Medicine at the Military Institute of Medicine—National Research Institute for the efficient collection of essential data for our study.

Conflicts of Interest: The authors declare no conflicts of interest.

References

1. Undersea & Hyperbaric Medical Society. Indications for Hyperbaric Oxygen Therapy. Available online: https://www.uhms.org/resources/hbo-indications.html (accessed on 10 January 2024).
2. Alexander, T.H.; Harris, J.P. Incidence of sudden sensorineural hearing loss. *Otol. Neurotol.* **2013**, *34*, 1586–1589. [CrossRef] [PubMed]
3. Byl, F.M. Seventy-six cases of presumed sudden hearing loss occurring in 1973: Prognosis and incidence. *Laryngoscope* **1977**, *87*, 817–825. [CrossRef] [PubMed]
4. Mattox, D.E.; Simmons, F.B. Natural history of sudden sensorineural hearing loss. *Ann. Otol. Rhinol. Laryngol.* **1977**, *86*, 463–480. [CrossRef] [PubMed]

5. Wu, H.; Wan, W.; Jiang, H.; Xiong, Y. Prognosis of Idiopathic Sudden Sensorineural Hearing Loss: The Nomogram Perspective. *Ann. Otol. Rhinol. Laryngol.* **2022**, *132*, 5–12. [CrossRef] [PubMed]
6. Xie, S.; Qiang, Q.; Mei, L.; He, C.; Feng, Y.; Sun, H.; Wu, X. Multivariate analysis of prognostic factors for idiopathic sudden sensorineural hearing loss treated with adjuvant hyperbaric oxygen therapy. *Eur. Arch. Otorhinolaryngol.* **2018**, *275*, 47–51. [CrossRef]
7. Sun, X.M.; Zhuang, S.M.; Xiao, Z.W.; Luo, J.Q.; Long, Z.; Lan, L.C.; Zhang, H.Q.; Zhang, G.P. Autoimmune thyroiditis in patients with sudden sensorineural hearing loss. *Laryngoscope Investig. Otolaryngol.* **2022**, *7*, 571–577. [CrossRef]
8. Huang, C.Y.; Li, D.S.; Tsai, M.H.; Chen, C.H.; Cheng, Y.F. The impact of acute tinnitus on listening effort: A study based on clinical observations of sudden sensorineural hearing loss patients. *Int. J. Environ. Res. Public Health* **2022**, *19*, 3661. [CrossRef] [PubMed]
9. Tisato, V.; Castiglione, A.; Ciorba, A.; Aimoni, C.; Silva, J.A.; Gallo, I.; D'aversa, E.; Salvatori, F.; Bianchini, C.; Pelucchi, S.; et al. LINE-1 global DNA methylation, iron homeostasis genes, sex and age in sudden sensorineural hearing loss (SSNHL). *Hum. Genom.* **2023**, *17*, 112. [CrossRef] [PubMed]
10. Dallan, I.; Fortunato, S.; Casani, A.P.; Bernardini, E.; Sellari-Franceschini, S.; Berrettini, S.; Nacci, A. Long-term follow up of sudden sensorineural hearing loss patients treated with intratympanic steroids: Audiological and quality of life evaluation. *J. Laryngol. Otol.* **2014**, *128*, 669–673. [CrossRef] [PubMed]
11. National Institutes of Health. *Sudden Deafness*; NIH Publication No. 00–4757; National Institutes of Health: Bethesda, MD, USA, 2000.
12. Chandrasekhar, S.S.; Do, B.S.T.; Schwartz, S.R.; Bontempo, L.J.; Faucett, E.A.; Finestone, S.A.; Hollingsworth, D.B.; Kelley, D.M.; Kmucha, S.T.; Moonis, G.; et al. Clinical Practice Guideline: Sudden Hearing Loss (Update). *Otolaryngol. Head Neck Surg.* **2019**, *161* (Suppl. S1), S1–S45. [CrossRef]
13. Joshua, T.G.; Ayub, A.; Wijesinghe, P.; Nunez, D.A. Hyperbaric Oxygen Therapy for Patients with Sudden Sensorineural Hearing Loss: A Systematic Review and Meta-analysis. *JAMA Otolaryngol. Head Neck Surg.* **2022**, *148*, 5–11. [CrossRef] [PubMed]
14. Undersea & Hyperbaric Medical Society. 14. Idiopathic Sudden Sensorineural Hearing Loss (New! Approved on October 8, 2011 by the UHMS Board of Directors). Published October 8, 2011. Available online: https://www.uhms.org/14-idiopathic-sudden-sensorineural-hearing-loss-new-approved-on-october-8-2011-by-the-uhms-board-of-directors.html (accessed on 16 October 2023).
15. Mathieu, D.; Marroni, A.; Kot, J. Tenth European Consesus Conference on Hyperbaric Medicine: Recommendations for accepted and non-accepted clinical indications and practice of hyperbaric oxygen treatment. *Diving Hyperb. Med.* **2017**, *47*, 24–32. [CrossRef] [PubMed]
16. Topuz, E.; Yigit, O.; Cinar, U.; Seven, H. Should hyperbaric oxygen be added to treatment in idiopathic sudden sensorineural hearing loss? *Eur. Arch. Otorhinolaryngol.* **2018**, *274*, 103–110. [CrossRef] [PubMed]
17. Gill, A.; Bell, C. Hyperbaric oxygen: Its uses, mechanisms of action and outcomes. *Qjm Int. J. Med.* **2004**, *97*, 385–395. [CrossRef] [PubMed]
18. Huo, Z.; Cheng, X.; Gu, J.; Hong, Y.; Wang, Z.; Zhang, Z. Prognostic factors for hearing outcomes in patients that undergo adjuvant hyperbaric oxygen therapy for sudden sensorineural hearing loss. *Laryngoscope Investig. Otolaryngol.* **2022**, *7*, 592–598. [CrossRef]
19. Kim, H.; Kong, S.; Kim, J.; Lee, H.; Choi, S.; Lee, I.; Oh, S. The Optimized Protocol of Hyperbaric Oxygen Therapy for Sudden Sensorineural Hearing Loss. *Laryngoscope* **2022**, *133*, 383–388. [CrossRef] [PubMed]
20. Krajčovičová, Z.; Meluš, V.; Zigo, R.; Matišáková, I.; Večeřa, J.; Králová, E. Hyperbaric oxygen therapy in treatment of sudden sensorineural hearing loss: Finding for the maximal therapeutic benefit of different applied pressures. *Undersea Hyperb. Med.* **2019**, *46*, 665–672. [CrossRef] [PubMed]
21. LeGros, T.L.; Murphy-Lavoie, H. HBO2 for sudden sensorineural hearing loss. *Undersea Hyperb. Med.* **2020**, *47*, 271–295. [CrossRef]
22. Rozbicki, P.; Usowski, J.; Siewiera, J.; Jurkiewicz, D. The Influence of Steroid Therapy on the Treatment Results in Patients with Sudden Sensorineural Hearing Loss. *J. Clin. Med.* **2022**, *11*, 6085. [CrossRef] [PubMed]
23. Hosokawa, S.; Sugiyama, K.; Takahashi, G.; Takebayashi, S.; Mineta, H. Prognostic factors for idiopathic sudden sensorineural hearing loss treated with hyperbaric oxygen therapy and intravenous steroids. *J. Laryngol. Otol.* **2017**, *131*, 77–82. [CrossRef]
24. Jadczak, M.; Rapiejko, P.; Kantor, I.; Szczygielski, K.; Usowski, J.; Piechocki, J.; Jurkiewicz, D. Evaluation of hyperbaric oxygen and pharmacological therapy in sudden hearing loss. *Otolaryngol. Pol.* **2007**, *61*, 887–891. [CrossRef] [PubMed]
25. Wang, Y.; Gao, Y.; Wang, B.; Chen, L.; Zhang, X. Efficacy and Prognostic Factors of Combined Hyperbaric Oxygen Therapy in Patients With Idiopathic Sudden Sensorineural Hearing Loss. *Am. J. Audiol.* **2019**, *28*, 95–100. [CrossRef] [PubMed]
26. Cavaliere, M.; De Luca, P.; Scarpa, A.; Strzalkowski, A.M.; Ralli, M.; Calvanese, M.; Savignano, L.; Viola, P.; Cassandro, C.; Chiarella, G.; et al. Combination of Hyperbaric Oxygen Therapy and Oral Steroids for the Treatment of Sudden Sensorineural Hearing Loss: Early or Late? *Medicina* **2022**, *58*, 1421. [CrossRef] [PubMed]
27. Rhee, T.-M.; Hwang, D.; Lee, J.-S.; Park, J.; Lee, J.M. Addition of Hyperbaric Oxygen Therapy vs Medical Therapy Alone for Idiopathic Sudden Sensorineural Hearing Loss: A Systematic Review and Meta-analysis. *JAMA Otolaryngol. Head Neck Surg.* **2018**, *144*, 1153–1161. [CrossRef] [PubMed]
28. Zolnierek, K.B.H.; Dimatteo, M.R. Physician communication and patient adherence to treatment: A meta-analysis. *Med. Care* **2009**, *47*, 826–834. [CrossRef] [PubMed]

29. Skarzynski, P.H.; Kolodziejak, A.; Gos, E.; Skarzynska, M.B.; Czajka, N.; Skarzynski, H. Hyperbaric oxygen therapy as an adjunct to corticosteroid treatment in sudden sensorineural hearing loss: A retrospective study. *Front. Neurol.* **2023**, *14*, 1225135. [CrossRef] [PubMed]
30. Eryigit, B.; Ziylan, F.; Yaz, F.; Thomeer, H.G.X.M. The effectiveness of hyperbaric oxygen in patients with idiopathic sudden sensorineural hearing loss: A systematic review. *Eur. Arch. Otorhinolaryngol.* **2018**, *275*, 2893–2904. [CrossRef] [PubMed]
31. Choi, Y.; Han, S.J.; Kim, S.K.; Hong, S.M. The therapeutic effect of hyperbaric oxygen therapy in patients with severe to profound idiopathic sudden sensorineural hearing loss. *Sci. Rep.* **2024**, *14*, 3321. [CrossRef]
32. Czerniejewska-Wolska, H.; Kałos, M.; Sekula, A.; Piszczatowski, B.; Rutkowska, J.; Rogowski, M.; Zadrożniak, M.; Szymański, M.S.; Klatka, J.; Durko, M.; et al. Quality of life and hearing after cochlear implant placement in patients over 60 years of age. *Otolaryngol. Pol.* **2015**, *69*, 34–39. [CrossRef]

audiology research

MDPI

Article

Middle Ear Active Implant Indications, Comparative Audiometric Results from Different Approaches, and Coupling with the Vibrant Soundbridge®: A Single Center Experience over More Than 20 Years

Joan Lorente-Piera *, Raquel Manrique-Huarte, Janaina P. Lima, Diego Calavia and Manuel Manrique

Department of Otorhinolaryngology, Clínica Universidad de Navarra, 31000 Pamplona, Spain; rmanrique@unav.es (R.M.-H.); jpatriciode@unav.es (J.P.L.); dcalaviag@unav.es (D.C.); mmanrqeu@unav.es (M.M.)
* Correspondence: jlorentep@unav.es; Tel.: +34-948-25-54-00

Abstract: Background: Middle ear active implants, such as the Vibrant Soundbridge (VSB), offer an alternative to reconstructive surgery and other implantable hearing aid systems for patients with conductive, mixed, or sensorineural hearing loss. The primary objective of this work is to describe the auditory results obtained with VSB in our patient cohort, measuring the auditory gain in terms of average tonal thresholds and spoken word discrimination at 65 dB. Secondly, auditory gain differences between different types of hearing loss, coupling to the ossicular chain compared to round and oval windows, and the impact of open versus more conservative surgical approaches, were analyzed. Methods: A cross-sectional observational study, with retrospective data collection, was conducted at a tertiary care center. Clinical and audiometric data pre- and post-implantation were included, from patients who underwent VSB device placement surgery between 2001 and 2024. Results: 55 patients with an average age of 62.58 ± 17.83 years and a slight preference in terms of the female gender (52.72%) were included in the study. The average gain in the PTA for all types of hearing loss was 41.56 ± 22.63 dB, while for sensorineural hearing loss (SNHL) the gain was 31.04 ± 8.80 dB. For mixed-conductive hearing loss (C-MHL) a gain of 42.96 ± 17.70 was achieved, notably, in terms of absolute values, at frequencies of 4000 and 6000 Hz, with gains reaching 49.25 ± 20.26 dB at 4 K and 51.16 ± 17.48 dB at 6 K. In terms of spoken word discrimination, for all types of hearing loss, an improvement of 75.20 ± 10.11% was achieved. However, patients with C-MHL exhibited an approximately 13% higher gain compared to those with SNHL (69.32 ± 24.58% vs. 57.79 ± 15.28%). No significant differences in auditory gain were found between open and closed surgical techniques, nor in the proportion of adverse effects, when comparing one technique with the other. Conclusions: The VSB is effective in improving hearing in patients with mixed, conductive, and sensorineural hearing loss, with significant gains at high frequencies, especially through the round window membrane approach. The choice of surgical technique should consider the patient's anatomical characteristics and specific needs in order to optimize auditory outcomes and minimize postoperative complications.

Keywords: middle ear active implant; Vibrant Soundbridge; hearing loss; cholesteatoma; hearing implants

1. Introduction

Active middle ear implants (AMEIs) are hearing systems designed to transmit mechanical energy to a vibratory component of the ossicular chain or directly to the fluids in the inner ear at the round window (RW) or oval window (OW), unlike the mechanism of action of conventional hearing aids [1]. These devices offer an alternative to reconstructive surgery and other implantable hearing aid systems, such as bone conduction implants or hearing aids. AMEIs are especially recommended for individuals who cannot use traditional solutions or whose hearing loss is beyond the range of other hearing systems. This may be due to medical contraindications, such as an external ear condition that contraindicates occluding the auditory canal with hearing aids, insufficient performance of these devices as measured by speech audiometry, or surpassing the indications for bone conduction with bone conduction implants.

Subjectively, patients report better sound quality, improved localization, and notably better speech intelligibility when using AMEIs compared to other devices, such as hearing aids [2]. However, they are costly and require surgery under general anesthesia for both installation and replacement, or for the repair of potential implant failures.

AMEIs like the Vibrant Soundbridge (VSB) have emerged as a viable alternative for patients with sensorineural, mixed, or conductive hearing loss. The VSB system is surgically implanted under the skin and connected to a vibratory component (the floating mass transducer, or FMT). In terms of indications, the original recommendation for sensorineural hearing loss involves coupling the VSB to the incus, on either the long process or the body of the incus. This is particularly advised for individuals with moderate to severe high-frequency hearing loss and speech discrimination of ≥50% at 65 dB, who are either dissatisfied with their hearing aids or experience limitations in their use, such as recurrent external otitis [3,4].

Conversely, coupling the VSB to the round window is indicated for patients with conductive or mixed hearing loss. This approach is particularly recommended for cases of chronic otitis media, cholesteatomatous mastoidectomy (using either open or closed techniques), or unsatisfactory otosclerosis surgery. Special caution is advised in these instances due to the potential lack of movement in the windows, which is necessary for intracochlear fluid vibration [5–7]. To optimize vibration in these situations, a manufacturer-provided coupler can be used, and fascia or cartilage can be placed between the FMT and the round window. Additionally, the VSB has been used in the round window for patients with malformations, whether it be external auditory canal atresia or ossicular chain malformations. The expected auditory gain with a FMT in the round window varies between 25 dB and 60 dB, while placement in the oval window can achieve 30 to 35 dB [2]. However, the greatest functional gain with AMEIs has been demonstrated with stapes coupling, achieving up to 65 dB.

Finally, it is important to note that the performance of the VSB system can vary based on individual anatomical differences, either intrinsic or due to surgical procedures to treat the underlying pathology, as well as the efficiency of the FMT coupling [8]. The evaluation of the need to use a coupler or coupling system depends on the surgeon's judgment, potentially introducing variability in surgical and auditory outcomes [9].

The primary objective of this study is to describe the auditory outcomes achieved with the VSB in our patient cohort, specifically measuring the auditory gain in pure tone thresholds at speech frequencies. Secondarily, we aim to confirm intergroup differences in the auditory gain among patients with different types of hearing loss (sensorineural vs. conductive–mixed hearing loss), comparing ossicular chain coupling to the RW and OW anchoring. Additionally, we seek to determine whether the placement of this middle ear active implant in a cavity treated with an open mastoidectomy technique versus a more conservative approach influences the audiometric outcomes.

2. Materials and Methods

2.1. Study Design

A cross-sectional observational study, with retrospective data collection, was conducted at a tertiary care center. This study was designed and carried out in accordance with the ethical guidelines in the Declaration of Helsinki of 1975. Written informed consent was obtained from all study participants.

2.2. Inclusion Criteria

Pre- and post-implantation data were collected from subjects who underwent surgery for the placement of a Vibrant Soundbridge VORP503 device (MED-EL, Innsbruck, Austria), between 2001 and 2024. The audiological indications for mixed–conductive hearing loss, as well as sensorineural hearing loss, are represented in Figure 1.

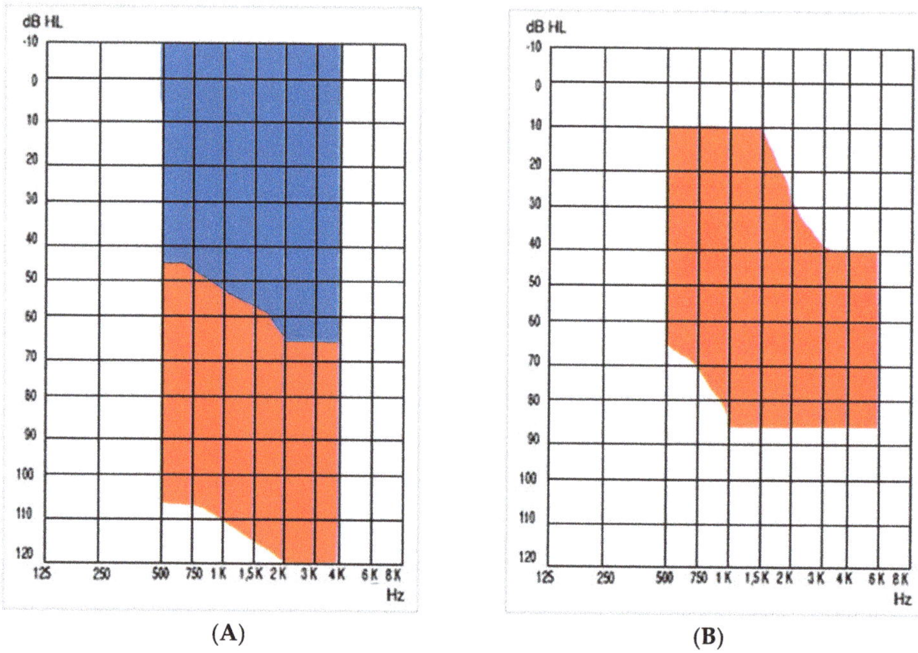

Figure 1. (**A**) shows the Vibrant Soundbridge indication for conductive or mixed hearing loss: the bone conduction threshold must fall within the blue shaded area on the chart, while the air conduction threshold should be within the red shaded area. (**B**) shows the indication for sensorineural hearing loss: the air conduction threshold must be within the red shaded area on the chart. In both cases, at least 50% speech understanding is required, using headphones, during an open-set word test. Courtesy of VSB MED-EL Co.

2.3. Surgical Procedure

In our study, two primary approaches were used for the placement of the FMT: either coupling to the ossicular chain (incus or stapes) or through round and oval windows. Generally, the most employed procedure is the standard approach through a mastoidectomy with posterior tympanotomy, followed by anchoring the transducer to one of the previously mentioned structures. Depending on the patient, stabilization is achieved using a coupler, along with the placement of fascia or cartilage interposed between the FMT and the ossicle, or the round or oval window.

However, it is important to note that, regarding the coupling at the incus, although classically the FMT is anchored to the long process of this ossicle, in some cases, the FMT is placed on the short process of the incus through an atticotomy. Examples of different approaches to get into the incus are shown in Figure 2 [2].

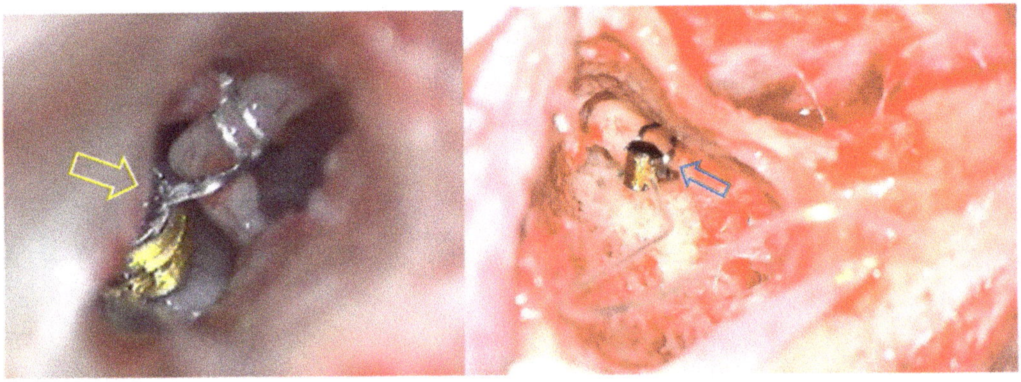

Figure 2. Surgery for the placement of the VSB using two different approaches. Firstly, in the left image, the yellow arrow shows the FMT anchored on the long process of the incus through a posterior timpanotomy. In the right image, the blue arrow shows the FMT anchored also on the long process of the incus, but in this case, through an extended atticotomy.

Additionally, regarding cholesteatoma resection techniques, two options were considered, namely the closed technique (canal wall up) or two types of open techniques: the classic or canal wall down, with or without closure of the external auditory canal, or in some cases, an alternative, such as on-demand techniques. These were used in a considerable number of patients in our cohort, specifically attic exposure–antrum exclusion (AE-AE), a technique that completely exposes the attic by drilling the superior wall of the external auditory canal and which excludes the antrum and mastoid by closing the aditus with cartilage grafts (Manrique-Huarte et al. [10]).

2.4. Follow-Up and Audiometric Studies

Postoperative follow-up of the implant includes medical appointments at one week, four weeks (implant activation), three months, six months, and one year. Additionally, continuous monitoring of the otological cause is maintained. Our study encompasses the medical history and audiometric analysis at the pre-implantation stage and compares it with one-year post-implant. It also studies the surgical details and potential complications.

The key variables for comparing auditory performance with the AMEI include pre- and post-implant average tonal thresholds (PTA) and the gain difference measured in decibels at 500, 1000, 2000, 4000, and 6000 Hz, with variables measured in terms of tonal audiometry. The decision to measure different frequencies, especially high frequencies, was due to the extensive knowledge that this type of implant provides an effective level of amplification, particularly at higher frequencies [3,4]. On the other hand, through speech recognition, the gain achieved with the VSB in terms of the percentage of discrimination at 65 dB was measured, both prior to implant placement and post-implant using free-field audiometry.

2.5. Statistical Study

Quantitative demographic data were presented using the mean, range, and standard deviation. The normality of the data distribution was assessed using the Shapiro–Wilk test and parametric methods were used.

To compare the gains in the PTA and the verbal discrimination between different groups, *t*-tests were used. The *t*-tests conducted were paired comparison tests, as they compared the differences in speech discrimination measures for each patient at two different times: before and after the placement of the VSB. The groups were categorized based on the surgical technique used (canal wall down with AE-AE vs. canal wall up) and the type of hearing loss (SNHL vs. C-MHL) in the group with ossicular chain coupling. In the case of the overall results and the coupling at the round and oval windows, no statistical comparisons were made due to the large differences in the sample sizes between them, making it difficult to demonstrate statistical significance. Finally, to determine which type of surgical approach was associated with a higher proportion of adverse effects, Fisher's exact test was conducted.

For the statistical analysis, a significance level of $p < 0.05$ was considered. All analyses were performed using RStudio 1.4.1106 software, ensuring the accuracy and reproducibility of the results.

3. Results

A total of 55 patients underwent Vibrant Soundbridge (VSB) implantation between 2001 and 2024. Of these subjects, 52.72% were women (n = 29), while the remaining 26 patients (47.28%) were men. All patients (100%) were regular users of the implant from the time of placement until the end of the follow-up. A summary of the demographic data is presented in Table 1.

Table 1. Summary of the demographic data of the patients included in this study.

	Demographic Description		
Age at treatment	62.58 ± 17.83 (12–87) years		
Gender	29 (52.72%) Women	26 (47.28%) Men	
Follow-up	11.54 ± 4.77 years (2.89 months–23.16 years)		
Ear	26 (47.28%) Left	26 (47.28%) Right	3 (5.45%) Bilateral

3.1. Etiologies and Overall Results

Regarding the etiologies of implantation, we found that, as seen in Figure 3, the most frequent audiometric pattern was mixed or conductive hearing loss in a total of 47 patients (85.45%). Among these, the most common cause was cholesteatomatous chronic otitis media (COM) in 20 patients (36.36%), followed by non-cholesteatomatous COM in 10 patients (18.18%), the presence of a retraction pocket in 5 patients (9.09%), and otosclerosis in 4 patients (7.27%). Less frequent causes included post-trauma with ossicular chain damage in three patients (5.45%) and keratosis obturans in two patients (3.64%). Malformations, both of the external and middle ear, accounted for four patients (7.27%), and the least frequent categories, each with one patient (1.82%), were post-radiotherapy necrosis in a patient with a history of nasopharyngeal carcinoma and iatrogenic external auditory canal stenosis.

On the other hand, among the eight patients with sensorineural hearing loss (14.54%), the most frequently found causes were presbycusis with poor hearing aid outcomes in five patients (9.09%), followed by streptomycin ototoxicity, genetic causes, and labyrinthitis, each with one patient (1.82%).

In this way, the average hearing situation of the patients included in the sample, prior to the placement of the VSB, was as follows: Considering the overall results for all types of hearing loss, we found that the pre-implantation PTA for all the frequency averages was 75.25 ± 20.68 dB, while post-implantation, it reached 33.70 ± 7.71 dB (a gain of 41.56 ± 22.63 dB). The comparison was statistically significant, with a p-value < 0.001.

For patients with sensorineural hearing loss, the pre-implantation PTA for all the frequency averages was 63.44 ± 13.41 dB, while post-implantation, it reached 32.4 ± 10.12 dB (a gain of 31.04 ± 8.80 dB). On the other hand, for patients with mixed or conductive hearing loss, the pre-implantation PTA for all the frequency averages was 82.59 ± 20.85 dB, while post-implantation, it rose to 39.63 ± 11.01 dB (a gain of 42.96 ± 17.70 dB). The comparison was not statistically significant, with a p-value = 0.080. A summary of the audiometric results for each type of hearing loss, by frequency, is shown in Table 2 and represented in Figure 4.

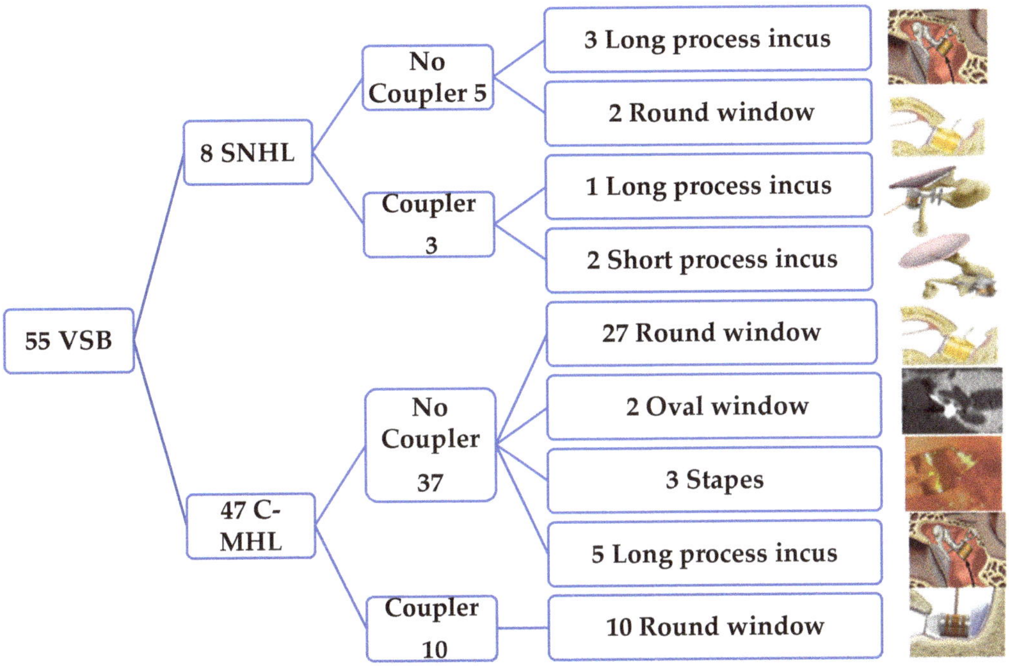

Figure 3. Summary of the sample distribution based on the type of hearing loss, the use of a coupler, and the FMT coupling location. The right column shows the situation both intraoperatively and in imaging tests, as well as representations that exemplify the versatility and different positions the implant can occupy, with or without a coupler, in the middle ear.

Table 2. Summary of the general audiometric results in patients with SNHL or C-MHL.

Frequency/dB HL	Sensorineural Hearing Loss (n = 8)			Conductive–Mixed Hearing Loss (n = 47)		
	AC Pre	BC Pre	AC VSB	AC Pre	BC Pre	AC VSB
500 Hz	44.48 ± 19.12	37.20 ± 28.31	26.67 ± 19.44	80.19 ± 26.44	44.07 ± 21.39	36.17 ± 22.41
1000 Hz	51.26 ± 16.88	40.09 ± 16.98	16.02 ± 12.77	85.79 ± 18.32	52.19 ± 18.90	31.91 ± 19.63
2000 Hz	67.77 ± 12.31	68.22 ± 15.38	27.31 ± 22.46	91.82 ± 11.08	62.21 ± 16.32	31.11 ± 15.44
4000 Hz	72.88 ± 18.33	67.85 ± 23.22	36.44 ± 17.36	102.24 ± 23.75	73.95 ± 12.12	47.22 ± 17.89
6000 Hz	77.23 ± 17.14	75.43 ± 19.78	38.22 ± 18.24	107.36 ± 19.11	82.29 ± 21.47	50.06 ± 21.07
Mean	62.72 ± 16.91	57.36 ± 21.49	28.53 ± 18.56	93.48 ± 20.57	62.54 ± 18.45	39.29 ± 19.67

On the other hand, we analyzed the speech discrimination percentage using speech audiometry at 65 dB. For all types of hearing loss, before implantation, the mean score was 11.35 ± 11.33%, while after the placement of the VSB, it was 86.56 ± 18.012%.

For sensorineural hearing loss, before implantation, the result was 22.12 ± 12.33%, while after the placement of the VSB, it was 79.91 ± 9.03%. This implies a gain of 57.79 ± 15.28%. Conversely, in the total patients with conductive or mixed hearing loss, the pre-implantation discrimination percentage was 11.15 ± 13.22%, whereas after the placement of the VSB, it was 80.47 ± 20.73%. This implies a gain of 69.32 ± 24.58%.

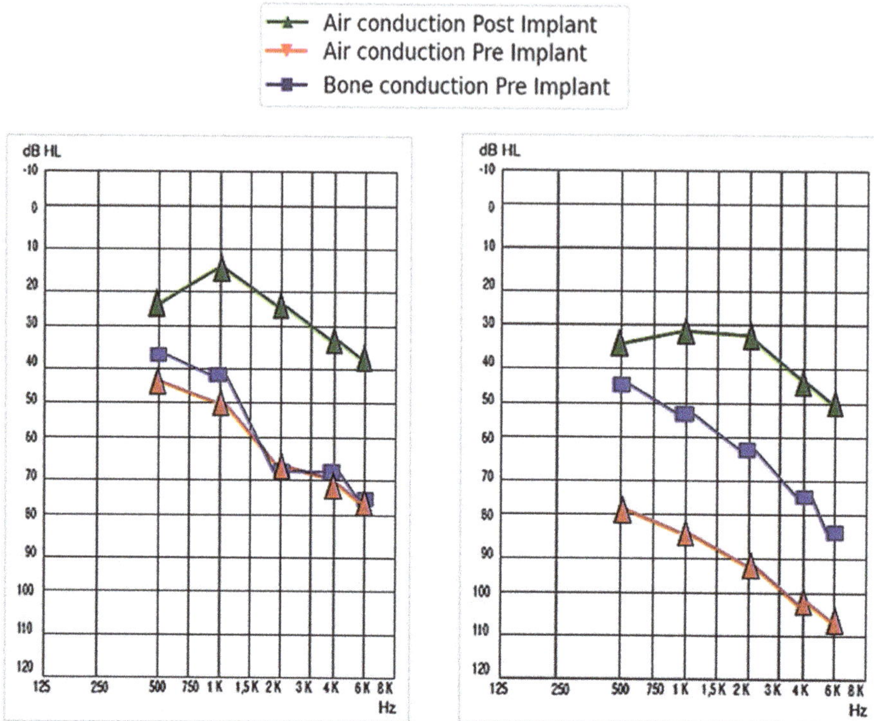

Figure 4. Representation of the audiometric situation pre- and post-VSB placement in patients with sensorineural hearing loss (**left** image) and mixed-conductive hearing loss (**right** image).

3.2. Surgical Anchorage and Auditory Results

3.2.1. Coupling in the Round and Oval Window

When studying the gain behavior based on anchorage, we found that out of the total implanted patients, 41 (74.54%) used coupling in the round or oval window, as described in Figure 2. Among these, 24.39% (n = 10) used a coupling system. Of these patients, 39 (95.12%) had conductive or mixed hearing loss, while the remaining two (4.88%) had sensorineural hearing loss.

Considering the overall results for patients with anchorage to the round or oval window, we found that the pre-implantation PTA for all the frequency averages was 79.02 $\pm$ 18.91 dB, while post-implantation, it reached 30.23 $\pm$ 7.34 dB (a gain of 48.79 $\pm$ 21.25 dB). The comparison was statistically significant, with a p-value < 0.001.

For patients with sensorineural hearing loss, the pre-implantation PTA for all the frequency averages was 64.50 $\pm$ 17.68 dB, while post-implantation, it reached 25.00 $\pm$ 7.07 dB (a gain of 39.50 $\pm$ 17.68 dB). On the other hand, for patients with mixed or conductive hearing loss, the pre-implantation PTA for all the frequency averages was 80.23 $\pm$ 18.85 dB, while post-implantation, it decreased to 30.67 $\pm$ 7.33 dB (a gain of 49.56 $\pm$ 20.19 dB). The comparison was not statistically significant, with a p-value = 0.449. A summary of the audiometric results for each type of hearing loss in patients who used round or oval window coupling, by frequency, is shown in Table 3 and represented in Figure 5.

Table 3. Summary of audiometric results in patients with SNHL or C-MHML using RW or OW coupling.

Frequency/dB HL	Sensorineural Hearing Loss (n = 2)			Conductive–Mixed Hearing Loss (n = 39)		
	AC Pre	BC Pre	AC VSB	AC Pre	BC Pre	AC VSB
500 Hz	15.50 ± 2.50	15.00	15.00	72.64 ± 21.20	43.22 ± 18.33	30.07 ± 8.24
1000 Hz	32.25 ± 1.88	10.25 ± 5.21	15 ± 2.50	86.55 ± 18.66	49.19 ± 9.65	28.19 ± 10.57
2000 Hz	60.25 ± 4.00	64.75 ± 3.22	45.00 ± 10.00	90.89 ± 14.44	67.24 ± 18.38	36.12 ± 12.24
4000 Hz	68.75 ± 3.25	68.50 ± 2.77	49.97 ± 1.52	96.00 ± 19.81	69.05 ± 10.18	38.33 ± 19.54
6000 Hz	75.00 ± 2.77	68.50 ± 3.12	50.73 ± 0.76	100.78 ± 19.16	71.30 ± 17.34	41.29 ± 11.89
Mean	50.75 ± 25.20	45.40 ± 27.03	35.94 ± 19.34	89.37 ± 9.63	60.06 ± 14.78	34.80 ± 12.50

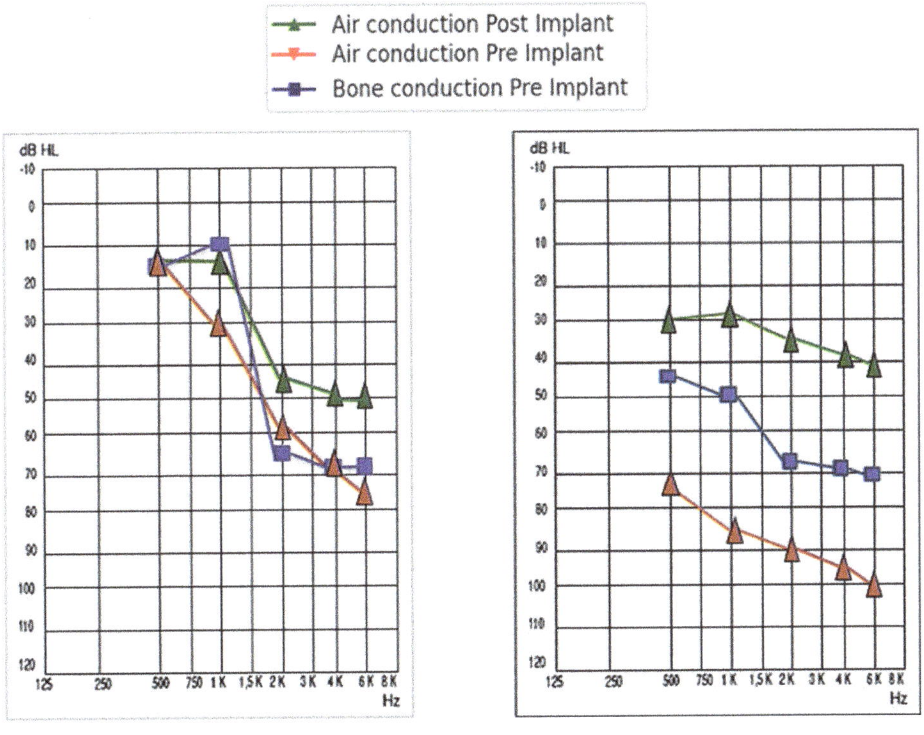

Figure 5. Representation of the audiometric situation pre- and post-VSB placement with round or oval window coupling in patients with sensorineural hearing loss (**left** image) and mixed-conductive hearing loss (**right** image).

When we analyzed the speech discrimination percentage using speech audiometry at 65 dB, we noticed that, for all types of hearing loss, before implantation, the main score was 7.42 ± 10.13%, while after the placement of the VSB, it was 87.73 ± 19.85%. This indicates an improvement of 80.31 ± 17.45%.

For sensorineural hearing loss, before implantation, the result was 25.00 ± 21.21%, while after the placement of the VSB, it was 95.00 ± 7.07%. This implies a gain of 70.00 ± 22.43%. Conversely, in the total number of patients with conductive or mixed hearing loss, the pre-implantation discrimination percentage was 5.96 ± 7.93%, whereas after the placement of the VSB, it was 87.13 ± 20.52%. This implies a gain of 81.17 ± 21.19%.

3.2.2. Ossicular Chain Coupling

In another portion of the sample, we found a total of 14 patients in whom ossicular chain coupling was used. Specifically, in 11 of them (20%), the coupling was carried out at the incus, mainly at the long process in 81.82% (n = 9) via posterior tympanotomy, while in the remaining 18.18% (n = 2), it was performed at the short process via extended atticotomy. These differences are illustrated in Figure 1. In the remaining three patients (21.42%), the FMT was anchored to the stapes. Similarly, the same proportion of patients (21.42%) used a coupler system involving the ossicles. Out of the 14 patients, 8 of them (57.14%) had mixed hearing loss, while the remaining 42.86% (n = 6) had sensorineural hearing loss.

Considering the overall results for the patients with ossicular chain anchorage, we found that the pre-implantation PTA for all the frequency averages was 67.98 ± 14.71 dB, while post-implantation, it reached 35.70 ± 9.13 dB (a gain of 32.28 ± 14.71 dB). The comparison was statistically significant, with a p-value < 0.001.

For patients with sensorineural hearing loss, the pre-implantation PTA for all the frequency averages was 62.22 ± 15.90 dB, while post-implantation, it reached 31.33 ± 9.83 dB (a gain of 30.88 ± 15.90 dB). On the other hand, for patients with mixed or conductive hearing loss, the pre-implantation PTA for all the frequency averages was 70.45 ± 14.04 dB, while post-implantation, it decreased to 37.57 ± 8.48 dB (a gain of 32.88 ± 14.04 dB). The comparison was not statistically significant, with a p-value of 0.753. A summary of the audiometric results for each type of hearing loss is presented in Figure 6 and Table 4.

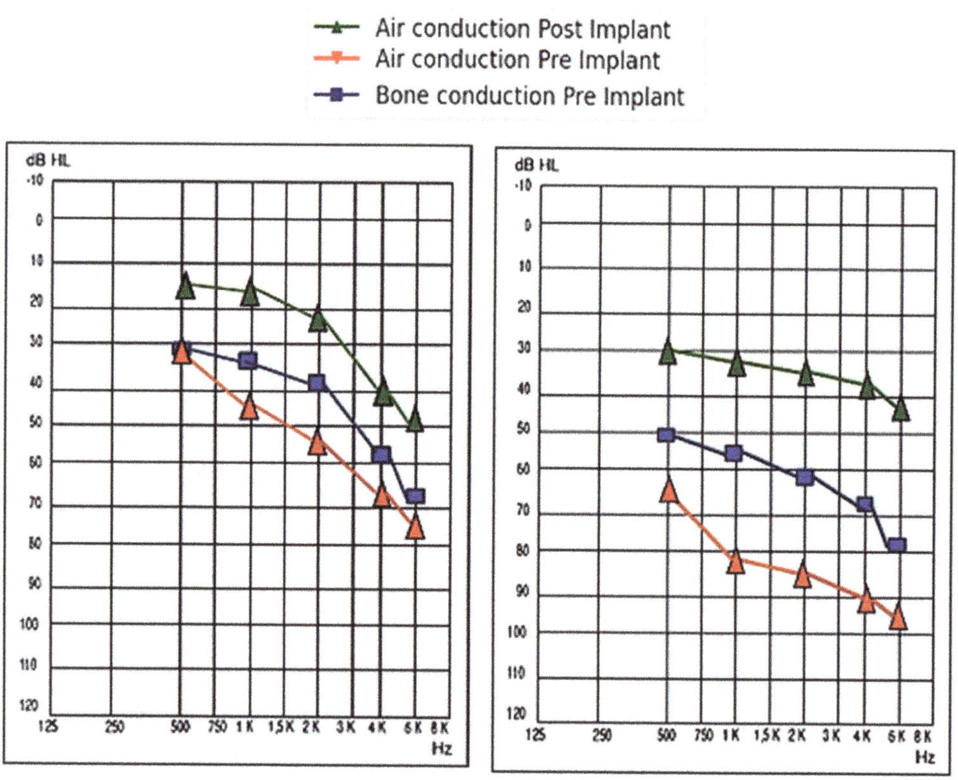

Figure 6. Representation of the audiometric situation pre- and post-VSB placement with incus or stapes coupling in patients with sensorineural hearing loss (**left** image) and mixed-conductive hearing loss (**right** image).

Table 4. Summary of the audiometric results in patients with SNHL or C-MHML using incus or stapes coupling.

Frequency/dB HL	Sensorineural Hearing Loss (n = 6)			Conductive–Mixed Hearing Loss (n = 8)		
	AC Pre	BC Pre	AC VSB	AC Pre	BC Pre	AC VSB
500 Hz	31.65 ± 8.11	30.08 ± 7.65	14.95 ± 11.23	63.52 ± 13.26	50.17 ± 6.96	30.18 ± 4.73
1000 Hz	43.57 ± 13.44	44.29 ± 12.19	16.02 ± 4.76	82.18 ± 7.44	56.37 ± 14.33	32.19 ± 12.54
2000 Hz	55.32 ± 19.22	53.69 ± 3.44	22.11 ± 8.06	84.96 ± 14.44	60.62 ± 10.72	37.26 ± 14.67
4000 Hz	66.82 ± 14.89	67.33 ± 9.21	41.57 ± 7.20	90.03 ± 20.18	67.23 ± 3.89	39.82 ± 3.28
6000 Hz	75.77 ± 11.06	73.85 ± 12.89	49.51 ± 11.04	92.65 ± 7.58	79.66 ± 14.30	43.59 ± 13.29
Mean	54.63 ± 13.34	53.85 ± 9.08	28.83 ± 8.46	82.67 ± 13.45	62.81 ± 10.04	34.84 ± 9.24

When we analyzed the speech discrimination percentage using speech audiometry at 65 dB, we noticed that, for all types of hearing loss, before implantation, the main score with ossicular chain anchorage was 17.85 ± 16.31%, while after the placement of the VSB, it was 84.55 ± 21.24%. This implies an improvement of 66.70 ± 17.45%, and the difference between both moments was statistically significant, with a p-value < 0.001.

For sensorineural hearing loss, before implantation, the result was 28.67 ± 21.79%, while after the placement of the VSB, it was 70.17 ± 27.41%. This implies a gain of 41.50 ± 22.43%. Conversely, in the total number of patients with conductive or mixed hearing loss, the pre-implantation discrimination percentage was 13.21 ± 11.37%, whereas after the placement of the VSB, it was 90.71 ± 15.30%. This implies a gain of 77.50 ± 21.19%. This difference was statistically significant, with a p-value < 0.001, after conducting t-tests.

3.3. Improvements in Speech Discrimination at 65 dB

The evolution in the percentage of discrimination at 65 dB is summarized in Figure 7.

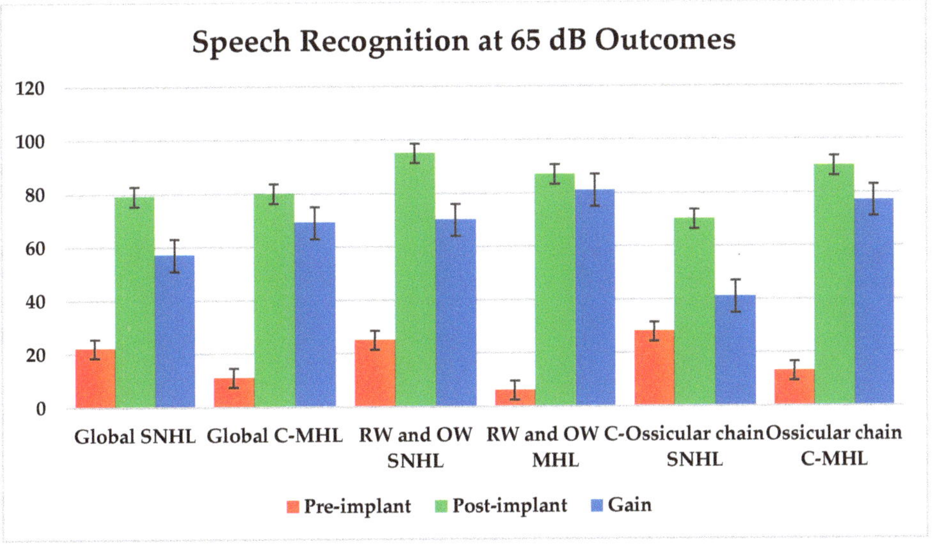

Figure 7. Representation of speech discrimination performance with different couplings and for various types of hearing loss. Error bars represent the 95% confidence interval, providing a visual representation of the variability and reliability of the data.

3.4. *Surgical Technique for Chronic Otitis Media and Auditory Results*

Regarding the surgical techniques used to treat complications derived from chronic otitis media (COM) in implanted patients, we found that in 21 cases (70% of patients with chronic otitis media), an open technique was used. This group included 16 cases of canal wall down and 5 cases of attic exposure–antrum exclusion (AE-AE). In the other group, five cases (30%) underwent a closed mastoidectomy technique or canal wall up.

For patients treated with an open technique and implanted with a VSB, the average pre-implantation PTA was 73.55 ± 16.79 dB, which, after the middle ear implant, became a PTA of 41.78 ± 19.02 dB, resulting in an average gain of 43.56 ± 19.01 dB. Regarding speech audiometry information, the average discrimination percentage at 65 dB in patients treated with this surgical technique, before the VSB placement, was 26.81 ± 6.67%. After implantation, it increased to 81.81 ± 7.41%, indicating a gain of 55.00 ± 7.81%.

In contrast, for patients who underwent a closed mastoidectomy surgical technique, an average PTA gain of 56.53 ± 10.57 dB was observed, as the pre-implantation PTA was 90.42 ± 17.53 dB and post-implantation it was 33.89 ± 6.96 dB. Similarly, the gain in terms of the discrimination at 65 dB was 55.11 ± 7.15%, since it was 25.0 ± 6.81% before the VSB implantation and 80.11 ± 6.56% afterwards.

When comparing the PTA gains and speech discrimination according to the surgical technique (open technique vs. canal wall up), we found that comparing the PTA gain between both techniques, the *p*-value was 0.159, indicating that there were no statistically significant differences. Similarly, the gain recorded with speech audiometry was not statistically significant, with a *p*-value of 0.187. A summary of the results according to different surgical techniques is presented in Table 5.

Table 5. Comparison of the audiometric results obtained with open and closed techniques, both in terms of pure tone audiometry and speech audiometry, with and without the use of an implant.

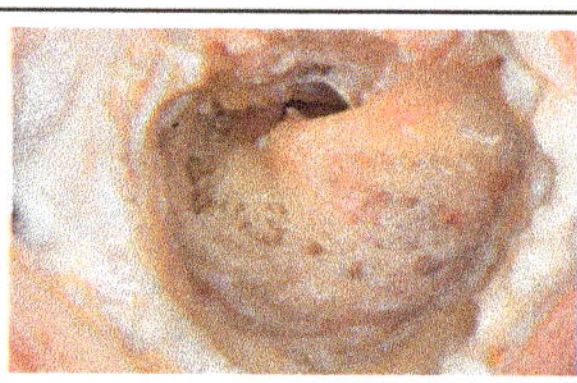	**Open Cavity (n = 21)**	**Canal Wall Up (n = 5)**	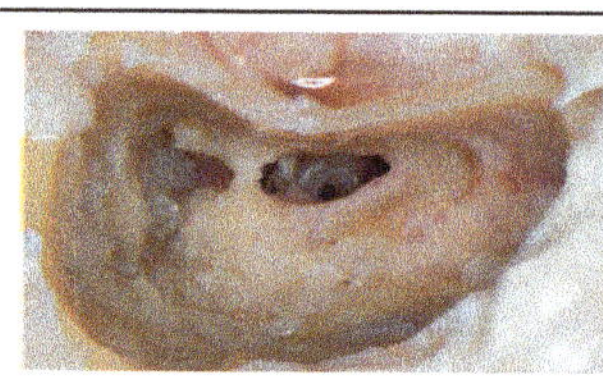
PTA pre-implant	75.33 ± 16.79	90.42 ± 17.53	PTA pre-implant
PTA post-implant	31.77 ± 8.91	33.89 ± 6.96	PTA post-implant
Gain	43.56 ± 19.01	56.53 ± 10.57	Gain
Speech intelligibility pre-implant	26.81 ± 6.67	25.00 ± 6.81	Speech intelligibility pre-implant
Speech intelligibility post-implant	81.81 ± 7.41	80.11 ± 6.56	Speech intelligibility post-implant
Gain	55.00 ± 7.81	55.11 ± 7.15	Gain

Complications and Adverse Effects

Finally, it was observed that a total of nine patients experienced adverse effects derived from the placement of the VSB. Four of them (44.44%) had to undergo reoperation due to cable migration and FMT displacement, with three of these patients having an open mastoidectomy cavity. Another four patients experienced pain in the area of the audioprocessor, which was managed with analgesics, while the remaining patient (11.11%) suffered a skin ulceration due to magnet overpressure, requiring retroauricular plasty for correction.

However, when we compared the risk of experiencing adverse effects between the two surgical techniques, Fisher's test result gave us a *p*-value of 0.356, indicating that there was no statistically significant relationship.

4. Discussion

From a global perspective, the results for this series of patients indicate the effectiveness of the VSB device, even when using different anchoring methods, as an outstanding treatment option in subjects with mixed–conductive and sensorineural hearing loss, with degrees of hearing loss ranging from moderate to severe. Furthermore, the results underscore the role of middle ear active implants as an alternative in conditions where a sufficiently satisfactory gain cannot be achieved with other devices, such as hearing aids, when bone conduction levels fall outside the range for bone-anchored implants, or even in the event of unsatisfactory stapedectomy surgeries in patients with otosclerosis. Similarly, the VSB option may be particularly attractive in cases of chronic otitis media with poor response to tympanoplasty, or in the presence of pathological findings in the external ear that prevent a hearing aid from fitting properly within the external auditory canal, exacerbating poor self-cleaning.

Firstly, the indications for VSB implantation in our cohort reflect the most common etiologies, with cholesteatomatous chronic otitis media being the most prevalent, ac-counting for 36.36% of cases, followed by non-cholesteatomatous chronic otitis media (18.18%) and the presence of a retraction pocket (9.09%). These data are consistent with the literature, where chronic otitis media is also highlighted as one of the main indications for this type of implant [11]. Additionally, other etiologies, such as otosclerosis and presbycusis, are also commonly indicated in both our work and in the literature for the use of the VSB.

Regarding the amplification achieved with the VSB, for all types of hearing loss, a gain of 41.56 ± 22.63 dB was reached. In SNHL, the gain was 31.04 ± 8.80 dB and 42.96 ± 17.70 dB in the case of mixed–conductive hearing loss. These values are almost the same as those reported by Luetje et al., who found an average gain of 31.40 dB at the long-term follow-up for the whole sample [12]. Similarly, other studies have also reported significant auditory gains of a similar magnitude with VSB implantation, particularly at higher frequencies, highlighting the effectiveness of this device in improving hearing in patients with mixed and sensorineural hearing loss [13,14]. In fact, in our study, gains reaching 32.71 ± 18.21 dB at 4000 Hz in SNHL and 49.25 ± 20.26 dB in C-MHL were observed, with this finding being even more pronounced at 6000 Hz, with gains of up to 39.43 ± 9.15 dB in SNHL and 51.16 ± 17.48 dB in C-MHL.

An interesting observation in our study is the notable amplification achieved with the placement of the FMT in the coupling of round and oval windows. This is particularly relevant in terms of average tonal thresholds, both in SNHL (32.00 ± 9.05 dB) and in C-MHL (47.11 ± 3.76 dB). This great efficiency is possibly due to the VSB's ability to better transmit vibrations to the cochlear fluids through the round window, thereby optimizing the auditory response [15,16]. Additionally, in these cases, there is an inversion of endolymphatic propagation, which goes from the round window to the oval window and not vice versa, as occurs in healthy subjects.

Similarly, in terms of the results provided by speech audiometry, measuring speech intelligibility at 65 dB, it was observed that, especially in patients with C-MHL, the gain was approximately 13% higher (76.64 vs. 63.00%) and was also statistically significant.

To try to understand the reason for this significant superiority when coupling the FMT to a RW or a OW, it could be explained by different phenomena: initially, by the ability to effectively transmit high-frequency vibrations through the round window [17–19], thereby improving audibility in these critical frequencies for speech comprehension. Secondly, the importance of greater amplification at high frequencies for consonant discrimination, in turn, has a positive and significant impact on speech intelligibility [20,21]. Subsequently, direct coupling of the FMT to the round window could minimize potential distortions that may occur with other anchoring points, such as the incus, and avoid possible mechanical interferences that can arise with other coupling points. Similarly, as described by Beltrame et al., the use of a coupling system during RW and OW implantation could further improve these results by providing additional stability and ensuring efficient vibration transmission [17].

Regarding surgical techniques, we did not find any significant differences in the auditory gain between open and closed techniques. This finding is consistent with other studies that also did not demonstrate any clear differences in auditory outcomes between the two techniques [22]. The choice of technique seems to depend more on the underlying pathology and the surgeon's preference than on the implant's efficacy itself [23].

However, in our work, although it did not reach statistical significance, a higher incidence of adverse effects was observed with the open technique. This finding can be attributed to the more invasive nature of this approach, which may increase the risk of postoperative complications, such as infections due to inefficacy in self-cleaning or a larger surface area of previously operated cavities that complicate cable coupling. Previous experiences [24] also indicate that more invasive procedures are associated with a higher rate of complications, reinforcing our findings. As observed in our study, patients undergoing open techniques showed a higher incidence of adverse effects, especially related to cable migration, compared to those who underwent a more conservative technique.

Study Limitations

Although the sample size is considerably large, with a total of 55 individuals, the heterogeneity in etiologies and demographic characteristics could influence the generalization of the results. Different etiologies may respond differently to VSB implantation, complicating the interpretation of the overall data.

Moreover, being a single-center study, variability in the choice of surgical techniques (open vs. closed) and FMT anchoring sites (incus vs. round window) may introduce an additional source of variation in the auditory results. Although an attempt was made to control these variables in the analysis, the inherent variability in individual surgical skills and preferences could have influenced the outcomes.

To conclude, another limitation is not having been able to conduct quality of life questionnaires for patients to express their subjective impressions and evaluations of the devices in everyday situations. Patient evaluation complements the results of audiometric tests. Despite the existence of questionnaires like the APHAB (Abbreviated Profile of Hearing Aid Benefit), a future challenge could be to consider a modification of this or a new version specifically for this type of implant.

5. Conclusions

This study reaffirms the effectiveness of the Vibrant Soundbridge implant in improving hearing in patients with mixed, conductive, and sensorineural hearing loss, with significant auditory gain, especially at higher frequencies, particularly through the round window membrane approach, possibly related to better transmission of vibrations to cochlear fluids, optimizing the amplification of critical frequencies for speech intelligibility.

Regarding surgical techniques, no significant differences in auditory gain were observed between open and closed techniques, although the open technique was associated with a high incidence of postoperative complications, requiring reoperation on several occasions.

Finally, the study highlights the need for an individualized approach to VSB implantation, considering the anatomical characteristics and specific auditory needs of each patient, to optimize the outcomes.

Author Contributions: Conceptualization, M.M. and J.L.-P.; methodology, R.M.-H. and J.L.-P.; software, J.L.-P.; validation, M.M. and J.L.-P. Formal analysis M.M. and J.L.-P.; investigation, J.L.-P., J.P.L. and R.M.-H.; resources, M.M. data curation, J.L.-P. and D.C.; writing—original draft preparation, J.L.-P.; writing—review and editing, J.L.-P. and R.M.-H.; visualization, J.P.L. and J.L.-P.; supervision, J.P.L. and M.M.; project administration, R.M.-H.; funding acquisition, not required. All authors have read and agreed to the published version of the manuscript.

Funding: This research received no external funding. No third-party funding was received for this research.

Institutional Review Board Statement: The study protocol was reviewed on 6 May 2024 and approved by ethics committee of Clínica Universidad de Navarra, approval number (CEI 2024.181). Even more importantly, this study was designed and performed in accordance with the ethical guidelines in the 1975 Declaration of Helsinki. Written informed consent was obtained from all patients in order to participate in the study. Written informed consent was obtained from the patient for publication of the details of their medical case and any accompanying images.

Informed Consent Statement: Informed consent was obtained from all subjects involved in the study.

Data Availability Statement: Data pertaining to this study can be shared upon request to the corresponding author.

Conflicts of Interest: The authors report that there are no conflicts of interest. The authors alone are responsible for the content and writing of the paper.

References

1. Beleites, T.; Neudert, M.; Bornitz, M.; Zahnert, T. Sound transfer of active middle ear implants. *Otolaryngol. Clin. N. Am.* **2014**, *47*, 859–891. [CrossRef]
2. Lassaletta, L.; Sánchez-Cuadrado, I.; Espinosa, J.M.; Batuecas, Á.; Cenjor, C.; Lavilla, M.J.; Cavallé, L.; Huartew, A.; Nuñez, F.; Manrique, M.; et al. Implantes activos de oído medio. *Acta Otorrinolaringol. Esp.* **2019**, *70*, 112–118. [CrossRef]
3. Sprinzl, G.M.; Riechelmann, H. Current trends in treating hearing loss in elderly people: A review of the technology and treatment options—A mini-review. *Gerontology* **2010**, *56*, 351–358. [CrossRef]
4. Zwartenkot, J.W.; Hashemi, J.; Cremers, C.W.R.J.; Mulder, J.J.S.; Snik, A.F.M. Active middle ear implantation for patients with sensorineural hearing loss and external otitis: Long-term outcome in patient satisfaction. *Otol. Neurotol.* **2013**, *34*, 855–861. [CrossRef] [PubMed]
5. Colletti, V.; Soli, S.D.; Carner, M.; Colletti, L. Treatment of mixed hearing losses via implantation of a vibratory transducer on the round window. *Int. J. Audiol.* **2006**, *45*, 600–608. [CrossRef]
6. Bittencourt, A.G.; Burke, P.R.; Jardim, I.D.S.; Brito, R.D.; Tsuji, R.K.; Fonseca, A.C.D.O.; Bento, R.F. Implantable and semi-implantable hearing aids: A review of history, indications, and surgery. *Int. Arch. Otorhinolaryngol.* **2014**, *18*, 303–310. [PubMed]
7. Dillon, M.T.; Buss, E.; Adunka, O.F.; Buchman, C.A.; Pillsbury, H.C. Influence of test condition on speech perception with electric-acoustic stimulation. *Am. J. Audiol.* **2015**, *24*, 520–528. [CrossRef] [PubMed]
8. Cremers, C.W.; O'Connor, A.F.; Helms, J.; Roberson, J.; Clarós, P.; Frenzel, H.; Profant, M.; Schmerber, S.; Streitberger, C.; Baumgartner, W.-D.; et al. International consensus on Vibrant Soundbridge® implantation in children and adolescents. *Int. J. Pediatr. Otorhinolaryngol.* **2010**, *74*, 1267–1269. [CrossRef] [PubMed]
9. Lenarz, T.; Zwartenkot, J.W.; Stieger, C.; Schwab, B.; Mylanus, E.A.M.; Caversaccio, M.; Kompis, M.; Snik, A.F.M.; D'hondt, C.; Mojallal, H. Multicenter study with a direct acoustic cochlear implant. *Otol. Neurotol.* **2013**, *34*, 1215–1225. [CrossRef] [PubMed]
10. Manrique, R.; Sanhueza, I.; Manrique, M. Aticoexposición-antroexclusión como técnica quirúrgica a la demanda para el tratamiento del colesteatoma. *Acta Otorrinolaringol. Esp.* **2013**, *64*, 22–30. [CrossRef]
11. Mosnier, I.; Sterkers, O.; Bouccara, D.; Labassi, S.; Bebear, J.-P.; Bordure, P.; Dubreuil, C.; Dumon, T.; Frachet, B.; Fraysse, B.; et al. Benefit of the Vibrant Soundbridge device in patients implanted for 5 to 8 years. *Ear Hear.* **2008**, *29*, 281–284. [CrossRef] [PubMed]
12. Luetje, C.M.; Brackman, D.; Balkany, T.J.; Maw, J.; Baker, R.S.; Kelsall, D.; Backous, D.; Miyamoto, R.; Parisier, S.; Arts, A. Phase III clinical trial results with the Vibrant Soundbridge implantable middle ear hearing device: A prospective controlled multicenter study. *Otolaryngol. Head Neck Surg.* **2002**, *126*, 97–107. [CrossRef] [PubMed]
13. Tjellström, A.; Luetje, C.M.; Hough, J.V.; Arthur, B.; Hertzmann, P.; Katz, B.; Wallace, D. Acute human trial of the floating mass transducer. *Ear Nose Throat J.* **1997**, *76*, 204–210. [CrossRef] [PubMed]
14. Ball, G.R.; Huber, A.; Goode, R.L. Scanning laser Doppler vibrometry of the middle ear ossicles. *Ear Nose Throat J.* **1997**, *76*, 213–222. [CrossRef] [PubMed]
15. Fredrickson, J.M.; Coticchia, J.M.; Khosla, S. Ongoing investigations into an implantable electromagnetic hearing aid for moderate to severe sensorineural hearing loss. *Otolaryngol. Clin. N. Am.* **1995**, *28*, 107–120. [CrossRef]
16. Maniglia, A.J.; Dolgin, S.R.; Ko, W.H.; Rosenbaum, M.L.; Zhang, R.X.; Montague, F.W. Electromagnetic implantable middle ear hearing device of the ossicular-stimulating type: Principles, designs, and experiments. *Ann. Otol. Rhinol. Laryngol.* **1988**, *97*, 3–16. [CrossRef]
17. Lim, D.; Stone, S.; Levin, B. Clinical performance of a round window floating mass transducer. *Otol. Neurotol.* **2011**, *32*, 744–752.
18. Hough, J.; Himelick, T.; Richard, G.; Dormer, K.; Vernon, J.; Meikel, M.; Ma, T.H.; Pe, G.R. A middle ear implantable hearing device for controlled amplification of sound in the human: A preliminary report. *Laryngoscope* **1987**, *97*, 141–151. [CrossRef]
19. Beltrame, A.M.; Martini, A.; Prosser, S.; Giarbini, N.; Streitberger, C. Coupling the Vibrant Soundbridge to cochlea round window: Auditory results in patients with mixed hearing loss. *Otol. Neurotol.* **2009**, *30*, 194–201. [CrossRef]

20. Stöver, T.; Lenarz, T. Vibrant Soundbridge: A new perspective in middle ear implants. *ORL J. Otorhinolaryngol. Relat. Spec.* **2009**, *71*, 309–316.
21. Colletti, V.; Soli, S.D.; Carner, M.; Colletti, L. Treatment of mixed hearing losses via implantation of a Vibrant Soundbridge: Audiometric outcomes in 21 patients. *Otol. Neurotol.* **2006**, *27*, 422–427.
22. Baumgartner, W.D.; Böheim, K.; Hagen, R.; Müller, J.; Lenarz, T.; Reiss, S.; Schlögel, M.; Mlynski, R.; Mojallal, H.; Colletti, V.; et al. The Vibrant Soundbridge for conductive and mixed hearing losses: European multicenter study results. *Acta Otolaryngol.* **2010**, *130*, 971–983.
23. Verhaegen, V.J.; Mulder, J.J.; Snik, A.F.; Mylanus, E.A. Audiological application criteria for implantable hearing devices: A clinical experience at the Nijmegen ORL clinic. *Otol. Neurotol.* **2012**, *33*, 1193–1199. [CrossRef] [PubMed]
24. Barbara, M.; Biagini, M.; Monini, S. Clinical application of the Vibrant Soundbridge™ in a series of patients with mixed hearing loss. *Acta Otorhinolaryngol. Ital.* **2014**, *34*, 294–298.

audiology research

MDPI

Article

Cochlear and Bone Conduction Implants in Asymmetric Hearing Loss and Single-Sided Deafness: Effects on Localization, Speech in Noise, and Quality of Life

Oana Astefanei [1,2,†], Cristian Martu [2,3], Sebastian Cozma [2,3] and Luminita Radulescu [1,2,3,*,†]

1 Doctoral School, Grigore T. Popa University of Medicine and Pharmacy, 700115 Iasi, Romania; oana.botezatu-astefanei@d.umfiasi.ro
2 ENT Clinic Department, Clinical Rehabilitation Hospital, 700661 Iasi, Romania; martu.cristian@umfiasi.ro (C.M.); sebastian.cozma@umfiasi.ro (S.C.)
3 Department of Otorhinolaryngology, Faculty of Medicine, Grigore T. Popa University of Medicine and Pharmacy, 700115 Iasi, Romania
* Correspondence: luminita.radulescu@umfiasi.ro
† These authors contributed equally to this work.

Abstract: Background: Single-sided deafness (SSD) and asymmetric hearing loss (AHL) impair spatial hearing and speech perception, often reducing quality of life. Cochlear implants (CIs) and bone conduction implants (BCIs) are rehabilitation options used in SSD and AHL to improve auditory perception and support functional integration in daily life. **Objective**: We aimed to evaluate hearing outcomes after auditory implantation in SSD and AHL patients, focusing on localization accuracy, speech-in-noise understanding, tinnitus relief, and perceived benefit. **Methods**: In this longitudinal observational study, 37 patients (adults and children) received a CI or a BCI according to clinical indications. Outcomes included localization and spatial speech-in-noise assessment, tinnitus ratings, and SSQ12 scores. Statistical analyses used parametric and non-parametric tests ($p < 0.05$). **Results**: In adult CI users, localization error significantly decreased from 81.9° ± 15.8° to 43.7° ± 13.5° ($p < 0.001$). In children, regardless of the implant type (CI or BCI), localization error improved from 74.3° to 44.8°, indicating a consistent spatial benefit. In adult BCI users, localization error decreased from 74.6° to 69.2°, but the improvement did not reach statistical significance. Tinnitus severity, measured on a 10-point VAS scale, decreased significantly in CI users (mean reduction: 2.8 ± 2.0, $p < 0.001$), while changes in BCI users were small and of limited clinical relevance. SSQ12B/C scores improved in all adult groups, with the largest gains observed in spatial hearing for CI users (2.1 ± 1.2) and in speech understanding for BCI users (1.6 ± 0.9); children reported high benefits across all domains. Head shadow yielded the most consistent benefit across all groups (up to 4.9 dB in adult CI users, 3.8 dB in adult BCI users, and 4.6 dB in children). Although binaural effects were smaller in BCI users, positive gains were observed, especially in pediatric cases. Correlation analysis showed that daily device use positively predicted SSQ12 improvement (r = 0.57) and tinnitus relief (r = 0.42), while longer deafness duration was associated with poorer localization outcomes (r = –0.48). **Conclusions**: CIs and BCIs provide measurable benefits in SSD and AHL rehabilitation. Outcomes vary with age, device, and deafness duration, underscoring the need for early intervention and consistent auditory input.

Keywords: single-sided deafness (SSD); asymmetric hearing loss (AHL); cochlear implant (CI); bone conduction implant (BCI); binaural hearing; localization; tinnitus suppression; self-reported outcomes

1. Introduction

Single-sided deafness (SSD) is defined as severe-to-profound sensorineural hearing loss (SNHL) in one ear while normal hearing is preserved in the contralateral ear. Asymmetric hearing loss (AHL) is characterized by an interaural threshold difference of ≥15 dB hearing loss (HL) between the ears, with the better ear threshold ranging from 30 to 55 dB, as determined by the pure-tone average of four frequencies (PTA4), and one ear presenting SNHL [1–3].

The auditory cortex integrates input from both cochlear nerves, processing sound intensity, duration, and frequency differences, which are essential for binaural hearing [4–6]. This central processing creates a three-dimensional perception of sound, enabling spatial localization and improved speech perception in noisy environments through binaural summation and the squelch effect [4–6]. In normal-hearing (NH) individuals, redundant auditory input from both ears eases the suppression and summation of signals, providing an advantage in speech processing in complex environments [4–6]. Sound localization relies on interaural time differences (ITDs) for low frequencies (<1500 Hz) and interaural level differences (ILDs) for high frequencies (>1500 Hz) [5]. In patients with SSD and AHL, localization is significantly impaired due to the absence of binaural cues, leading to increased azimuth estimation errors [1,2,4–6]. These individuals are unable to separate sound from noise when spatially distinct sources are present (the squelch effect) and lack binaural summation due to unilateral input loss. The head shadow effect further obstructs sound transmission to the hearing ear, compromising auditory perception [4–6]. Consequently, monaural hearing induces cortical auditory modifications and adaptive changes in signal processing, as binaural mechanisms are disrupted [4,6].

The ability to perceive and understand speech in complex environments, localize sound sources, and filter background noise is crucial for daily functioning, particularly in social interactions and communication. When auditory input from one ear is compromised, these processes become significantly impaired, leading to increased listening effort, auditory fatigue, and difficulties in communication, ultimately affecting social engagement and professional performance [7].

Until the early 2000s, normal or near-normal hearing in one ear was considered sufficient for effective communication. However, research has since proven the significant and often-underestimated impact of asymmetric hearing loss. Unlike other sensory impairments, the effects of asymmetric hearing loss are less noticeable, which leads to the under-recognition of individuals' needs.

To address these challenges, various auditory technologies have been developed, including implantable hearing devices such as cochlear implants (CIs) and bone conduction implants (BCIs) [2,8–14]. Cochlear implantation restores auditory perception in individuals with SSD and AHL by directly stimulating the cochlear nerve, bypassing damaged hair cells, and re-establishing neural input to the auditory cortex [4]. This intervention enhances binaural cues, mitigates the head shadow effect, improves spatial hearing, and helps speech perception in noise, provided the auditory nerve remains functional. Although CI users generally exhibit reduced localization ability compared to normal-hearing individuals, adaptation occurs over time [15–17]. These findings suggest that true binaural hearing is achievable only with a CI, despite its first indication being for intractable tinnitus in the affected ear. Severe tinnitus (rated 6–7 out of 10) was a primary factor in implant choice, as CIs are believed to not only restore binaural hearing, but also alleviate tinnitus perception [18,19]. Cochlear implantation in adults with SSD or AHL significantly improves speech perception, tinnitus control, sound localization, and quality of life (QOL) [20–26].

Bone conduction implants serve as an alternative treatment, particularly for SSD patients who are not CI candidates [11–14]. These devices reroute auditory signals through bone conduction, improving sound awareness and reducing the head shadow effect. While BCIs may enhance speech recognition in noise, they do not restore binaural hearing, and their impact on sound localization is limited. In patients with SSD, a BCI is used in a CROS configuration (BCI-CROS), where sounds from the deaf side are transmitted to the normal-hearing cochlea. Although this input reaches the same auditory pathway with a slight delay, it enhances access to environmental sounds without reactivating the impaired side, making it a suitable option when cochlear implantation is contraindicated. However, BCIs are recommended for a subset of patients, particularly those prioritizing speech perception in noise, but who are ineligible for a CI due to hearing loss characteristics (e.g., onset, duration) or personal preference [27–29].

An essential aspect of SSD and AHL management is finding the etiology of hearing loss. Various causes include inner ear anomalies, head trauma, Ménière's disease, vestibular schwannoma, ischemia, autoimmune disorders, and infections; however, the etiology of hearing loss often remains unknown [30]. Management approaches differ significantly between congenital or early-onset cases and those who acquire hearing loss after language development—whether in children or adult—highlighting the importance of accurately determining the onset to guide appropriate intervention strategies [21]. Idiopathic post-lingual sudden SNHL is one of the conditions that benefits from CIs. In congenital/early-onset SSD, caution is necessary when selecting rehabilitation solutions (CI, BCI, CROS), as cochlear nerve deficiency (CND) or cochlear nerve hypoplasia appears to be the most prevalent cause [31]. Since cochlear nerve function is a key prognostic factor for CI success, proper candidate choice is imperative [2].

The most common etiology of pediatric SSD is cochlear nerve deficiency, although the condition itself remains relatively rare. High-resolution temporal bone imaging is essential for assessing cochlear implantation candidacy [32,33]. When cochlear implantation is contraindicated due to cochlear nerve deficiency or severe inner ear malformations, bone conduction implants (BCIs) may remain anatomically viable, providing an alternative rehabilitative strategy in selected cases. A systematic review and meta-analysis found that cochlear implantation in children with SSD was associated with clinically meaningful improvements in audiological and patient-reported outcomes, with shorter durations of deafness linked to better outcomes [34].

The eligibility criteria for cochlear implantation in adult-onset SSD populations continue to evolve, with several previous contraindications now being reconsidered [2,35,36]. The duration of auditory deprivation remains a major point of discussion. The relationship between the duration of auditory deprivation and implant outcomes has been extensively documented. For instance, a study from 2013 demonstrated a significant inverse correlation between the duration of deafness and speech recognition performance in a large cohort of adult CI users, with the most pronounced declines observed after 10 years of deprivation [37]. The inherent variability among patients needs a nuanced approach, recognizing individual ability to tolerate and integrate CI technology. This underscores the importance of comprehensive evaluation in deciding CI candidacy and planning interventions [2,31,35,36,38].

When comparing CIs with BCIs, discrepancies become clearer in noisy listening environments [39,40]. A meta-analyzer had shown that CIs provide substantial advantages in sound localization, tinnitus suppression, and overall quality of life assessment, whereas

BCIs perform better in speech discrimination in noisy settings and in assessing quality of life related to background noise perception [13].

Regarding MRI compatibility, cochlear implants are generally MRI-conditional up to 1.5 T or 3 T, depending on the model and safety measures. For bone conduction systems, active transcutaneous implants allow 3 T imaging without magnet removal, while percutaneous devices typically have lower compatibility and may cause imaging artifacts due to their direct skin penetration.

The implementation of auditory technologies can significantly enhance the quality of life for individuals with SSD and AHL, aiding social and professional integration [41–43]. Regarding the benefits of these devices, the recent consensus on SSD highlights three essential outcome domains: the impact on social situations, group conversations in noisy environments, and spatial orientation [44]. These recommended outcome domains serve as a minimum standard but do not restrict clinical studies from evaluating additional measures. Five other outcome domains—listening effort, one-on-one conversations in general noise, awareness of sound, device usage, and listening in complex situations—were also named in the final consensus session. The primary outcome domains align with the first consensus group's recommendations [1], which served as the foundation for the present study, alongside five other secondary measures.

2. Materials and Methods

This prospective observational study was conducted at the ENT Clinic, within the Department of Otorhinolaryngology and the Audiology Department, with the aim of evaluating auditory rehabilitation outcomes in both adult and pediatric patients with SSD and AHL. This study included patients eligible for auditory implants, such as CIs and BCIs, based on the specific indication and contraindication of each device (patients with prolonged deafness or congenital perilingual hearing loss received BCIs). This selection strategy also reflects differing cortical implications: while a CI reactivates the previously deprived auditory pathway, a BCI (in a CROS setup) leverages the intact pathway, potentially avoiding the effects of cortical reorganization observed in long-term asymmetry.

The study method (the AHL/SSD audiological criteria and outcome measures) follows the recommendations of the unified framework for SSD/AHL studies published in 2017 by the international consensus group [1] and is aligned with the approach used in recent long-term outcome evaluations, such as the study by Távora-Vieira et al. (2019) [45].

Device selection was a collaborative process involving both physician recommendations and patient preferences, guided by national guidelines and manufacturer recommendations, to ensure the best, individualized treatment approach. Pre-procedural counseling was conducted by a multidisciplinary team to establish realistic expectations and support informed decision-making. Interventions were chosen based on clinical and audiological characteristics, with treatment decisions tailored to each patient's audiologic diagnosis, individual pathogenesis, and the duration of hearing loss. In alignment with individualized care principles, randomization was not applied. This personalized approach not only enhanced the relevance of this study by reflecting real-world clinical practice, but also ensured ethical integrity by prioritizing patient autonomy in the decision-making process.

Patient outcomes were systematically evaluated following rehabilitation to assess the effectiveness of the selected interventions. Participants, all native Romanian speakers with speech recognition <60% at 60 dB SPL in the poorer ear, were grouped based on the following clinical and audiological criteria:

SSD: hearing loss of at least 70 dBHL in the affected ear with an audiometric threshold of ≤30 dBHL in the contralateral ear.

AHL: pure-tone average (PTA4) thresholds of 70 dB in the poorer ear and between 31 and 55 dBHL in the contralateral ear.

All patients underwent imaging evaluations using MRI or CT to rule out anatomical anomalies and confirm their eligibility for cochlear implantation or bone conduction implantation. These investigations enabled the assessment of auditory nerve presence, exclusion of auditory nerve tumors, identification of progressive lesions, and evaluation of anatomical compatibility with the selected device. MRI was primarily used in patients with sudden or progressive sensorineural hearing loss to exclude retrocochlear pathologies, such as vestibular schwannoma, and to confirm the presence of the cochlear nerve. In these cases, imaging played a crucial role in determining the indication for implantation, ensuring that the auditory structures were suitable for electrical stimulation. CT was conducted to evaluate the condition of the temporal bone and cochlear anatomy, which is necessary for assessing structural compatibility for implantation. For BCI candidates, this imaging modality allowed the evaluation of temporal bone thickness and the identification of potential anatomical variations that could influence device placement.

All implant decisions in this study were made according to the criteria set by the National Cochlear Implantation Program. In line with these guidelines, device selection was based on clinical, audiological, and imaging data, including the onset and duration of deafness, speech understanding, and anatomical findings on CT or MRI. In the SSD group, all patients met the inclusion criteria for the affected ear, while the contralateral ear provided preserved hearing and speech understanding. Imaging was systematically performed to confirm cochlear nerve presence and anatomical suitability for implantation. While electrophysiological tests, such as electrically evoked auditory brainstem responses (eABRs) and electrically evoked auditory late responses (eALRs), were not applied in this cohort, they may be valuable in future clinical protocols to support implant candidacy decisions, particularly in patients with uncertain neural integrity and functionality. As demonstrated in recent studies, eABR may also be used intraoperatively to verify auditory nerve activation and assess functional electrode placement, especially when neural response is uncertain preoperatively [46,47]. Additionally, OTOPLAN software version 3.1.0 was selectively used for individualized surgical planning in CI and BCI candidates, to secure the placement of the hearing implant in relation to sensitive anatomical landmarks and to optimize audiological outcomes [48].

Outcome Measures

Baseline (T0) Assessments:

Pure-tone audiometry (PTA4): hearing thresholds measured at 0,5, 1, 2, and 4 KHz.

Localization accuracy: sound source localization.

SSQ12A scale: speech, spatial hearing, quality of hearing (0–10 scale).

Tinnitus severity: visual analog scale (VAS, 0–10).

Follow-up (T1) assessments were conducted once for each patient, between 12 and 24 months after implant activation.

PTA4: aided for poorer ear and unaided/aided for better ear in AHL thresholds.

Speech-in-noise tests (SRT50): Assessed head shadow effect, release from masking, binaural squelch, and summation. Aided and unaided conditions.

Localization accuracy: aided and unaided conditions.

SSQ12B/C: post-intervention quality of hearing changes (−5 to +5 scale).

Tinnitus impact: aided and unaided assessment via VAS.

The estimated duration of device use was based on self-reported data from patients.

Audiological Evaluation and Hearing Thresholds

The audiological assessment for implantation candidacy included measuring pure-tone audiometry thresholds across frequencies ranging from 0.25 to 8 kHz for each ear in a standard audiometric booth. At T0, word recognition scores were taken as the percentage of correctly identified words at 60 dB SPL. Equinox 2.0 audiometer software, version 2.12.3 (Interacoustics®, Denmark), was used for conducting pure-tone and speech audiometry. TDH39 headphones were used for pure-tone thresholds and speech recognition tests. During follow-up appointments, PTA thresholds in the better ear were monitored to ensure compliance with SSD and AHL criteria at T1. For AHL subjects using a conventional hearing aid in the contralateral ear, assessments were conducted while aided. Audiological gain at T1 was assessed using free-field stimuli from a loudspeaker placed 1 m in front of the subject, with the better ear masked or occluded.

Speech Perception in Noise Assessment

Speech perception in noise was evaluated using a speech-in-noise test (Interacoustics® A/S, Middelfart, Denmark with synthetic sentences, each containing five semantically unpredictable words. This test measured SRT50, defined as the signal-to-noise ratio (SNR), in dB at which the subject correctly recognized 50% of the presented stimuli. This study used a sentence score, with 50% of sentences correctly recognized. In training sessions, participants were presented one list in quiet conditions and another list with noise at SNR 0. The lists of 10 sentences were randomly presented and designed to have similar intelligibility. The background noise was set to 65 dB SPL, while the speech level was modified according to subject responses. The tests were performed under the following presentation configurations:

S_0N_0: speech and noise are presented from a single front-facing loudspeaker.

$S_0N_{SSD/AHL}$: speech presented from the front, noise from the deaf side.

$S_{SSD/AHL}N_{AH}$: speech presented from the SSD/AHL side, noise from the contralateral acoustic hearing (AH) side.

The sentence test was administered both with the device activated and without it at T1. Any positive difference in dB between the unaided and aided condition indicates an improvement. Improvement was calculated using the following parameters:

Head shadow effect: SRT $S_{SSD/AHL}N_{AH}$ unaided/SRT $S_{SSD/AHL}N_{AH}$ aided.

Release from masking: SRT S_0N_0 unaided/SRT $S_0N_{SSD/AHL}$ aided.

Binaural squelch: SRT $S_0N_{SSD/AHL}$ aided/SRT $S_0N_{SSD/AHL}$ aided.

Binaural summation: SRT S_0N_0 unaided/SRT S_0N_0 aided.

Sound Localization Evaluation

The accuracy of sound localization was evaluated using a setup with 7 speakers placed in a semicircle spanning 180°, with each speaker positioned 30° apart. Participants were directed to maintain head stability, and responses were assessed in terms of localization error and bias, both measured in degrees. The stimuli consisted of randomly presented white noise bursts, each with 20 ms rise and fall times. Two noise signals (unfiltered and filtered CCITT sound) were randomly presented at 65, 70, and 75 dBA for each speaker. Each stimulus was presented once, totaling 42 presentations (7 speakers × 3 levels × 2 signals). Each listening condition test lasted approximately 2–3 min. The localization measures analyzed were the root mean square (RMS) error between the indicated and actual speaker angles. An RMS error ≤15° is considered normal for hearing. A lower RMS error indicates better localization accuracy. Localization measurements took place in a semi-anechoic chamber with sound-attenuating walls and flooring for free-field testing. The average background noise level in the chamber was 41.05 dBA, as measured using a PCE-322A sound level meter (measurement range: 30 dB to 130 dB, resolution: 0.1 dB). The same chamber was used for the SRT50 evaluation.

Speech, Spatial, and Qualities of Hearing Scale (SSQ12)

The Speech, Spatial, and Qualities of Hearing Scale (SSQ12) consists of three subscales evaluating speech understanding, spatial hearing, and sound quality, with a scoring range from 0 (unable to perform the indicated action) to 10 (perfect hearing perception). Subscale scores provide insights into the specific disabilities most affected by asymmetric hearing. The overall SSQ score was determined by averaging all the responses provided. SSQ12B and SSQ12C assessed self-reported changes after rehabilitation intervention, with scoring ranging from −5 to +5, allowing the identification of improvements or declines in hearing-related quality of life. The questionnaires were filled out in paper format. Participants could request clarification from the research team. Evaluated parameters included total SSQ12A score, total SSQ12B/C score, and subscale SSQ12B/C scores (speech, spatial, qualities).

Tinnitus Assessment

Tinnitus severity was measured in both CI and BCI subjects using a visual analog scale (VAS). A score of 10 indicated maximum disability, while 0 signified no tinnitus-related handicap.

Statistical analyses were conducted in Python using descriptive and inferential methods to evaluate auditory rehabilitation outcomes. Patients were grouped by hearing loss type (SSD or AHL), and subgroup analyses were performed separately for adults and children where appropriate. Tinnitus analyses were restricted to adults.

Parametric tests (e.g., *t*-tests, ANOVA, ANCOVA) and non-parametric alternatives (e.g., Wilcoxon signed-rank test, Mann–Whitney U test) were selected based on data distribution. The significance threshold was set at $p < 0.05$. Post hoc effect sizes (Cohen's d) and statistical power (1−β) were computed for each comparison to assess the robustness of observed effects. Bonferroni correction was applied for multiple comparisons when necessary. Estimations were performed using Stata MP 16 and Python 3.13 software packages.

3. Results

3.1. Patients

In the CI-implanted adult group (n = 18), 13 patients had SSD (mean age: 42 years), and 5 had AHL (mean age: 44.2 years, subject 14–subject 18). In the BCI-implanted group of adults, five patients had perilingual, possibly congenital, hearing loss (mean age: 32.8 years), while four had postlingual hearing loss (mean age: 50.7 years). A pediatric cohort (n = 9, age range: 9–16 years) was also included, comprising five patients who received a CI for postlingual hearing loss and four who received a BCI for perilingual hearing loss. Table 1a,b present the demographic characteristics of the patients and the underlying causes of their hearing loss. The results indicate that CI recipients had a significantly shorter duration of asymmetric hearing loss before implantation compared to BCI users. On average, CI users had lived with hearing asymmetry for 5.4 years, while BCI users had a mean duration of 19.5 years. In pediatric patients, implantation occurred significantly earlier (mean: 12.7 years).

Table 1. (**a**) Demographic characteristics of adult participants. (**b**) Demographic characteristics of pediatric participants.

(a)

Subject ID	Gender	Age at Implant (Years)	Etiology	Onset	Duration of Deafness (Years)	Electrode CI Type/BCI System	Follow-Up Period (Months)
S1	F	52.0	trauma	postlingual	1.0	Cochlear Slim Straight	16.0
S2	M	18.0	viral infection	postlingual	8.0	MED-EL FLEX 28	16.0
S3	F	49.0	Scohl-vest	postlingual	2.0	MED-EL FLEX 28	12.0
S4	F	30.0	Scohl-vest	postlingual	4.0	MED-EL FLEX 28	18.0
S5	M	49.0	trauma	postlingual	15.0	Cochlear Slim Straight	16.0
S6	F	52.0	trauma	postlingual	2.0	Cochlear Slim Straight	14.0
S7	F	56.0	Scohl-vest	postlingual	8.0	Cochlear Slim Straight	14.0
S8	M	50.0	Scohl-vest	postlingual	5.0	Cochlear Slim Straight	16.0
S9	M	42.0	trauma	postlingual	2.0	MED-EL FLEX 28	14.0
S10	F	35.0	Scohl-vest	postlingual	4.0	MED-EL FLEX 28	12.0
S11	M	47.0	viral infection	postlingual	1.0	MED-EL FLEX 28	12.0
S12	F	33.0	Scohl-vest	postlingual	9.0	Cochlear Slim Straight	18.0
S13	M	33.0	schwannoma	postlingual	2.0	MED-EL FLEX 28	12.0
S14	F	47.0	Scohl-vest	postlingual	9.0	MED-EL FLEX 28	14.0
S15	F	54.0	otospongiozsis	postlingual	7.0	Cochlear Slim Straight	16.0
S16	F	45.0	otospongiozsis	postlingual	5.0	MED-EL FLEX 28	16.0
S17	F	52.0	Scohl-vest	postlingual	1.0	Cochlear Slim Straight	14.0
S18	F	23.0	ototoxicity	postlingual	13.0	Digisonic SP EVO	24.0
S19	M	63.0	viral infection	postlingual	25.0	Cochlear Baha 5	14.0
S20	F	37.0	labyrinthitis	postlingual	10.0	Cochlear Baha 5	16.0
S21	M	52.0	labyrinthitis	postlingual	3.0	Cochlear Baha 5	14.0
S22	M	51.0	trauma	postlingual	0.5	MED-EL Bonebridge	12.0
S23	M	35.0	unknown	perlingual	35.0	MED-EL Bonebridge	12.0
S24	M	54.0	unknown	perlingual	54.0	MED-EL Bonebridge	14.0
S25	F	25.0	unknown	perlingual	25.0	MED-EL Bonebridge	12.0
S26	M	30.0	unknown	perilingual	30.0	MED-EL Bonebridge	12.0
S27	F	20.0	unknown	perilingual	20.0	MED-EL Bonebridge	12.0

(b)

Subject ID	Gender	Age at Implant (Years)	Etiology	Onset	Duration of Deafness (Years)	Electrode Type CI/BCI System	Follow-Up Period (Months)
S1	M	16.0	viral infection	postlingual	8.0	Cochlear Slim Straight	16.0
S2	M	13.0	unknown	postlingual	6.0	MED-EL FLEX 28	12.0
S3	F	12.0	unknown	postlingual	5.0	Digisonic SP EVO	24.0
S4	M	9.0	unknown	postlingual	6.0	MED-EL FLEX 28	12.0
S5	F	13.0	labyrinthitis	postlingual	2.0	MED-EL FLEX 28	16.0
S6	M	10.0	unknown	perilingual	10.0	MED-EL Bonebridge	12.0
S7	F	15.0	unknown	perilingual	15.0	MED-EL Bonebridge	12.0
S8	F	15.0	unknown	perilingual	15.0	MED-EL Bonebridge	14.0
S9	M	11.0	unknown	perilingual	11.0	MED-EL Bonebridge	14.0

Note: CI: cochlear implant; BCI: bone conduction implant.

Although not used as a formal grouping variable, clinical history showed varied pre-implant auditory stimulation. Most adult SSD patients reported sporadic and unsatisfactory hearing aid use, and none had used a CROS device. Among the BCI users with congenital or perilingual onset, only two had trialed hearing aids without sustained benefit. AHL patients demonstrated more consistent hearing aid use, especially in the better ear, with four still using one at the time of evaluation. These observations provide relevant context regarding prior auditory input.

3.2. OUTCOMES

3.2.1. Pure-Tone Audiometry (PTA4)

Figure 1a illustrates the individual evolution of PTA4 thresholds (poorer ear) from baseline (T0) to follow-up (T1 aided) after auditory implantation. The figure separates children and adults to provide a clearer view of hearing outcomes by age group. Each line represents one subject's change in PTA4 thresholds, reflecting the degree of functional gain achieved. All patients showed substantial improvements in the aided condition (T1), with consistently lower PTA4 values compared to the unaided baseline. Figure 1b shows the evolution of PTA4 thresholds in the better ear for AHL subjects, measured at baseline (T0, unaided) and at follow-up (T1, in the best aided condition). At T1, most individuals were assessed while using a hearing aid in the better ear, except for one who was evaluated while unaided. These results underline the importance of optimal hearing aid fitting and regular use in patients with AHL undergoing auditory rehabilitation.

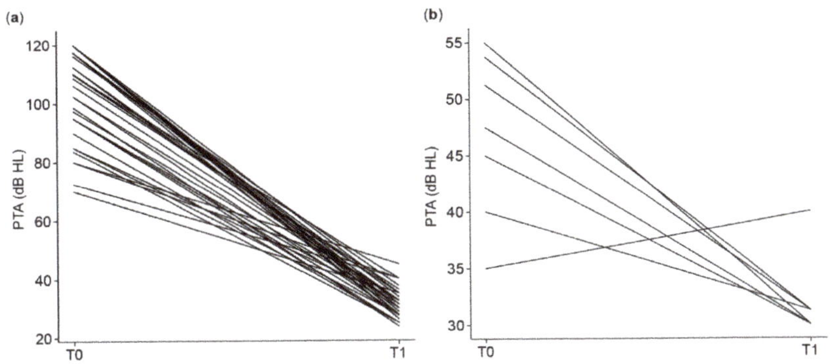

Figure 1. PTA in the poorer (implanted) ear at baseline and follow-up (**a**). PTA in the better ear (AHL subjects) at baseline and follow-up (**b**). (**a**) Individual PTA4 thresholds (dB HL) in the poorer ear at baseline (T0) and follow-up (T1 aided), across all participants. Each line represents one subject, illustrating the change in hearing threshold following cochlear or bone conduction implantation. (**b**) Individual PTA4 thresholds (dB HL) in the better ear of AHL patients at baseline (T0) and follow-up (T1, best aided condition).

Figure 2 provides a comparative analysis of PTA4 thresholds between CI and BCI users and quantitatively compares these groups. Statistically significant improvements were seen for both CI ($p < 0.001$) and BCI ($p = 0.0002$) groups (Wilcoxon signed-rank test). Postoperative thresholds achieved approximately 30 dB HL, confirming substantial auditory rehabilitation success in both implant types, with notably stronger results in CI users. The variation in individual responses suggests differences in baseline hearing, auditory adaptation, and amplification effects.

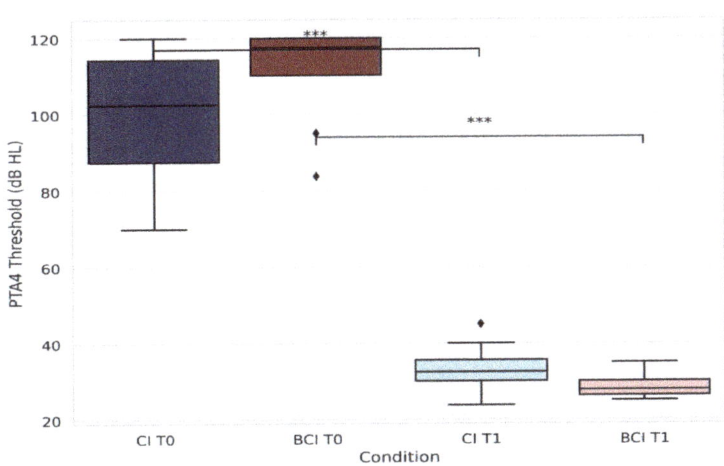

Figure 2. Comparative analysis of PTA4 thresholds (CI vs. BCI users). Boxplot showing PTA4 thresholds in the poorer ear at T0 and T1 for the CI and BCI groups, separately. Both CI (navy/light blue) and BCI (dark red/light coral) users showed statistically significant improvement post-implantation. Asterisks show significance: *** $p < 0.001$. Diamonds represent outliers.

3.2.2. Localization Accuracy (RMS)

Localization accuracy was evaluated using the root mean square (RMS) error in degrees across three listening conditions: unaided baseline (T0), unaided follow-up (T1 unaided), and aided follow-up (T1 aided). The RMS value reflects the average angular deviation between the presented and perceived sound source locations, with lower values showing better spatial hearing.

To assess within-subject improvements, statistical comparisons were performed using paired *t*-tests or Wilcoxon signed-rank tests, depending on normality. Normality was assessed using the Shapiro–Wilk test. Cohen's d was calculated to find effect sizes, and power analyses were conducted to evaluate the robustness of the findings.

Across the full cohort (excluding n = four cases with missing T0 data), localization improved significantly from T0 (mean = 77.9° ± 13.8°) to T1 aided (mean = 44.6° ± 18.1°), as confirmed with a paired t-test ($p < 0.001$, d = 1.176, power = 0.9998). These results show a large and reliable improvement in spatial hearing following auditory implantation.

CI users showed consistent and substantial improvements, while BCI users showed more variable or modest improvements. These differences were further supported by statistical tests conducted within each subgroup.

Among adult CI users, RMS T0 was 81.9° ± 15.8° (55.5–108.3°), and RMS T1 aided was 43.7° ± 13.5° (18.5–69.6°), showing a significant improvement. Among adult BCI users, RMS T0 was 74.6° ± 12.1° (62.3–101.1°), while RMS T1 aided was 69.2° ± 16.3° (47.7–90.6°). Wilcoxon signed-rank tests revealed statistically significant improvements in CI users between T0 and T1 aided (z = 4.029, $p < 0.01$) and between T1 unaided and T1 aided (z = 4.180, $p < 0.01$). Among the pediatric recipients, significant improvements were seen both from T0 to T1 aided (median: 74.3° → 44.8°, $p = 0.016$) and from T1 unaided to T1 aided ($p = 0.012$), as confirmed by Wilcoxon tests. These findings were consistent across children with both CIs and BCIs, reinforcing the positive impact of early auditory implantation on spatial hearing development. No significant changes were seen in BCI users (T0 vs. T1 aided: $p = 0.255$; T1 unaided vs. T1 aided: $p = 0.190$). Localization performance across the four subgroups—adult CI users, adult BCI users, children with CIs, and children with BCIs—is shown in Figure 3. While statistically significant improvements were observed in adult CI users and in the pooled pediatric group, subgroup analyses in pediatric CI and BCI recipients did not reach significance individually, likely due to the limited sample size in each category (n < 5).

Figure 4 compares RMS performance in adult CI users with SSD versus CI users with AHL. SSD users showed significant improvements from T0 to T1 aided ($p < 0.001$) and from T1 unaided to T1 aided ($p < 0.001$). No statistically significant difference was found between SSD and AHL users at T1 aided ($p = 0.197$). This may reflect genuinely similar final performances or could be due to the limited sample size. Although AHL users did not show statistically significant changes across conditions, their mean RMS values followed a similar pattern of reduction.

The analysis of onset type among adult BCI users showed similar mean RMS values at T1 aided between perilingual and postlingual cases (t = 0.23, $p = 0.823$, d = −0.17; Mann–Whitney U = ns). However, due to the small sample size in this subgroup, the statistical power was low, and the absence of a significant difference should not be interpreted as evidence of no effect. These observations remain exploratory and do not allow firm conclusions regarding the influence of onset timing on localization outcomes in BCI users.

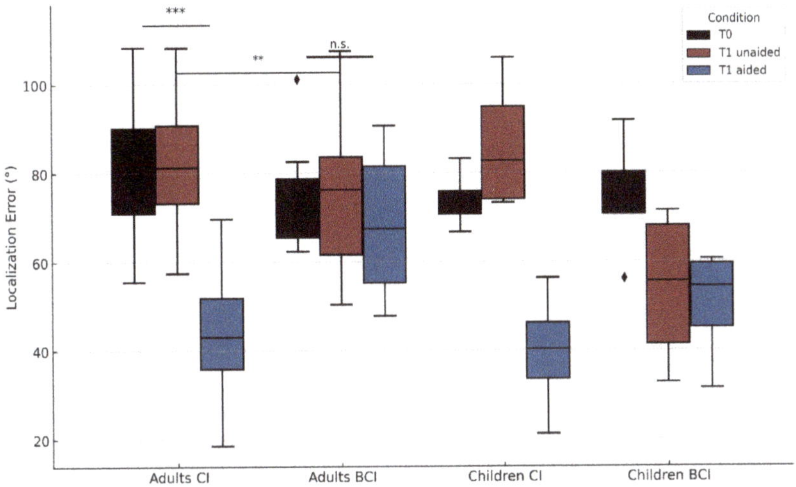

Figure 3. Localization performance across conditions. Boxplots showing RMS localization error in four subgroups (Adults CI, Adults BCI, Children CI, Children BCI) across three listening conditions: baseline (T0), T1 unaided, and T1 aided. Diamonds represent outliers. Asterisks indicate statistical significance within or between groups (** $p < 0.01$, *** $p < 0.001$). "n.s." indicates non-significant differences.

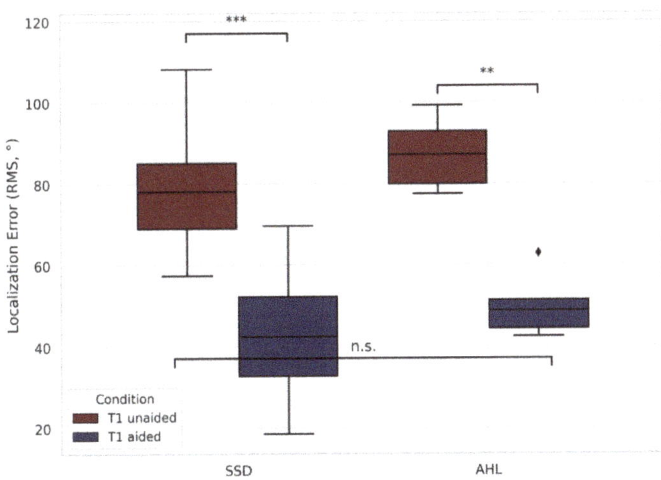

Figure 4. Boxplots of localization error (RMS, °) at follow-up unaided (T1), and with the device activated (T1 aided) in cochlear implant users with single-sided deafness (SSD) and asymmetric hearing loss (AHL). Outliers are represented by black diamonds (♦), defined as values outside 1.5 times the interquartile range Asterisks indicate statistical significance within or between groups (** $p < 0.01$, *** $p < 0.001$), "n.s." indicates non-significant differences.

Figure 5 further illustrates individual trajectories in children by hearing loss type and device. Subjects showed improved RMS error post-implant, with some variability, supporting the notion that auditory implants help children regardless of etiology or device type.

Together, these results prove that cochlear implants offer large and statistically robust improvements in localization, particularly in adults, while BCI users showed less consistent gains.

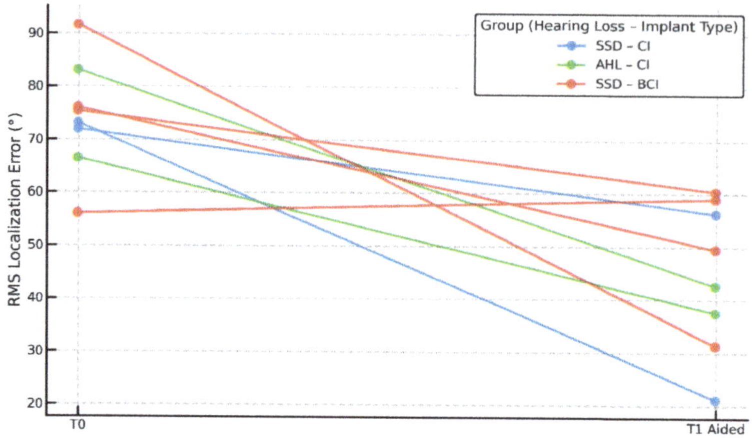

Figure 5. Individual localization outcome from baseline to follow-up in children. Line plot showing RMS localization error at baseline (T0) and follow-up (T1 aided) for each subject, separated by implant type. Most subjects demonstrated improved localization accuracy at follow-up. One BCI user exhibited a higher RMS error at T1, indicating a deterioration in spatial performance.

3.2.3. Speech Perception in Noise

Statistical comparisons were performed using Welch's t-tests for independent group comparisons (e.g., SSD patients vs. AHL patients, CI users vs. BCI users), and one-sample t-tests were performed for within-group comparisons against zero improvement. Significance was set at $p < 0.05$. Post hoc effect sizes (Cohen's d) and statistical power (1–β) were computed for each comparison to assess the robustness of observed effects. No corrections for multiple comparisons were applied, as the post hoc tests were hypothesis-driven.

Across the entire cohort, the mean binaural effects were as follows: head shadow effect = 4.7 ± 3.1 dB (range: −1.8 to 10.8), release from masking = 0.6 ± 3.2 dB (range: −6.0 to 6.6), binaural squelch = 1 ± 3.6 dB (range: −9.8 to 8.4), and binaural summation = 2.5 ± 3.7 dB (range: −2.4 to 12.6). One-sample t-tests confirmed significant improvements for head shadow ($p < 0.001$, d = −0.54, power = 0.99) and binaural summation ($p < 0.001$, d = 0.69, power = 0.99), while release from masking and binaural squelch did not reach significance.

When subgroup analysis was performed, CI SSD adults showed a head shadow effect of 4.9 ± 4 dB and binaural summation of 2.8 ± 3.6 dB, while adult BCI users showed scores of 3.8 ± 2.5 dB and 1.89 ± 2.92 dB, respectively. In children, all effects were positive, with notable improvements in head shadow (4.6 ± 3.1 dB), release from masking (3.3 ± 2.6 dB), and binaural squelch (2.7 ± 3 dB).

Although all binaural effects were numerically positive in each subgroup, none of the one-sample t-tests reached statistical significance (all $p > 0.05$). Calculated power values ranged from 0.05 to 0.33, underscoring the limited statistical strength of these subgroup analyses. Therefore, while the observed values are consistent with potential benefit, the current data do not permit reliable confirmation at the subgroup level.

No significant differences were seen between adult CI and adult BCI users for any of the four effects (all $p > 0.4$). These findings are summarized in Figure 6, which displays the distribution of all binaural effects across groups. Notably, comparisons between binaural effects in the overall cohort revealed that the head shadow effect was significantly stronger than all other effects (all $p < 0.01$), having the largest mean improvement and highest statistical power (d = −0.54, power = 0.99). Head shadow consistently appeared as the most effective binaural mechanism in CI, BCI, and pediatric users alike. The binaural squelch effect was present in some individuals but was less consistent overall, with the group-level gains being smaller and more variable.

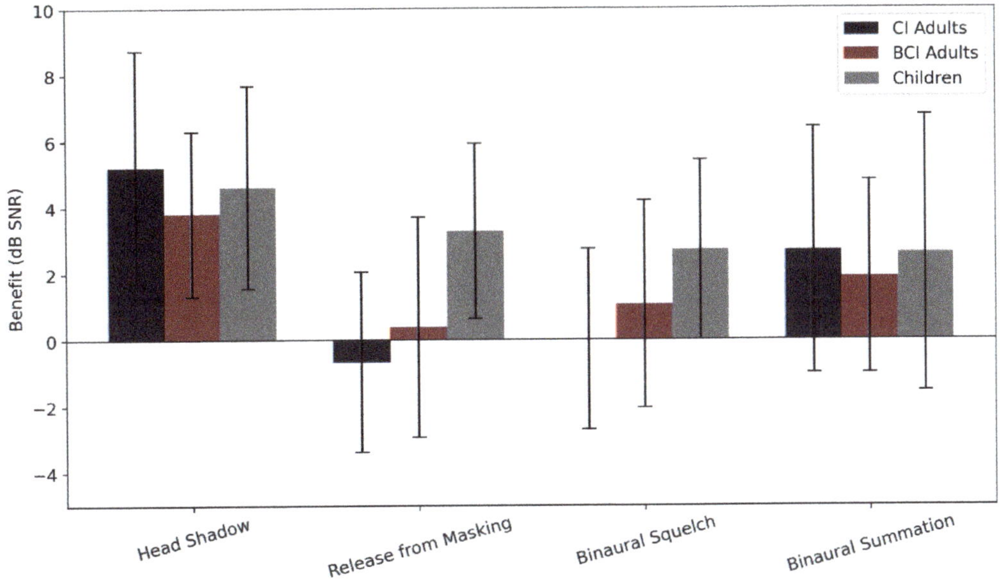

Figure 6. Binaural effects by group. The boxplots illustrate the distribution of four binaural effects—head shadow effect, release from masking, binaural squelch, and binaural summation—across three groups: CI SSD adults, BCI adults, and children. Each effect is expressed as the SRT improvement in the dB signal-to-noise ratio SNR (positive values indicate auditory benefit). The horizontal reference line at 0 dB denotes no change. Boxes represent interquartile ranges (IQRs), whiskers extend to 1.5 × IQR.

The variability within each group was substantial for all effects, as reflected in the large standard deviations (Figure 7). These differences likely reflect both subject-specific characteristics and differences in device performance and auditory adaptation. On average, children showed the greatest overall binaural benefit, particularly in the squelch and summation conditions, while CI SSD adults showed a strong head shadow advantage, but minimal benefit in central binaural integration.

Statistical comparisons between groups (Figure 8) revealed that children performed significantly better than CI SSD adults for release from masking ($t = 3.04$, $p = 0.007$, $d = 1.54$). The difference with adult BCI users did not reach statistical significance ($t = 2.10$, $p = 0.059$, $d = 1.14$), although mean values remained higher in the pediatric cohort. While this finding may reflect an enhanced capacity to extract speech from spatially separated noise, it should be interpreted with consideration of the key clinical differences between groups. The pediatric group included both CI and BCI users, with either congenital/perilingual or acquired hearing loss. Nonetheless, due to earlier implantation, even children with congenital or early-onset deafness experienced significantly shorter durations of auditory deprivation compared to adults. In contrast, several adult BCI users had long-standing perilingual or postlingual deafness, potentially limiting the plasticity of their auditory pathways. These differences likely contributed to the observed advantage in pediatric performance.

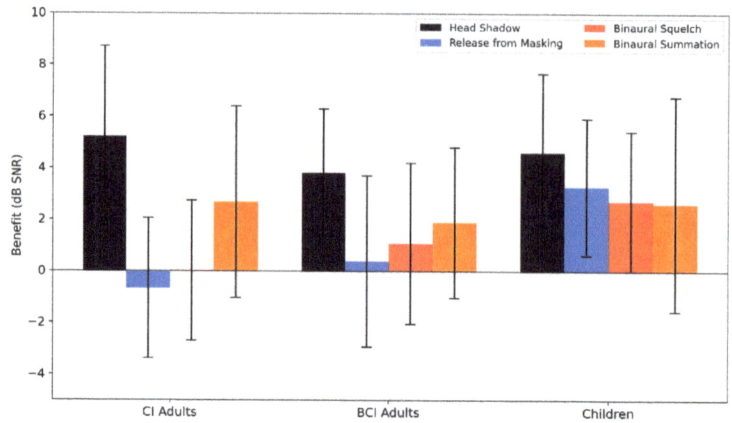

Figure 7. Binaural benefit patterns within groups. Bar plot showing the average improvement in speech reception threshold (SRT, in dB signal-to-noise ratio) for each of the four binaural effects—head shadow, release from masking, binaural squelch, and binaural summation—within each participant group: adults with CI, adults with BCI, and children. Each bar shows the mean benefit with standard deviation. The head shadow effect consistently appeared as the most prominent binaural advantage across all groups, as also confirmed statistically in the main cohort ($p < 0.01$).

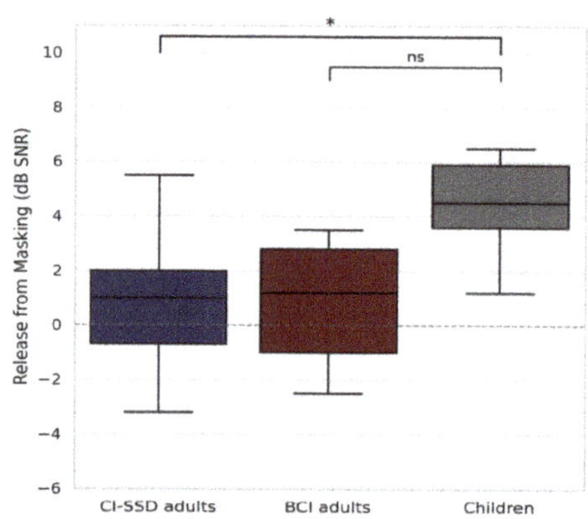

Figure 8. Release from masking by group. Children showed significantly greater release from masking compared to CI-SSD adults (t = 3.04, p = 0.007). The difference between children and adult BCI users did not reach statistical significance (t = 2.10, p = 0.059). Values are expressed in dB SNR, with higher values indicating better ability to extract speech from spatially separated noise. Asterisks indicate statistical significance within or between groups (* $p < 0.05$), "n.s." indicates non-significant differences.

A comparative analysis of adult CI users with SSD versus AHL was also conducted using Welch's t-tests. No statistically significant differences were found (head shadow: t = −0.752, p = 0.463, d = −0.27; release from masking: t = 0.887, p = 0.394, d = 0.39; binaural squelch: t = 0.440, p = 0.673, d = 0.23; binaural summation: t = 0.177, p = 0.865, d = 0.10). Power analyses for these comparisons were low (range: 0.05–0.11), suggesting limited ability to detect differences. Despite this, the results suggest that AHL patients may experience comparable binaural benefits following cochlear implantation, reinforcing the relevance of CI for both SSD and AHL profiles.

3.2.4. Tinnitus Severity

Tinnitus severity was evaluated in adult patients (≥18 years) using a visual analog scale (VAS, 0–10). To reflect the overall impact of auditory implants on the tinnitus burden in the population, all adults were included in the analysis, regardless of baseline tinnitus presence. Only T0 and T1 aided values were considered, excluding T1 unaided due to lack of control over implant-off duration.

Among cochlear implant (CI) users (n = 18), tinnitus severity decreased from a mean of 5.67 at T0 to 1.78 at T1 aided. A Wilcoxon signed-rank test confirmed a significant reduction ($p = 0.0001$, r = 0.71), with a high effect size and statistical power (1–β = 0.96). In the BCI group (n = 9), tinnitus scores decreased from 1.89 to 0.56 (mean reduction 1.6 ± 0.9), but this change was not statistically significant ($p = 0.25$, r = 0.50, power ≈ 0.30).

Although CI users showed a greater mean reduction (2.8 ± 2.0), a Mann–Whitney test comparing tinnitus improvement between CI and BCI users did not reach significance ($p = 0.371$) (Figure 9). Importantly, no new cases of tinnitus were seen after implantation, and all individuals with perilingual onset (n = 4) consistently reported VAS = 0 at both time points. This suggests that the tinnitus burden in this population was restricted to postlingual onset.

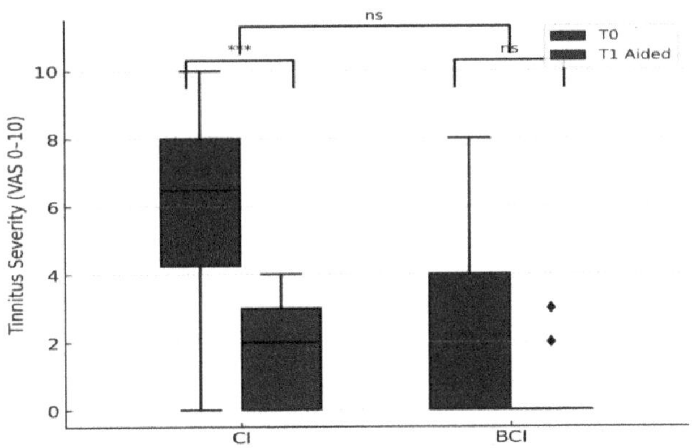

Figure 9. Tinnitus severity before and after implantation in adult users of CIs and BCIs. The boxplots show tinnitus severity at baseline (T0) and at follow-up with the device activated (T1 aided). Diamonds represent individual values. Asterisks indicate statistically significant differences (*** $p < 0.001$); ns = not significant.

A subgroup comparison between CI users showed no significant difference in tinnitus improvement between AHL and SSD cases ($p = 0.7872$), indicating that tinnitus relief is similarly achievable in both types of asymmetric hearing loss.

These findings highlight the role of cochlear implants in alleviating tinnitus burden in adults, particularly among those with pre-existing symptoms. While BCI users showed a favorable trend, the effect was not statistically robust, and interpretation is limited by sample size. Clinically, tinnitus was typically reported in the poorer-hearing or deaf ear, especially in SSD patients, which is consistent with the focus of our analysis on the implant-aided side. In AHL cases, bilateral or diffuse tinnitus was described more often. However, tinnitus laterality was not coded systematically and was therefore not included as a variable in the analysis.

3.2.5. Self-Reported Hearing Outcomes—SSQ12

Self-reported hearing outcomes were assessed using the SSQ12A at baseline and SSQ12B/C to evaluate perceived benefit after implantation. Among adults, baseline SSQ12A scores were slightly higher in BCI users (5.2 ± 2.1) compared to CI users (4.5 ± 2.1), though the difference was not statistically significant (p = 0.37). Within the adult CI group, SSD patients reported higher initial scores than AHL patients (4.8 ± 1.9 vs. 3.5 ± 2.5), but this difference also did not reach statistical significance (p = 0.32). In children, baseline SSQ12A scores were comparable between CI and BCI users, with no significant differences.

Following auditory rehabilitation, all participants reported significant perceived improvements across the SSQ12B/C scale. Mean total improvement scores were 1.7 ± 0.9 in adult CI users, 1.4 ± 0.5 in adult BCI users, and 1.9 ± 0.5 in children, with pediatric participants reporting the highest overall benefit. The difference between children and adult BCI users was statistically significant (p = 0.0035, Bonferroni-corrected p = 0.0105), while the comparisons between children and adult CI users, and between adult CI users and adult BCI users, were not significant.

To further explore the perceived benefit of implantation, SSQ12B/C subscale scores were analyzed separately for the three domains: speech, spatial, and qualities. Figure 10 illustrates these improvements across adult CI users, adult BCI users, and pediatric users. In the speech subscale, children reported the greatest gains (2.1 ± 0.7), followed by adult BCI users (1.6 ± 0.9) and adult CI users (1.5 ± 0.9). No significant difference was observed between adult CI and BCI users (p = 0.8808, Bonferroni p = 1.000). In the spatial subscale, adult CI users showed the largest benefit (2.1 ± 1.2), closely followed by children (2.0 ± 1.0), while adult BCI users reported lower gains (1.3 ± 0.8). The difference between adult CI and BCI users approached statistical significance (p = 0.0547, Bonferroni p = 0.1641). For sound qualities, children again reported the highest benefit (1.6 ± 0.6), followed by adult CI users (1.5 ± 1.0) and adult BCI users (1.2 ± 0.5), with no significant difference between adult groups (p = 0.2439, Bonferroni p = 0.7318).

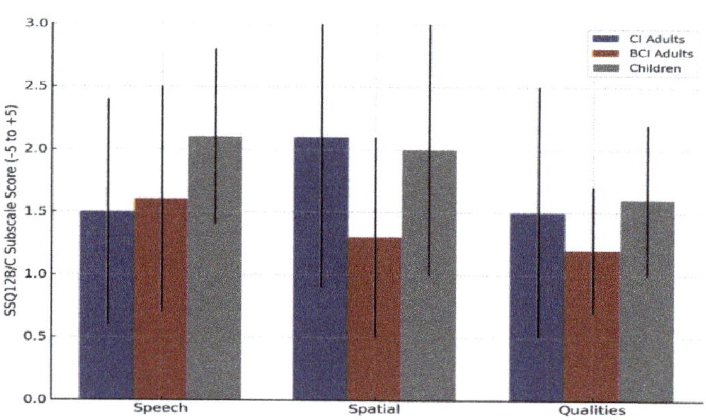

Figure 10. SSQ12B/C subscale improvements following auditory rehabilitation. Bar chart showing mean perceived improvement (± SD) on the SSQ12B/C subscales (speech, spatial, qualities) across three groups: adults with a cochlear implant (CI), adults with a bone conduction implant (BCI), and pediatric users. All groups reported subjective benefits from implantation.

3.2.6. Correlations and Device Use

Although not the focus of this study, we explored correlations between key clinical outcomes and individual characteristics such as daily device use and the duration of deafness. These analyses were conducted to gain a better understanding of the variability in patient response within our initial cohort of individuals with asymmetric or unilateral hearing loss.

Daily device use varied by age and implant type. These values represent the total daily time the implant was worn and powered on, as reported by the patients, regardless of environmental sound levels. Therefore, "device use" in this context should be interpreted as a general indicator of use rather than a measure of auditory input or sound exposure. CI users generally reported longer daily use compared to BCI users. Among adults with a CI, the mean daily use was 7.7 h (range: 1.5–12.0), while children with a CI showed the highest usage (mean: 8.0 h/day; range: 2.0–12.0). BCI users reported lower use, with adult BCI users averaging 5.3 h/day (range: 1.0–10.0), and children with BCI averaging 7.5 h/day (range: 2.0–12.0). These patterns suggest that younger users, especially those with a CI, tend to maintain more consistent auditory stimulation, which is likely supported by structured rehabilitation programs and caregiver involvement.

A significant negative correlation was found between RMS localization error in the aided condition and SSQ12B/C spatial scores ($r = -0.35$, $p = 0.037$), indicating that better localization accuracy is associated with greater perceived spatial benefit. Additionally, improvement in RMS performance (T1 unaided–T1 aided) positively correlated with the full SSQ spatial score ($r = 0.432$, $p = 0.009$), reinforcing the relationship between objective gains and subjective experience of spatial hearing.

Daily use of the auditory device was positively correlated with overall SSQ12B/C improvement ($r = 0.569$, $p < 0.001$), as well as with each subscale: speech ($r = 0.45$, $p = 0.006$), spatial ($r = 0.41$, $p = 0.013$), and qualities ($r = 0.50$, $p = 0.002$). These associations highlight the role of consistent auditory stimulation in enhancing self-reported hearing outcomes. A significant correlation was observed between longer durations of deafness and higher RMS error in the aided condition ($r = 0.44$, $p = 0.007$), suggesting that prolonged auditory deprivation may negatively impact localization ability. However, no significant correlation was found between daily use and RMS T1 aided performance ($r = -0.23$, $p = 0.17$), indicating that while consistent use is beneficial, it may not fully compensate for deficits related to auditory deprivation.

Daily device use also correlated moderately with tinnitus reduction ($r = 0.42$, $p = 0.011$), while it was inversely correlated with the duration of deafness ($r = -0.476$, $p = 0.003$). These findings support the hypothesis that earlier and consistent use may facilitate tinnitus relief, possibly through auditory masking or neuroplastic mechanisms.

Binaural squelch was the only speech-in-noise parameter that significantly correlated with the SSQ12 scores, showing strong associations with both the SSQ12B/C total score ($r = 0.585$, $p = 0.0002$) and the speech subscale ($r = 0.505$, $p = 0.0017$). This suggests that patients who derive greater benefit from binaural squelch also report enhanced speech understanding and overall hearing improvement. In contrast, other binaural measures, such as head shadow, release from masking, and binaural summation, did not show statistically significant correlations with SSQ12 scores.

ANCOVA analyses showed no significant influence of age or device use on head shadow effect, release from masking, or binaural summation. However, daily device use significantly predicted binaural squelch performance ($p = 0.048$), suggesting that auditory experience may enhance spatial filtering capabilities. A regression model for adult CI users indicated a trend-level effect of daily use on RMS T1 aided scores ($\beta = -2.05$, $p = 0.07$), explaining 33.1% of the variance ($R^2 = 0.331$, $p = 0.0218$). The duration of deafness was not a significant predictor in this model ($\beta = 0.48$, $p = 0.098$). Bootstrap analysis for subjects using their device $\geq$8 h/day yielded an estimated mean RMS T1 aided of 50.2° (95% CI: 41.2–59.6°), indicating moderate spatial accuracy with high usage. To better contextualize this result, we examined the baseline and unaided scores in the same subgroup (n = 15). The mean RMS error was 82.8° ± 14.1° at baseline (T0), 82.7° ± 13.9° at T1 unaided, and 50.3° ± 19.7° at T1 aided, with an average unaided-to-aided gain of 32.5° ± 21.6°. When stratified by device, CI users (n = 11) showed substantial benefit (mean improvement = 41.4° ± 17.1°), while BCI users (n = 4) showed minimal change (7.9° ± 10.3°), suggesting that the group-level accuracy was primarily driven by CI users.

These findings collectively emphasize the complex interplay between auditory experience, perceptual outcomes, and residual neural plasticity (Figure 11). Among the binaural effects, binaural squelch demonstrated the strongest link between objective performance and subjective benefit, suggesting that it may represent the most functionally relevant marker of binaural integration in this population.

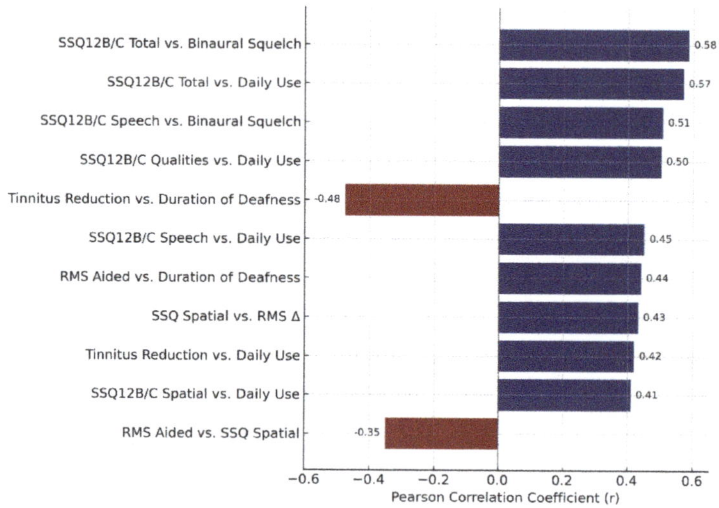

Figure 11. Correlations between auditory outcomes and patient characteristics.

Horizontal bar plot displaying Pearson correlation coefficients (r) for statistically significant relationships ($p < 0.05$) between clinical and auditory outcomes. Positive correlations are shown in dark blue (e.g., consistent device use and SSQ12 subscales), while negative correlations are shown in burgundy (e.g., the duration of deafness and localization error). The strongest associations were observed between binaural squelch and both the SSQ12 total and speech subscale scores, highlighting its functional relevance in patient-reported benefit.

4. Discussion

This study aimed to evaluate the outcomes of auditory rehabilitation in individuals with SSD and AHL following cochlear implantation or bone conduction implantation, based on standard clinical indications. We focused on improvements in hearing thresholds, localization, speech-in-noise performance, tinnitus relief, and subjective hearing experience, while examining the influence of patient-specific variables and binaural processing effects.

Improvements in PTA4 thresholds in the implanted ear confirmed restored access to sound for both CI and BCI users. AHL patients also showed minor improvements in their better ear, likely due to the adjusted contralateral hearing aid settings, highlighting the importance of bilateral management. These findings are consistent with prior reports on auditory restoration in asymmetrical hearing loss.

Localization improved significantly post-implantation, especially in CI users. The RMS localization error dropped across the CI users. This aligns with previous studies showing RMS gains of 25–35° following the use of CIs by SSD patients [15,21], although outcomes rarely reach normal-hearing accuracy [20] (Oh et al. Randomized controlled trials have similarly confirmed CIs' superiority over BCD and CROS solutions for spatial hearing restoration [24,40]).

BCI users, particularly adults, demonstrated smaller and more variable spatial gains. Among adult CI users, the SSD and AHL subgroups achieved comparable aided RMS values (~44°), though only SSD users improved significantly across all listening conditions, supporting previous findings [45]. Children, regardless of implant type, showed consistent improvement in localization, with average RMS reductions of ~30°. This may reflect neuroplastic compensation in the developing auditory system, even in the absence of formal training [32,34].

The duration of deafness correlated with poorer localization outcomes, reinforcing the value of early intervention [37]. A subgroup of high-use CI recipients (≥8 h/day) showed better aided localization (mean RMS = 50.2°), suggesting a possible dose–response relationship between daily stimulation and spatial accuracy. However, this pattern should be interpreted with caution given the small sample size and lack of stratification shown in Figure 4, which reflects group-level averages rather than usage-based subgroups. Importantly, daily use alone did not significantly correlate with aided RMS scores, indicating that consistent exposure may support—but not guarantee—spatial adaptation. These observations align with evidence emphasizing the role of early and sustained auditory input in optimizing spatial hearing outcomes (Santopietro et al., 2024) [33].

From a clinical perspective, localization is one of the most functionally relevant auditory abilities, contributing to sound awareness, safety, and communication in complex environments. The restoration of this ability through cochlear implantation confirms that spatial hearing is not only achievable, but also generalizable across different user groups, especially when intervention is timely. The discrepancy between CI and BCI outcomes, particularly in adults, underlines the limitations of passive acoustic transmission in supporting the encoding of spatial cues and stresses the importance of tailoring device selection to auditory goals. In children, the results suggest that developmental neuroplasticity may support more flexible integration of auditory input, potentially bypassing some of the mechanical limitations associated with BCIs.

Binaural effect analysis revealed that head shadow was the most consistent benefit across groups. This effect is driven by simple acoustic separation, based on the attenuation of sound intensity as it travels around the head from one ear to the other, rather than by true binaural integration. As such, it can be accessed regardless of age or device type. These results are in line with previous reports emphasizing that head shadow is an acoustic phenomenon largely independent of neural synchrony [27].

Binaural summation showed modest but consistent improvements, suggesting that access to bilateral stimulation provides perceptual advantages even in asymmetric listeners. Binaural squelch, which depends more on central auditory integration, was present only in select individuals and reached notable levels, primarily in children. A moderate-to-strong correlation between binaural squelch and SSQ12B/C scores ($r > 0.5$) further supports its relevance in subjective spatial benefit, in line with prior observations [21]. These results are consistent with multicenter studies reporting large interindividual variability in binaural integration following CI use (Marx et al., 2021; Wesarg et al., 2024) [27,28].

Release from masking demonstrated the most group-dependent variability. While children and BCI users showed positive effects, CI-SSD users exhibited no measurable benefit. This likely reflects reduced access to spatial unmasking cues in postlingually implanted CI users, possibly due to mismatched input timing, spectral differences, or insufficient binaural experience. The significant difference observed between children and CI SSD users ($p = 0.007$) underscores the importance of early auditory rehabilitation and greater plasticity during development.

Quantitative comparisons showed that CI SSD adults had the strongest binaural effects. Adult BCI users showed lower mean values for head shadow and summation, and limited benefit in summation and squelch—likely due to the lack of synchronous neural input between bone and air conduction pathways. Children showed positive values across all four effects, with notable improvements in head shadow, release from masking, and binaural squelch, reflecting meaningful perceptual gains during development.

Despite these findings, one-sample t-tests did not reach statistical significance within any subgroup (all $p > 0.05$), and power values ranged from 0.05 to 0.33, indicating limited ability to confirm the observed effects statistically. These findings align with previous studies reporting high interindividual variability in binaural outcomes [27,28]. No significant differences were observed between SSD and AHL adults with CIs for any of the four binaural effects (head shadow: $p = 0.463$; summation: $p = 0.865$; squelch: $p = 0.673$; release from masking: $p = 0.394$). While statistical power was low, the similarity in average values supports the hypothesis that cochlear implantation offers comparable binaural benefits for both asymmetry profiles.

ANCOVA revealed that neither age nor daily device use significantly influenced head shadow, summation, or release from masking. However, daily use was associated with greater binaural squelch ($p = 0.048$), suggesting that auditory training and consistent device exposure may enhance central binaural integration.

While no significant correlation was found between daily device use and aided RMS performance (r = −0.23, $p = 0.17$), clinical guidelines, such as those proposed by Dillon et al., suggest that consistent use of 8 h or more per day is associated with more effective auditory rehabilitation. This threshold was used in our bootstrap analysis. In comparison, Roger et al. [49] proposed a slightly higher threshold of 9 h/day when examining differences in speech-in-noise outcomes, which may indicate a gradual continuum rather than a fixed boundary. Although the current study did not stratify patients based on that specific cut-off due to sample size limitations, our results support the idea that more consistent use may enhance certain auditory outcomes, particularly binaural integration, as reflected in the significant association with binaural squelch. Future studies with larger samples should further examine the relationship between usage intensity and spatial or speech-in-noise performance.

The tinnitus analysis, which was restricted to adults, demonstrated significant suppression with device activation. CI users showed greater average reduction than BCI users, particularly in SSD with postlingual onset. This improvement was likely due to the cochlear input reversing central hyperactivity [20,50]. A moderate correlation between daily use and tinnitus relief further supports the value of consistent stimulation. These results align with systematic reviews reporting meaningful and sustained tinnitus suppression following cochlear implantation [18,21]. While speculative, these findings may suggest a neuromodulatory effect dependent on afferent stimulation and device type. Further research is needed to clarify the underlying mechanisms and to identify predictors of tinnitus relief across different clinical profiles.

Subjective hearing improvements, assessed via SSQ12, were substantial. This correlation should be interpreted in light of the prior literature. Blamey et al. [37] proposed a staged model of auditory performance decline, emphasizing that outcomes are shaped by both the duration and severity of hearing loss [37]. In addition, studies such as that by An et al. [51] indicate that prior auditory stimulation—even when inconsistent—may help preserve auditory processing and improve post-implantation outcomes. However, given that most patients in our cohort had little or no consistent history of hearing aid or CROS use, it is likely that they did not benefit from such protective effects, which may partly explain the observed relationship between deafness duration and spatial accuracy. The SSQ12B/C total improved, with the greatest gains observed in speech understanding, followed by sound quality and spatial perception. CI users showed greater gains in spatial subscales than BCI users, consistent with superior spatial resolution via electrical stimulation [39,40]. Children reported the largest gains in speech understanding, reflecting age-related neural plasticity (Santopietro et al., 2024; Benchetrit et al., 2021) [33,34].

Importantly, subjective outcomes correlated with objective measures, including binaural squelch and localization, affirming the real-life relevance of these effects. Daily device use was positively associated with SSQ12 improvements, supporting the need for active engagement. These findings emphasize the psychosocial and functional value of auditory rehabilitation, particularly when personalized and initiated early. The alignment between patient-reported outcomes and behavioral improvements has been confirmed in multiple trials investigating CI effectiveness in SSD (Sydlowski et al., 2022; Oh et al., 2023) [20,25].

Correlation and regression analyses provided additional insights. SSQ12B/C spatial scores negatively correlated with RMS error in the aided condition ($r = -0.35$) and positively with RMS improvement ($r = 0.43$), confirming the link between spatial hearing accuracy and subjective benefit. Daily device use showed significant positive correlations with overall SSQ12B/C improvement ($r = 0.57$) and with each subscale (speech: $r = 0.45$; spatial: $r = 0.41$; qualities: $r = 0.50$). Tinnitus relief also correlated with daily use ($r = 0.42$), while the duration of deafness was negatively associated with it ($r = -0.48$), reinforcing the importance of early and consistent auditory input.

Binaural squelch demonstrated the strongest relationship with SSQ12 spatial perception ($r > 0.5$), underscoring its clinical relevance. Regression analysis in adult CI users showed that daily use explained 33.1% of variance in the aided RMS scores, though the effect was marginal ($p = 0.07$). The duration of deafness did not significantly predict outcomes. These observations, though exploratory, suggest that while certain auditory outcomes are influenced by individual use patterns, others depend more on timing and the duration of sensory deprivation.

These correlations were not the focus of this study and should be interpreted cautiously, particularly given the cohort size and observational design. Nonetheless, they support emerging evidence on the role of patient-specific variables in shaping auditory rehabilitation outcomes and offer valuable directions for further investigation.

4.1. Study Strengths

This study provides clinical evidence about auditory rehabilitation with cochlear implants and bone conduction devices. The longitudinal design and inclusion of unselected patients strengthen its clinical relevance, ensuring that results reflect real-world auditory outcomes.

4.2. Limitations and Potential Biases

Several limitations and potential sources of bias should be considered when interpreting these findings. This study was conducted in a single tertiary referral center, which may limit the generalizability of results to broader clinical settings. Small sample sizes, particularly in the pediatric and BCI subgroups, reduce statistical power and increase the likelihood of type II error. Clinical heterogeneity in etiology, onset age, and device type (CIs vs. BCIs) may have influenced outcomes. Although subjective outcome measures such as SSQ12 and tinnitus ratings were collected using validated tools, their reliance on self-reporting introduces potential response bias. The SSQ12 questionnaire was formally validated in Romanian, while tinnitus severity was assessed via a VAS scale, which—though conceptually validated—is not based on a standardized tinnitus-specific inventory. Furthermore, unaided assessments at T1 may have been affected by uncontrolled variation in implant-off durations, introducing potential measurement bias. While clinical history of prior hearing aid user or CROS use was collected, it was not used as a grouping variable in the analysis. Observer bias was minimized through the use of standardized test protocols, but cannot be entirely excluded. These limitations underscore the need for cautious interpretation, especially when comparing subgroups with differing clinical profiles. Nonetheless, statistically significant improvements were demonstrated in core auditory domains, supporting the clinical relevance of the findings in real-world rehabilitation scenarios [37,49,51].

Finally, the observational design of this study inherently limits causal inferences. All implant decisions were made by the clinical team based on national program criteria and patient-specific factors, without randomization or blinding. Despite these limitations, statistically robust effects were observed in several key domains (e.g., localization, binaural squelch, SSQ12 improvement), supporting the overall consistency and relevance of the findings.

While many aspects of auditory rehabilitation—particularly regarding the efficacy of cochlear implantation in SSD and AHL—have been clarified through large-scale, multicenter studies, key questions remain. Future research should go beyond outcome validation and focus on establishing a deeper understanding of individual variability in spatial and binaural performance. This includes exploring how neural plasticity, age at onset, and the duration and type of auditory deprivation influence the extent of functional restoration.

Special attention should be given to the differential effects of CI and BCI systems on auditory integration, especially in pediatric and perilingual-onset populations, where neurodevelopmental dynamics may modulate outcomes in ways that are not yet fully understood. The interaction between residual hearing and device input and the role of structured auditory training are also promising avenues for optimization.

Finally, the growing interest in the neuromodulatory impact of implants—such as tinnitus suppression and perceptual recalibration—highlights the need for integrative research bridging clinical audiology, cognitive neuroscience, and patient-reported outcomes. Addressing these challenges will not only improve patient selection and rehabilitation protocols, but may also open new frontiers in auditory neuroscience.

5. Conclusions

This study demonstrates that both cochlear implants (CIs) and bone conduction implants (BCIs), when selected according to clinical criteria, offer measurable auditory benefits in cases of single-sided deafness and asymmetric hearing loss. CI users, especially adults, achieved superior improvements in spatial hearing and tinnitus suppression, while BCI users showed more variable gains with favorable outcomes, particularly in pediatric cases.

By analyzing real-world outcomes across distinct indication profiles, this study emphasizes the importance of individualized implant selection, accounting for anatomical constraints, onset timing, and the duration of deprivation. These findings support current clinical guidelines and underline the value of early and tailored intervention strategies.

In clinical practice, careful patient profiling remains key to optimizing the benefits of auditory implants, particularly in complex asymmetric hearing scenarios.

Author Contributions: Conceptualization, O.A. and L.R.; methodology, O.A.; software, O.A.; validation, C.M., S.C. and L.R.; formal analysis, O.A.; investigation, O.A.; resources, C.M.; data curation, S.C.; writing—original draft preparation, O.A.; writing—review and editing, L.R.; visualization, C.M. and S.C.; supervision, L.R.; project administration, O.A.; funding acquisition, L.R. All authors have read and agreed to the published version of the manuscript.

Funding: This research received no external funding.

Institutional Review Board Statement: This study was approved by the Institutional Ethics Committee of the University of Medicine and Pharmacy "Grigore T. Popa" Iași (no. 260/18 January 2023), granted for the doctoral research *"Rehabilitation with implantable devices for people with asymmetric hearing"*. The research was conducted ethically, with all study procedures performed in accordance with the requirements of the World Medical Association's Declaration of Helsinki.

Informed Consent Statement: Informed consent was obtained from all subjects involved in the study.

Data Availability Statement: The data are not publicly available due to institutional restrictions but may be provided by the corresponding author upon reasonable request and with permission from the hosting institution.

Acknowledgments: The authors would like to thank MED-EL for providing the equipment used for the localization ability assessment, as well as the dedicated statistical software. This support was offered in kind and did not involve any financial contribution.

Conflicts of Interest: The authors declare no conflicts of interest. MED-EL provided equipment and statistical software for the localization assessment only. MED-EL had no role in the design of the study; in the collection, analyses, or interpretation of data; in the writing of the manuscript; or in the decision to publish the results. The support was limited to localization testing and did not extend to other evaluation instruments used in the study.

Abbreviations

AHL	Asymmetric hearing loss
BCI	Bone conduction implant
CI	Cochlear implant
CROS	Contralateral routing of signals
dB HL	Decibel hearing level
dB SNR	Decibel signal-to-noise ratio
eABR	Electrically evoked auditory brainstem response
eALR	Electrically evoked auditory late response
HL	Hearing loss
MRI	Magnetic resonance imaging
PTA	Pure-tone average
RMS	Root mean square (localization error)
SPN	Speech-in-noise
SRT	Speech reception threshold
SSD	Single-sided deafness
SSQ12	Speech, Spatial, and Qualities of Hearing Scale–12-item version
TIN	Tinnitus score
VAS	Visual analog scale

S_0N_0	Speech and noise presented frontally (0° azimuth)
S_0N_AHL/SSD	Speech frontally, noise at impaired side (AHL/SSD)
S_AHL/SSD N_0	Speech at impaired side, noise frontally
S_AHL/SSD N_NH	Speech at impaired side, noise at normal-hearing ear
NAH	Normal-acoustic hearing ear (used in spatial test notation)

References

1. Van de Heyning, P.; Távora-Vieira, D.; Mertens, G. Towards a unified testing framework for single-sided deafness studies: A consensus paper. *Audiol. Neurotol.* **2017**, *21*, 391–398. [CrossRef]
2. Dillon, M.T.; Kocharyan, A.; Daher, G.S.; Carlson, M.L.; Shapiro, W.H.; Snapp, H.A.; Firszt, J.B. American Cochlear Implant Alliance Task Force Guidelines for Clinical Assessment and Management of Adult Cochlear Implantation for Single-Sided Deafness. *Ear Hear.* **2022**, *43*, 1605–1619. [CrossRef] [PubMed]
3. Kay-Rivest, E.; Irace, A.L.; Golub, J.S.; Svirsky, M.A. Prevalence of single-sided deafness in the United States. *Laryngoscope* **2022**, *132*, 1652–1656. [CrossRef]
4. Dhanasingh, A.; Hochmair, I. CI in single-sided deafness. *Acta Otolaryngol.* **2021**, *141* (Suppl. S1), 82–105. [CrossRef]
5. Zheng, Y.; Swanson, J.; Koehnke, J.; Guan, J. Sound localization of listeners with normal hearing, impaired hearing, hearing aids, bone-anchored hearing instruments, and cochlear implants: A review. *Am. J. Audiol.* **2022**, *31*, 819–834. [CrossRef] [PubMed]
6. Snapp, H.A.; Ausili, S.A. Hearing with one ear: Consequences and treatments for profound unilateral hearing loss. *J. Clin. Med.* **2020**, *9*, 1010. [CrossRef] [PubMed]
7. Lucas, L.; Katiri, R.; Kitterick, P.T. The psychological and social consequences of single-sided deafness in adulthood. *Int. J. Audiol.* **2017**, *57*, 21–30. [CrossRef]
8. Zeitler, D.M.; Dorman, M.F. Cochlear implantation for single-sided deafness: A new treatment paradigm. *J. Neurol. Surg. B Skull Base* **2019**, *80*, 178–186. [CrossRef]
9. Arndt, S.; Laszig, R.; Aschendorff, A.; Hassepass, F.; Beck, R.; Wesarg, T. Cochlear implant treatment of patients with single-sided deafness or asymmetric hearing loss. *HNO* **2017**, *65* (Suppl. S2), 98–108. [CrossRef]
10. Firszt, J.B.; Reeder, R.M.; Holden, L.K.; Dwyer, N.Y. Results in adult cochlear implant recipients with varied asymmetric hearing: A prospective longitudinal study of speech recognition, localization, and participant report. *Ear Hear.* **2018**, *39*, 845–862. [CrossRef]
11. Pantaleo, A.; Murri, A.; Cavallaro, G.; Pontillo, V.; Auricchio, D.; Quaranta, N. Single-sided deafness and hearing rehabilitation modalities: Contralateral routing of signal devices, bone conduction devices, and cochlear implants. *Brain Sci.* **2024**, *14*, 99. [CrossRef] [PubMed]
12. Ontario Health (Quality). Implantable devices for single-sided deafness and conductive or mixed hearing loss: A health technology assessment. *Ont. Health Technol. Assess. Ser.* **2020**, *20*, 1–165.
13. Donato, M.; Santos, R.; Correia, F.; Escada, P. Single-sided deafness: Bone conduction devices or cochlear implantation? A systematic review with meta-analysis. *Acta Otorrinolaringol.* **2020**, *72*, 101–108. [CrossRef] [PubMed]
14. Kitterick, P.T.; Smith, S.N.; Lucas, L. Hearing instruments for unilateral severe-to-profound sensorineural hearing loss in adults: A systematic review and meta-analysis. *Ear Hear.* **2016**, *37*, 495–507. [CrossRef] [PubMed]
15. Thompson, N.J.; Dillon, M.T.; Buss, E.; Rooth, M.A.; Richter, M.E.; Pillsbury, H.C.; Brown, K.D. Long-term improvement in localization for cochlear implant users with single-sided deafness. *Laryngoscope* **2022**, *132*, 2453–2458. [CrossRef]
16. Sullivan, C.B.; Al-Qurayshi, Z.; Zhu, V.; Liu, A.; Dunn, C.; Gantz, B.J.; Hansen, M.R. Long-term audiologic outcomes after cochlear implantation for single-sided deafness. *Laryngoscope* **2020**, *130*, 1805–1811. [CrossRef]
17. Speck, I.; Challier, P.; Wesarg, T.; Jakob, T.F.; Aschendorff, A.; Hassepass, F.; Arndt, S. Is the cochlear implant a successful long-term solution for single-sided deaf and asymmetric hearing-impaired patients? *Eur. Arch. Otorhinolaryngol.* **2021**, *278*, 3257–3265. [CrossRef]
18. Idriss, S.A.; Reynard, P.; Marx, M.; Mainguy, A.; Joly, C.-A.; Ionescu, E.C.; Assouly, K.K.S.; Thai-Van, H. Short- and long-term effect of cochlear implantation on disabling tinnitus in single-sided deafness patients: A systematic review. *J. Clin. Med.* **2022**, *11*, 5664. [CrossRef]
19. Mertens, G.; De Bodt, M.; Van de Heyning, P. Cochlear implantation as a long-term treatment for ipsilateral incapacitating tinnitus in subjects with unilateral hearing loss up to 10 years. *Hear. Res.* **2016**, *331*, 1–6. [CrossRef] [PubMed]
20. Oh, S.J.; Mavrommatis, M.A.; Fan, C.J.; DiRisio, A.C.; Villavisanis, D.F.; Berson, E.R.; Schwam, Z.G.; Wanna, G.B.; Cosetti, M.K. Cochlear implantation in adults with single-sided deafness: A systematic review and meta-analysis. *Otolaryngol. Head Neck Surg.* **2023**, *168*, 131–142. [CrossRef]
21. Daher, G.S.; Kocharyan, A.; Dillon, M.T.; Carlson, M.L. Cochlear implantation outcomes in adults with single-sided deafness: A systematic review and meta-analysis. *Otol. Neurotol.* **2023**, *44*, 297–309. [CrossRef] [PubMed]

22. Wazen, J.J.; Kim, C.S.; Ortega, C.; King, T.; Schwartz, S.R.; Zeitler, D.M. Benefits of unilateral cochlear implantation in adults with asymmetric hearing loss: Audiologic and patient-related outcome measures. *Am. J. Otolaryngol.* **2024**, *45*, 104138. [CrossRef] [PubMed]
23. Morelli, L.; Fancello, V.; Gaino, F.; Cagliero, G.; Caruso, A.; Sanna, M. Cochlear implantation in single-sided deafness: A single-center experience of 138 cases. *Eur. Arch. Otorhinolaryngol.* **2023**, *280*, 4427–4432. [CrossRef]
24. van Heteren, J.A.A.; Wendrich, A.W.; Peters, J.P.M.; Grolman, W.; Stokroos, R.J.; Smit, A.L. Speech perception in noise after cochlear implantation for single-sided deafness: A randomized clinical trial. *JAMA Otolaryngol. Head Neck Surg.* **2025**, *151*, 211. [CrossRef] [PubMed]
25. Sydlowski, S.A.; Farrokhian, N.; Carrozza, M.; Jamis, C.; Woodson, E. (Even off-label) cochlear implantation in single-sided deafness and asymmetric hearing loss results in measurable objective and subjective benefit. *Otol. Neurotol.* **2022**, *43*, e895–e902. [CrossRef]
26. Deep, N.L.; Spitzer, E.R.; Shapiro, W.H.; Waltzman, S.B.; Roland, J.T., Jr.; Friedmann, D.R. Cochlear implantation in adults with single-sided deafness: Outcomes and device use. *Otol. Neurotol.* **2021**, *42*, 414–423. [CrossRef]
27. Wesarg, T.; Kuntz, I.; Jung, L.; Wiebe, K.; Schatzer, R.; Brill, S.; Aschendorff, A.; Arndt, S. Masked speech perception with bone conduction device, contralateral routing of signals hearing aid, and cochlear implant use in adults with single-sided deafness: A prospective hearing device comparison using a unified testing framework. *Audiol. Neurotol.* **2024**, *29*, 271–289. [CrossRef]
28. Marx, M.; Mosnier, I.; Venail, F.; Mondain, M.; Uziel, A.; Bakhos, D.; Lescanne, E.; N'Guyen, Y.; Bernardeschi, D.; Sterkers, O.; et al. Cochlear implantation and other treatments in single-sided deafness and asymmetric hearing loss: Results of a national multicenter study including a randomized controlled trial. *Audiol. Neurotol.* **2021**, *26*, 414–424. [CrossRef]
29. Kurihara, S.; Ganaha, A.; Nakamura, T.; Kubuki, K.; Saruwatari, E.; Matsui, K.; Takahashi, K.; Tono, T. Pros and cons of a bone-conduction device implanted in the worse hearing ear of patients with asymmetric hearing loss. *Front. Audiol. Otol.* **2024**, *2*, 1362443. [CrossRef]
30. Usami, S.-I.; Kitoh, R.; Moteki, H.; Nishio, S.-Y.; Kitano, T.; Kobayashi, M.; Watanabe, K. Etiology of single-sided deafness and asymmetrical hearing loss. *Acta Oto-Laryngol.* **2017**, *137* (Suppl. S565), S2–S7. [CrossRef]
31. Arndt, S.; Prosse, S.; Laszig, R.; Wesarg, T.; Aschendorff, A.; Hassepass, F. Cochlear implantation in children with single-sided deafness: Does aetiology and duration of deafness matter? *Audiol. Neurotol.* **2015**, *20* (Suppl. S1), 21–30. [CrossRef] [PubMed]
32. Dewyer, N.A.; Smith, S.; Herrmann, B.; Reinshagen, K.L.; Lee, D.J. Pediatric single-sided deafness: A review of prevalence, radiologic findings, and cochlear implant candidacy. *Ann. Otol. Rhinol. Laryngol.* **2022**, *131*, 233–238. [CrossRef]
33. Santopietro, G.; Fancello, V.; Fancello, G.; Bianchini, C.; Pelucchi, S.; Ciorba, A. Cochlear implantation in children affected by single-sided deafness: A comprehensive review. *Audiol. Res.* **2024**, *14*, 77–85. [CrossRef] [PubMed]
34. Benchetrit, L.; Ronner, E.A.; Anne, S.; Cohen, M.S. Cochlear implantation in children with single-sided deafness: A systematic review and meta-analysis. *JAMA Otolaryngol. Head Neck Surg.* **2021**, *147*, 58–69. [CrossRef] [PubMed]
35. Hamed, N.; Alajmi, N.; Alkoblan, F.I.; Alghtani, Y.A.; Abdelsamad, Y.; Alhussien, A.; Alhajress, R.I.; Alhabib, S.F. The chronological evolution of cochlear implant contraindications: A comprehensive review. *J. Clin. Med.* **2024**, *13*, 2337. [CrossRef]
36. Kurz, A.; Rak, K.; Hagen, R.; Ehrmann-Müller, D. Evaluating the decision for cochlear implantation in individuals with single-sided deafness (SSD): Implementing the SSD consensus protocol into clinical routine. *Otol. Neurotol.* **2020**, *41*, 727–735. [CrossRef]
37. Blamey, P.; Artieres, F.; Başkent, D.; Bergeron, F.; Beynon, A.; Burke, E.; Dillier, N.; Dowell, R.; Fraysse, B.; Gallégo, S.; et al. Factors affecting auditory performance of postlinguistically deaf adults using cochlear implants: An update with 2251 patients. *Audiol Neurotol.* **2013**, *18*, 36–47. [CrossRef]
38. Johnson, B.R.; Dillon, M.T.; Thompson, N.J.; Richter, M.E.; Overton, A.B.; Rooth, M.A.; Davis, A.G.; Dedmon, M.M.; Selleck, A.M.; Brown, K.D. Benefits of cochlear implantation for older adults with asymmetric hearing loss. *Laryngoscope* **2025**, *135*, 352–360. [CrossRef]
39. Peters, J.P.M.; van Heteren, J.A.A.; Wendrich, A.W.; van Zanten, G.A.; Grolman, W.; Stokroos, R.J.; Smit, A.L. Short-term outcomes of cochlear implantation for single-sided deafness compared to bone conduction devices and contralateral routing of sound hearing aids: Results of a randomised controlled trial (CINGLE-trial). *PLoS ONE* **2021**, *16*, e0258610. [CrossRef]
40. van Heteren, J.A.A.; van Oorschot, H.D.; Wendrich, A.W.; Peters, J.P.M.; Rhebergen, K.S.; Grolman, W.; Stokroos, R.J.; Smit, A.L. Sound localization in single-sided deafness: Outcomes of a randomized controlled trial on the comparison between cochlear implantation, bone conduction devices, and contralateral routing of signals hearing aids. *Trends Hear.* **2024**, *28*, 23312165241287092. [CrossRef]
41. Marx, M.; Mounié, M.; Mosnier, I.; Venail, F.; Mondain, M.; Uziel, A.; Bakhos, D.; Lescanne, E.; N'guyen, Y.; Bernardeschi, D.; et al. Cost-utility of cochlear implantation in single-sided deafness and asymmetric hearing loss: Results of a randomized controlled trial. *Eur. J. Health Econ.* 2024, *in press*.

42. Lindquist, N.R.; Holder, J.T.; Patro, A.; Cass, N.D.; Tawfik, K.O.; O'Malley, M.R.; Bennett, M.L.; Haynes, D.S.; Gifford, R.H.; Perkins, E.L. Cochlear implants for single-sided deafness: Quality of life, daily usage, and duration of deafness. *Laryngoscope* **2023**, *133*, 2362–2370. [CrossRef]
43. Lee, S.W.; Yuen, H.W.; Low, D.; Kamath, S.; Chua, K.W.D. The functional impact of implantable hearing devices in patients with single-sided deafness. *Proc. Singapore Healthc.* **2023**, *32*. [CrossRef]
44. Katiri, R.; Hall, D.A.; Hoare, D.J.; Fackrell, K.; Horobin, A.; Hogan, N.; Buggy, N.; Van de Heyning, P.H.; Firszt, J.B.; Bruce, I.A.; et al. The Core Rehabilitation Outcome Set for Single-Sided Deafness (CROSSSD) study: International consensus on outcome measures for trials of interventions for adults with single-sided deafness. *Trials* **2022**, *23*, 764. [CrossRef]
45. Távora-Vieira, D.; Rajan, G.P.; Van de Heyning, P.; Mertens, G. Evaluating the long-term hearing outcomes of cochlear implant users with single-sided deafness. *Otol. Neurotol.* **2019**, *40*, e575–e580. [CrossRef]
46. Polterauer, D.; Mandruzzato, G.; Neuling, M.; Polak, M.; Müller, J.; Hempel, J.M. Evaluation of auditory pathway excitability using a pre-operative trans-tympanic electrically evoked auditory brainstem response under local anesthesia in cochlear implant candidates. *Int. J. Audiol.* **2023**, *62*, 1176–1186. [CrossRef]
47. Radeloff, A.; Shehata-Dieler, W.; Rak, K.; Müller, L.; Schmidt, J.; Knorr, S.; Wagner, I.; Dietz, A.; Huber, A.; Fuchs, C.; et al. Intraoperative monitoring using electrically evoked auditory brainstem responses (eABR) in cochlear implant surgery: Clinical experience. *Otol Neurotol.* **2021**, *42*, e287–e293.
48. Hempel, J.M.; Zimmermann, L.; Arnoldner, C.; Dhanasingh, A.; Polterauer, D.; Müller, J. Influence of cochlear coverage on speech perception in single sided deafness, bimodal, and bilateral implanted cochlear implant patients. *Eur. Arch. Otorhinolaryngol.* **2024**, *281*, 5197–5206. [CrossRef]
49. Roger, E.; Smith, Z.; Tan, A.; Keller, M. Predicting hearing aid outcomes using machine learning. *Audiol. Neurotol.* **2025**, *30*, 101–110. [CrossRef]
50. Mertens, G.; Desloovere, C.; De Bodt, M.; Van de Heyning, P. Tinnitus and audiological outcomes after cochlear implantation in patients with single-sided deafness. *Otol. Neurotol.* **2016**, *37*, 38–43.
51. An, Y.H.; Ahn, J.H.; Han, J.J.; Hong, Y.T.; Chung, J.W. Impact of hearing aid use on cochlear implant outcomes in adults with asymmetric hearing loss. *Int. Arch. Otorhinolaryngol.* **2022**, *26*, e541–e547. [CrossRef]

audiology research

MDPI

Article

Renewed Concept of Mastoid Cavity Obliteration with the Use of Temporoparietal Fascial Flap Injected by Injectable Platelet-Rich Fibrin after Subtotal Petrosectomy for Cochlear Implant Patients

Aleksander Zwierz [1,*], Krystyna Masna [1], Paweł Burduk [1], Stephan Hackenberg [2] and Matthias Scheich [2]

[1] Department of Otolaryngology, Phoniatrics and Audiology, Faculty of Health Sciences, Ludwik Rydygier Collegium Medicum, Nicolaus Copernicus University, 85-067 Bydgoszcz, Poland; krymasna@gmail.com (K.M.); pburduk@wp.pl (P.B.)

[2] Department of Otorhinolaryngology, Plastic, Aesthetic and Reconstructive Head and Neck Surgery, University Hospital Würzburg, 97080 Würzburg, Germany; hackenberg_s@ukw.de (S.H.); scheich_m@ukw.de (M.S.)

* Correspondence: aleksanderzwierz@gmail.com

Abstract: Background: The subtotal petrosectomy procedure may be useful for cochlear implantation in selected patient groups. Although it is highly effective, complications can arise, which may have economic implications for the patient due to the high cost of the device. Therefore, several authors have attempted to identify the most effective concept for obliteration. **Methods:** We present a pilot descriptive study of application techniques for obliterating cavities after subtotal petrosectomy using a temporoparietal fascial flap (TPFF) modified with injectable platelet-rich fibrin (IPRF+) for three cochlear implant (CI) patients. **Results:** Our concept preserves important anatomical structures, such as the temporalis muscle, which covers the CI receiver–stimulator. Injection of IPRF+ also increases the available tissue volume for obliteration and enhances its anti-inflammatory and regenerative potential. **Conclusions:** To the best of our knowledge, the use of TPFF for filling the cavity has not been adopted for CI with SP and for blind sac closure. Our literature review and our experience with this small group of patients suggest that this procedure, when combined with IPRF+ injections, may reduce the risk of potential infection in the obliterated cavity, particularly when used with CI. This technique is applicable only in cases when the surgeons are convinced that the middle ear cavity is purged of cholesteatoma.

Keywords: subtotal petrosectomy; cochlear implant; obliteration; temporoparietal facial flap; IPRF

1. Introduction

Cochlear implantation via the trans-mastoid approach through the facial recess has become the standard procedure for treating patients with profound sensorineural hearing loss. However, there is a dispute among researchers regarding the management of chronic ear discharge with or without cholesteatoma. The debate centers on whether to eradicate the underlying pathology, cover the electrode, and leave the cavity open, or to perform other challenging approaches, such as via the middle cranial fossa or through subtotal petrosectomy (SP) [1,2]. Szymański, in particular, reviewed the results of "covering techniques" performed by Olgun and Roehm. These techniques involved wrapping the electrode cable into the patient's dense tissues and resulted in a major complication rate of 14–19%, mainly due to electrode cable disruption. Therefore, he strongly discouraged the use of these techniques [2]. Moreover, he did not recommend the use of "bypass techniques" and electrode insertion from the diseased middle ear [2]. The only recommended technique was subtotal petrosectomy performed with external auditory canal (EAC) closure, since it isolates and seals the surgical cavity from the external environment, consequently leading to a lower risk of infection and CSF leak prevention, as well as providing a good exposure of the round window [3].

Bone dust, abdominal fat, cartilage, muscle, local flaps, and hydroxyapatite, among other things, have been used to fill the cavity in the SP procedure [4]. Since all these obliterative materials vary in the scope of available volume, vascularity, resorption rate, scarring, and damage to the donor site, identifying their advantages and disadvantages may help determine their indication of use.

A one-stage cochlear implant (CI) implantation within an infected middle ear cavity, affected by a chronic inflammatory process, necessitates a scrupulous cleansing of the inflammatory cavity. Additionally, it requires the utilization of tissues endowed with a robust blood supply, preferably local flaps, to effectively obliterate the cavity. In this context, the temporoparietal fascial flap (TPFF) emerges as an optimal choice. Positioned in close proximity to the ear cavity, the TPFF boasts a vascular pedicle arrangement conducive to rotational adjustments without compromising vascular flow. Notably, the TPFF is distinguished by its status as the thinnest pedunculated flap in humans, and its harvesting is devoid of any visible tissue defects [5].

To enhance the regenerative potential of this procedure, we incorporated injectable platelet-rich fibrin (IPRF+), an agent manifesting significant clinical utility. The advantageous impact of IPRF+ on expediting wound healing, mitigating postoperative hematoma, edema, and pain, and even addressing connective tissue defects is substantiated by a myriad of studies across diverse medical domains [6]. Its widespread application spans dermatology, where it is utilized for skin regeneration and the treatment of various wounds, exerting influence on angiogenesis and facilitating skin recovery post-irradiation [7–10]. The angiogenic properties of IPRF extend its utility to enhancing the survival of free skin grafts and fostering muscle regeneration [11,12]. IPRF has found extensive application in dentistry, with numerous studies attesting to its superiority in treating gingival recession, interdental deficiencies, and promoting healing after flap harvesting [13,14]. Furthermore, the antimicrobial activity of IPRF, as affirmed by Straub's study, adds another layer of efficacy to its multifaceted utility [15].

IPRF+ administration, being a time-efficient and cost-effective procedure, holds the potential to significantly influence treatment outcomes. Thus, in the pursuit of augmenting the effectiveness of postoperative healing, achieving the requisite tissue volume to fill the entire postoperative cavity with a flap, and preempting infections, we judiciously employed a temporoparietal fascial flap injected with IPRF+.

2. Materials and Methods

Herein, we present our concept of cochlear implantation in cases of SP procedure with cavity obliteration using the temporoparietal fascial flap (TPFF) (Byrd, 1980) augmented with injectable platelet-rich fibrin (IPRF+). The technique was used in three patients in the last 2 years. The affirmative feedback received thus far urged us to present a pilot descriptive study of implementation of this surgical treatment.

Initially, receiver–stimulator placement was planned on the skin. A wide retroauricular incision was then made, and a continued vertical incision was traced from the root of the helix towards the superior temporal line. The incision was lined up to the superior margin of the planned TPFF, based on both the parietal and frontal branches of the superficial temporal artery (STA), as identified by Doppler imaging or by palpation. Usually, the STA is located 2 cm superiorly and anteriorly from the EAC, running along with one or two veins located above the artery. The skin incision was then carried down to the TPFF and the mastoid periosteum. After identification of the EAC posterior wall, a C-shaped periosteal flap was created 5 mm posterior from the EAC, and a posteriorly horizontal incision along the linea temporalis was performed. Following this, the periosteal flaps were prepared, and a subperiosteal pocket for the receiver–stimulator was created. The mastoid and middle ear cavity were then cleared from the pathological tissue by mastoidectomy with complete exenteration of pneumatic cells and identification of the vertical facial nerve segment. Afterwards, the facial recess was opened, and if present, the incudostapedial joint was disconnected. The skin of the posterior and anterior external auditory bony canal was horizontally incised and lifted, and the posterior canal wall with the tympanic membrane, malleus, and incus were removed. After removing the underlying pathology and all of the middle ear mucosa, the Eustachian tube was obliterated with the free muscle tissue, and the skin of the EAC was everted in its ostium and then sutured with 3-0 absorbable sutures, supported by the inverted cartilage of the EAC. Following this, the TPFF was prepared. The anterior and posterior scalp flaps were elevated through meticulous sharp dissection in the subdermal plane, taking care to continue the dissection slightly below the hair follicles to leave a thin layer of subcutaneous fibrofatty tissue to prevent local alopecia. The STA was then identified 0.5–1 cm anterior to the root of the helix, and the dissection was continued peripherally along the vessel to prepare the entire area of the flap. Afterwards, the flap was raised caudally from the loose areolar tissue and was tailored to enter the open cavity in the anterior–superior direction (Figure 1). Subsequently, the round window niche was identified, the round window was exposed, the receiver–stimulator was fixed, the round window was opened, the electrode was inserted into the cochlea, and then the opening was sealed. Moreover, prior to insertion, 10 mL of blood was collected in each of the six sterile IPRF+ 13 mL tubes, and underwent centrifugation at 700 rpm for 5 min (Duo Quattro PRF centrifuge). Following this, the superficial part of the liquid was taken using a syringe, which gave approximately 8 mL of IPRF+. The TPFF was then evenly injected with IPRF+ and rotated so that IPRF+ filled the entire cavity. After approximately 20 min of stiffness, the temporalis muscle, periosteal flap, subcutaneous tissue, and skin were all sutured. Lastly, pressure dressing was applied for 48 h.

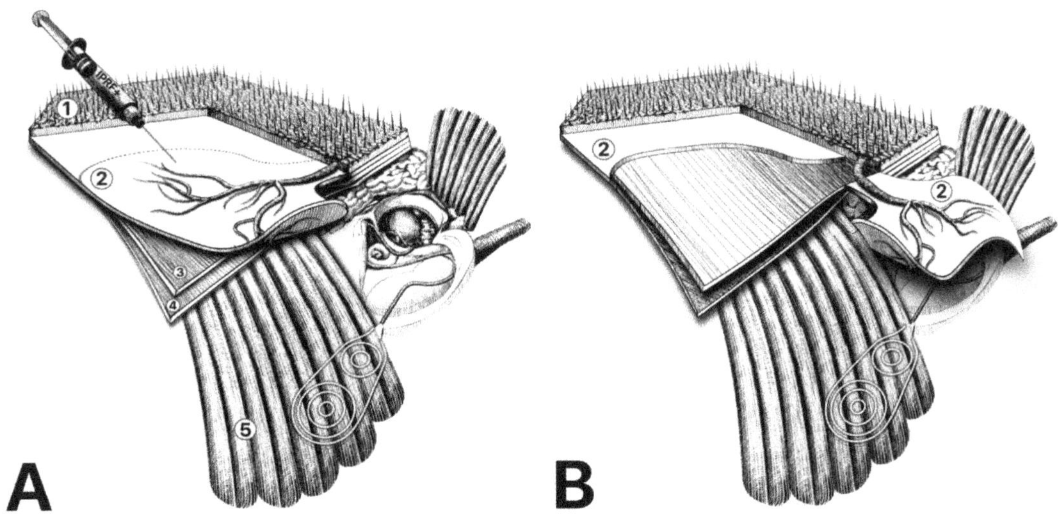

Figure 1. (**A**) Flap preparation and IPRF+ injection. Anatomic layers of the temporoparietal region: 1—skin and subcutaneous tissue, 2—temporoparietal fascia, 3—loose areolar tissue, 4—temporalis muscle fascia, 5—temporalis muscle. (**B**) Temporoparietal fascial flap rotated into subtotal petrosectomy cavity.

3. Results

3.1. Case 1

A 59-year-old man was admitted to our clinic with a history of bilateral chronic otitis media with cholesteatoma. His right ear was operated on many years ago and a canal wall down procedure was performed. The inflammation caused deafness in the right ear with cochlear ossification (Figure 2). After many years, left-side cholesteatoma gradually destroyed the left ear, impaired the hearing, and finally caused complete deafness. We performed left-side SP with mastoid cavity obliteration with a temporoparietal fascial flap injected by injectable platelet-rich fibrin and a one-stage CI procedure. A full insertion with the cochlear implant placed in the scala tympani was achieved (Figure 3). After rehabilitation, the patient developed audiological performance of open-set word testing with the range of 90%. We present very good aesthetic results of the obliteration obtained by the usage of TPFF injected with IPRF+ (Figure 4). We did not observe any complications within period of 15 months.

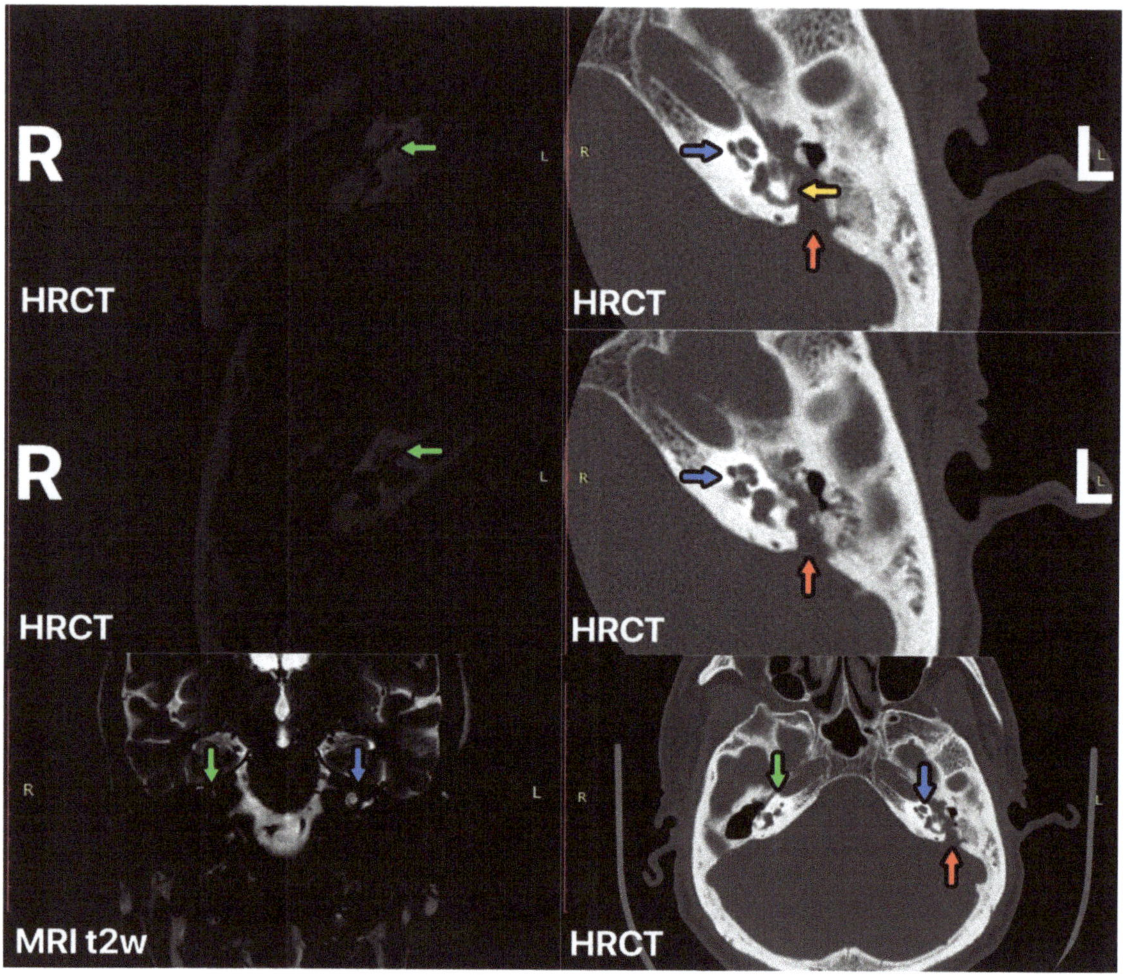

Figure 2. HRCT and MRI of the ear before SP surgery. Right cochlear ossification—green arrow, left cochlear—blue arrow, posterior fossa destruction by cholesteatoma—red arrow, lateral semicircular canal destruction—yellow arrow.

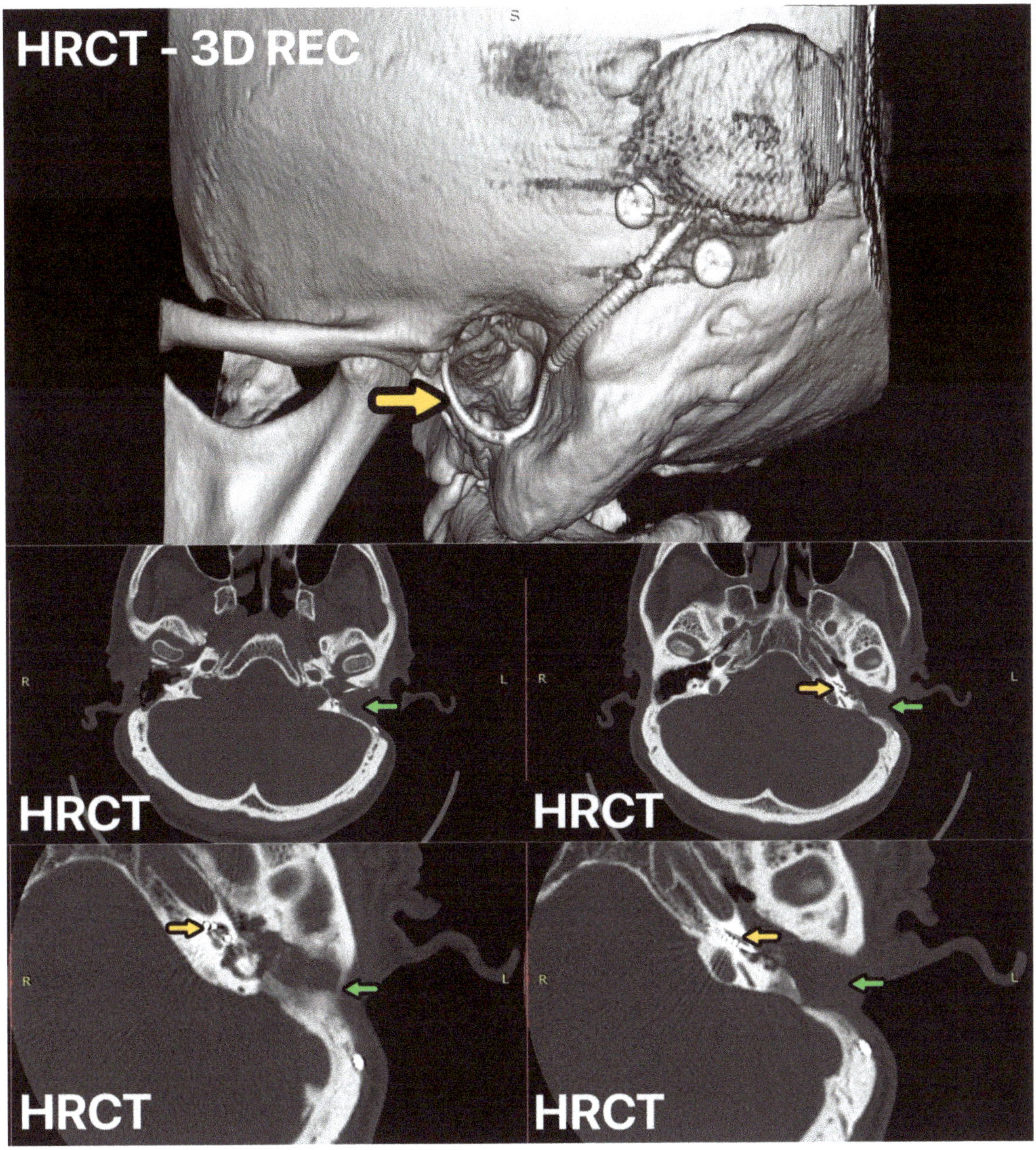

Figure 3. HRCT of the left ear 12 months after surgery, CI electrode—yellow arrow, mastoid cavity obliterated with temporoparietal fascial flap (TPFF) injected with injectable platelet-rich fibrin (IPRF+)—green arrow.

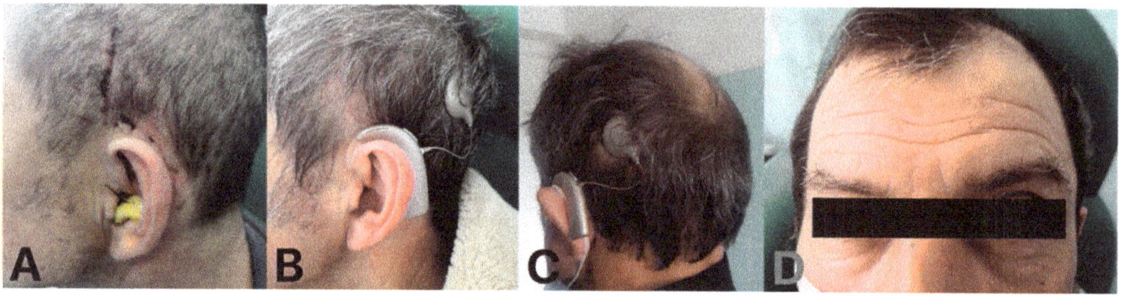

Figure 4. (**A**) Patient #1 after 3 weeks, (**B**,**C**) after 12 months, (**D**) full symmetry of the head.

3.2. Case 2

A 68-year-old man, who had experienced bilateral deafness, was admitted to the clinic. Several years prior, he had undergone surgery on his right ear due to chronic otitis media with cholesteatoma. The procedure involved a canal wall down ear surgery and tympanic membrane reconstruction; however, ossiculoplasty was not performed during this operation (Figure 5). At that time, the patient had already developed right-sided conductive hearing loss in the right ear, which was effectively managed with a hearing aid. He experienced progressive bilateral sensorineural hearing loss, rendering bilateral hearing aids ineffective for a period of 4 years. There was stated discharge from the right ear but without cholesteatoma recurrence. As a result, the patient became a candidate for right-sided cochlear implantation. A one-stage procedure was executed, involving subtotal petrosectomy and cochlear implantation. A temporoparietal fascial flap obliteration with augmentation using injectable platelet-rich fibrin was also performed during the procedure (Figure 6). The postoperative course proceeded without complications, characterized by rapid tissue healing and the absence of fistulas or wound-related inflammation.

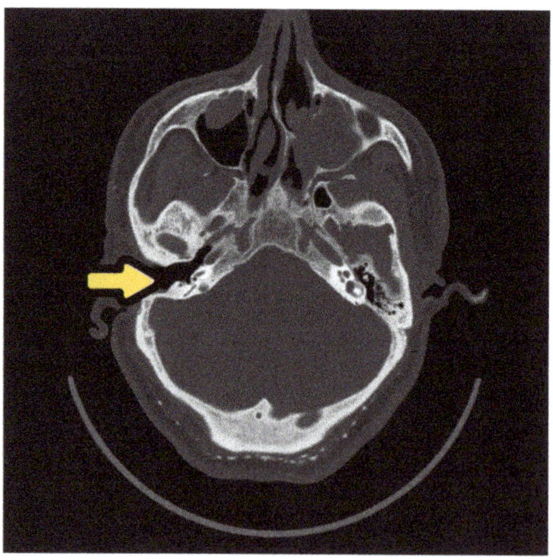

Figure 5. HRCT of the ear before SP and CI procedure. Open right-ear cavity after first ear surgery—yellow arrow.

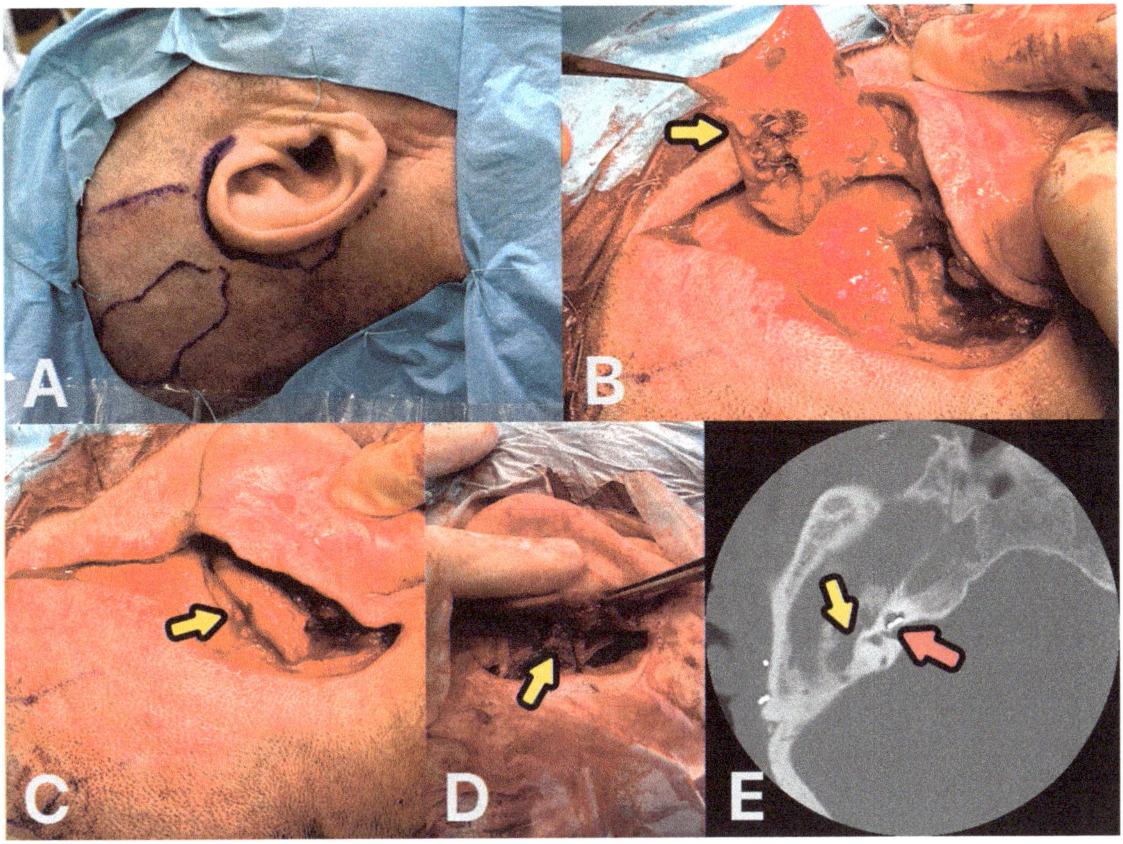

Figure 6. Surgical steps of the obliteration. (**A**) Planning of the surgery. (**B**) Harvesting of the temporoparietal fascial flap—yellow arrow. (**C**) Temporoparietal fascial flap rotated to subtotal petrosectomy cavity—yellow arrow. (**D**) Ear closing—yellow arrow. (**E**) Control CT scan 12 months after surgery, obliterated cavity—yellow arrow. CI electrode in the cochlea—red arrow.

3.3. Case 3

A 69-year-old man sought admission to the clinic due to sudden right-sided deafness and dizziness that had persisted for two months. Computed tomography revealed the presence of an extensive cholesteatoma in the tympanic cavity and mastoid region, with associated destruction of the lateral semicircular canal, categorizing it as a type III labyrinth fistula according to the Dornhoffer and Milewski classification (Figure 7). Given the potential risk of cochlear fibrosis subsequent to cholesteatoma removal from the lateral semicircular canal, a one-stage surgical intervention was planned. This consisted of a lateral petrosectomy with obliteration using a temporoparietal fascial flap (TPFF) augmented with 2 mL of injectable platelet-rich fibrin (IPRF+), along with simultaneous cochlear implantation (Figure 7). In this case as well, healing progressed properly, and the patient rapidly gained the ability to utilize the cochlear implant.

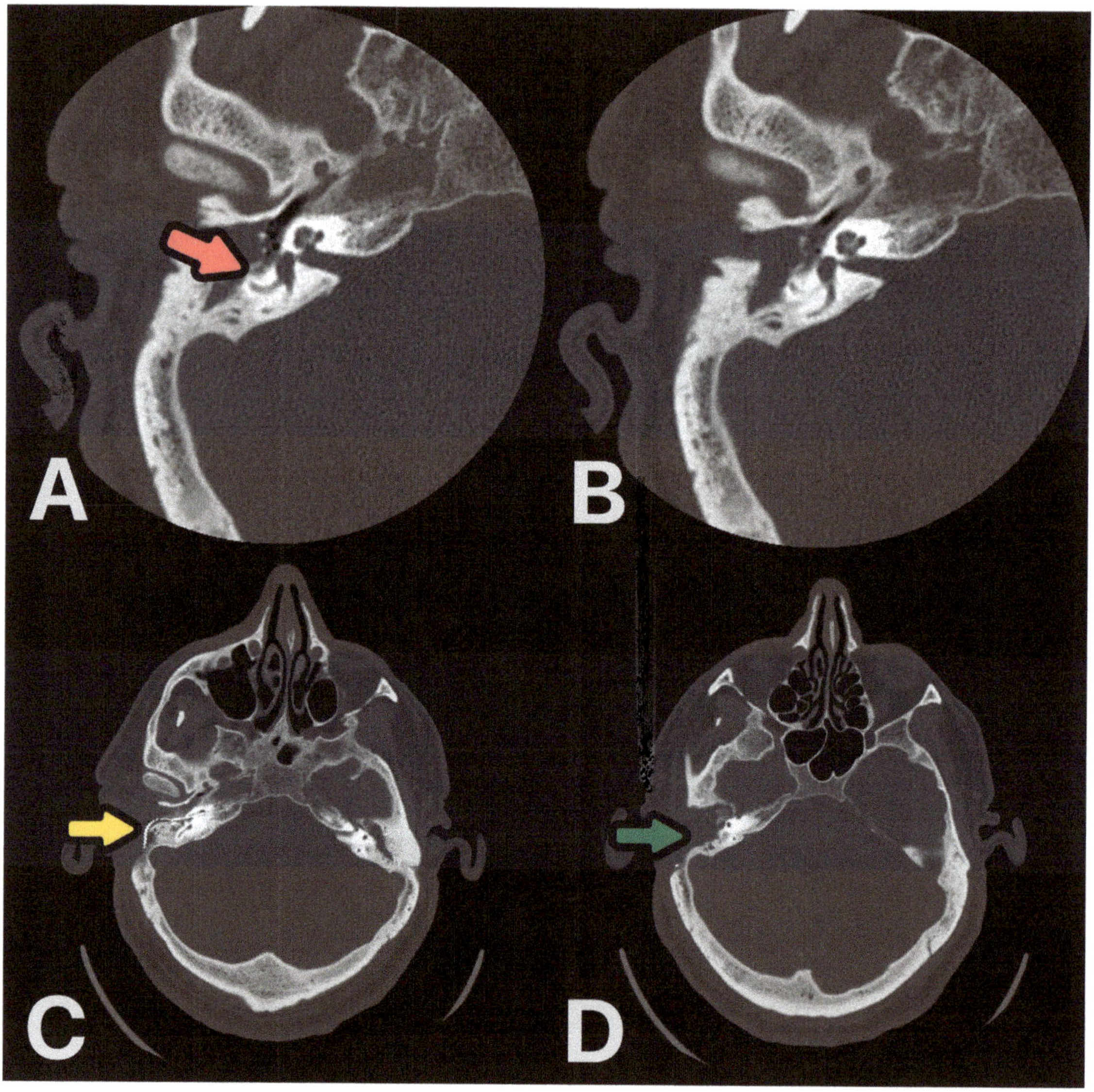

Figure 7. (**A**,**B**) HRCT scans before surgery: destruction of the lateral semicircular canal and posterior canal wall—magenta arrow. (**C**,**D**) Control HRCT scans 6 months after procedure: CI electrode—yellow arrow, ear obliterated—green arrow.

It is particularly important to precisely remove the pathology in order to minimize the risk of cholesteatoma recurrence. In each of the described cases, we were convinced during the surgery that the cholesteatoma was completely removed; if this was not the case, we were always prepared to put a dummy electrode and perform the procedure in two stages. All patients are still under our medical supervision.

4. Discussion

The idea of subtotal petrosectomy for pathological ear treatment has been established for the past few decades. It was first described by Mosher in 1911; its concept was then retaken and modified by Rambo in 1958, was finally named by Ugo Fisch in 1965, and was further modified by other famous and experienced ear surgeons, such as Gacek and Palva [4]. Notably, the procedure described by Rambo did not involve closure of the external auditory canal, since he explained that its closure minimizes ear discharge. With these developments over the years, SP has become an effective method for eliminating recurrent ear infections, removing large tumors, obliterating the middle ear and mastoid, and eliminating the possibility of intracranial spread from infections, always with the possibility of CI implantations in difficult cases [4].

Regarding the filling used for SP, Rambo reported the use of the temporalis muscle for obliteration, while in 1976, Gacek presented the use of abdominal fat and an inferiorly based muscle pedicle [4]. Brizgalis suggested that the temporalis muscle flaps in SP need to be small enough to allow overfilling of the large cavity to compensate for its gradual postoperative shrinkage [1]. However, Bartells has reported complaints of severe pain above the ear and cases of necrosis following temporalis muscle flap creation [16]. On the other hand, free tissue grafts, such as abdominal fat, cartilage or bony palate, lack vascularity and are subject to resorption [17]. Particularly, Yung noted postoperative infections and fat necrosis in a number of patients obliterated with abdominal fat [18], which was consistent with our findings and that of other studies. Moreover, Bernardeschi reported that 8% of minor complications at the donor site were abdominal hematomas [19]. Giulia D'Angelo similarly presented one case of seroma and one case of hematoma in 32 patients who underwent SP with abdominal fat grafting [20]. In these cases, other sources of free grafts are recommended as an alternative, such as fat or temporalis muscle. In 1996, Chenay introduced an interesting concept of using the pedicled TPFF for cavity obliteration in the SP procedure [21]. TPFF has been found to have a beneficial effect on the healing and acceptance of free skin grafts for mastoid obliteration due to its resistance to bending and compression as a result of the large diameter of the pedicle vessels [17,22]. Therefore, based on the results of Chenay and Yung, the author of this article used TPFF for obliteration after the SP procedure [18,21]. However, problems regarding the flap's maximal evaluable volume for cavity obliteration and postoperative muscle shrinkage were noted. The TPFF, in particular, has a flat surface (150 cm^2) and is the thinnest in the human body pedicle flap (2 mm), only providing a volume of 30 mL, which may be a limitation for its use. For this reason, we used up to 8 mL IPRF+ injections to increase the flap volume, given its high vascularity and regenerative ability [23]. IPRF+ is a second-generation, fully autologous, blood-derived biomaterial with a three-dimensional fibrin meshwork that is widely used in dentistry, dermatology, and orthopaedics [24]. Furthermore, IPRF+ preparation is easy and requires a basic instrument set without biochemical blood handling [25]. IPRF+ is widely used due to its high regenerative potential from its plates and lymphocytes, which deliver growth factors. Moreover, it consists of type-1 collagen, making it useful in various surgical conditions [24,26], and its anti-inflammatory role in wound healing is also essential for postsurgical recovery [27]. In summary, it is important to note the advantages and disadvantages of the commonly used SP obliteration materials. Although fat has a high volume, it has poor vascularization and has a tendency for inflammation and absorption (Figure 8). On the other hand, the temporalis muscle flap has a lower volume availability that is needed for rotation, which creates a situation of incomplete coverage of the receiver–stimulator. The flap also has a tendency to shrink, but it has good vascularity, providing efficient anti-inflammatory resistance. Lastly, TPFF injected with IPRF+ demonstrates all the advantages of these two reconstructive materials, while providing the best cosmetic effect.

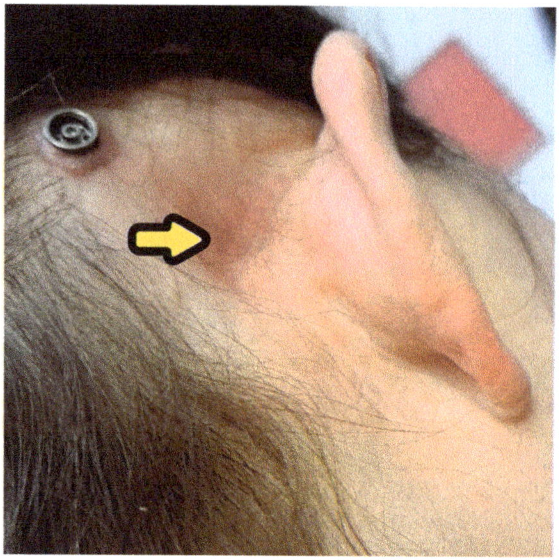

Figure 8. Patient 12 months after SP with external auditory canal closure and fat obliteration. Yellow arrow shows a depression caused by absorption of fat.

The first cases of SP and cochlear implantation were reported by Bendet and Issing in 1998 [28,29]. SP and CI placements are especially useful in the treatment of chronic ear disease with or without cholesteatoma, cerebrospinal fluid (CSF) leakage, middle and inner ear malformations, cochlear obliteration, and ossifications requiring partial drilling in cases of difficult insertion [2,4,30]. Szymański, in accordance with Fisch's teaching techniques, proposed two variants of surgery, depending on whether the ear has been previously operated or not [2]. In unoperated patients, the gap was closed using fat covered with free fascia graft from the temporalis muscle and the musculoperiosteal flap. For previously operated patients, fat coverage using the temporalis muscle rotated inferiorly was recommended [2]. Despite the good results in the second patient group, the receiver–stimulator was not completely covered by the temporalis muscle, which may have possibly impacted the extrusion of the receiver–stimulator. Moreover, although Polo reported a low rate of major complications (6.37%) in 110 cases of SP and CI insertion performed by the Grupo Otologico in Piazenza [3], a reduction of this incidence should be attempted, both for the patient's health and for the economic burden due to the cost of the device. Specifically, the major complications of SP and CI included fat infection, sac closure breakdown, entrapped cholesteatoma, and extrusion of the CI electrode or the receiver–stimulator [31]. If these procedures are performed with care, external canal skin closure would prevent its breakdown. This is equally important in second-layer closure with cartilage, which was performed using the Grupo Otologico principles, resulting to no cases of blind sac breakdown [32,33]. In contrast, Leung reported one case of blind sac breakdown among 17 patients who underwent Melbourne SP procedures, emphasizing again the importance of performing with care [30]. Additionally, meticulous surgical techniques have reduced the risk of cholesteatoma recurrence in SP to 1.5% [4], which is less in comparison to that of the canal wall down procedure (1.5–15%), as described by Prasad. In Leung's and D'Angelo's SP patients with CI, cholesteatoma recurrence was not observed; however, the follow-up periods were too short to reach a definitive conclusion in both studies [20,30]. In contrast to these studies, Altunia reported an 8% complication rate of fat inflammation that required CI removal [31]. Given these reported complications, the proposed obliteration with well-vascularized TPFF and IPRF+ injections should reduce the incidence of inflammation and accelerate the healing process. Furthermore, device migration and exposure may occur, moving or rotating the temporalis muscle flap and resulting in complications. This was seen in Leung, who strongly preferred temporalis muscle flap obliteration, reporting one case of potential exposure among the 17 reported operations [30]. Interestingly, Hernandez proposed the application of the other concepts in three of his cases [33]. In his attempt to avoid all complications related to obliteration, he proposed a controversial technique of SP and CI with ear canal and Eustachian tube obliteration, but without mastoid obliteration [34].

The use of the presented technique in all of the above cases resulted in favorable outcomes, with complete ear obliteration achieved without postoperative infections or wound breakdowns. As a result, middle-ear pathology was successfully resolved, cochlear implants were securely positioned, hearing was restored, there was no evidence of head asymmetry, and a satisfactory cosmetic outcome was achieved. During the different periods of treated patient observation, from 9 to 15 months, we did not observe the occurrence of severe symptoms such as headache and local soft tissue inflammation, which may indicate a possible recurrence of cholesteatoma. We scheduled a follow-up MRI 1.5 T (Non-Echo Planar Diffusion-Weighted Imaging) 1.5 years after the procedure, bearing in mind that MRI scans are sometimes deteriorated by artifacts and had limited applicability on the CI side [35].

5. Conclusions

To the best of our knowledge, the concept of using TPFF to fill the cavity has not been adopted for CI with SP and for blind sac closure. The combination of this procedure with IPRF+ injections may reduce the risk of potential infection in the obliterated cavity, which is especially important when the procedure is performed with CI. Our concept preserves important anatomical structures such as the temporalis muscle, which covers the CI receiver–stimulator and may prevent extrusion complications. Injection of IPRF+ also seems to increase the volume of tissue available for obliteration and enhances its anti-inflammatory and regenerative potential. Compared to the use of fat, TPFF with IPRF+ injections may reduce the incidence of necrosis, tissue absorption, and poor cosmetic effects, such as retro auricular holes and abdominal scars. Moreover, raising of the TPFF, the thinnest pedicled flap, does not change the shape of the head (Figure 4).

In addition, obliteration with TPFF and IPRF+ injections may still be used in patients who had previously undergone ear surgery with other local muscular obliteration, including Palva flaps and superiorly or inferiorly based muscular pedicle flaps [21,23].

It should be emphasised that this technique is applicable only in the case when the surgeons are convinced that middle ear cavity is purged of cholesteatoma.

Author Contributions: Conceptualization, A.Z.; methodology, A.Z.; software, A.Z.; validation, P.B., formal analysis, A.Z. and M.S.; investigation, A.Z.; resources, A.Z. and K.M.; data curation, K.M.; writing—original draft preparation, A.Z.; writing—review and editing, A.Z. and MS.; visualization, K.M.; supervision, P.B. and S.H.; project administration, P.B. All authors have read and agreed to the published version of the manuscript.

Funding: This research received no external funding.

Institutional Review Board Statement: This article describes the stage of the case at the time of treatment adopted in accordance with current standards. Consent from the Ethics Committee was not required.

Informed Consent Statement: Informed consent was obtained from all subjects involved in the study.

Data Availability Statement: All data are available for request.

Acknowledgments: We would like to thank Martyna Pszenniak for graphics. Special thanks to Renata Skowrońska from the Polish Historical Mission in Würzburg for supporting the cochlear implant development program in the Department of Otolaryngology, Phoniatrics and Audiology,

Faculty of Health Sciences, Ludwik Rydygier Collegium Medicum, Nicolaus Copernicus University, Bydgoszcz, Poland.

Conflicts of Interest: The authors declare no conflicts of interest.

References

1. Birzgalis, A.R.; Farrington, W.T.; O'Keefe, L. Reconstruction of Discharging Mastoid Cavities Using the Temporalis Myofascial Flap. *Clin. Otolaryngol. Allied Sci.* **1994**, *19*, 70–72. [CrossRef]
2. Szymański, M.; Ataide, A.; Linder, T. The Use of Subtotal Petrosectomy in Cochlear Implant Candidates with Chronic Otitis Media. *Eur. Arch. Otorhinolaryngol.* **2016**, *273*, 363–370. [CrossRef]
3. Polo, R.; Del Mar Medina, M.; Arístegui, M.; Lassaletta, L.; Gutierrez, A.; Aránguez, G.; Prasad, S.C.; Alonso, A.; Gavilán, J.; Sanna, M. Subtotal Petrosectomy for Cochlear Implantation: Lessons Learned After 110 Cases. *Ann. Otol. Rhinol. Laryngol.* **2016**, *125*, 485–494. [CrossRef]
4. Prasad, S.C.; Roustan, V.; Piras, G.; Caruso, A.; Lauda, L.; Sanna, M. Subtotal Petrosectomy: Surgical Technique, Indications, Outcomes, and Comprehensive Review of Literature. *Laryngoscope* **2017**, *127*, 2833–2842. [CrossRef]
5. Zwierz, A.; Masna, K. Surgical Outcomes of Using Temporoparietal Fasciocutaneus and Temporoparietal Pedicle Flap for Auricular Reconstruction. *J. Int. Adv. Otol.* **2022**, *15*, 426–432. [CrossRef]
6. Cieslik-Bielecka, A.; Choukroun, J.; Odin, G.; Dohan Ehrenfest, D.M. L-PRP/L-PRF in esthetic plastic surgery, regenerative medicine of the skin and chronic wounds. *Curr. Pharm. Biotechnol.* **2012**, *13*, 1266–1277. [CrossRef]
7. Beaudoin, P.L.; Carles, G. Template for Diced Cartilage with Platelet-Rich Fibrin (PRF) in Rhinoplasty: An Easy Solution for Millimetric Camouflage of the Full Dorsal Esthetic Unit. *Facial Plast. Surg.* **2023**, *39*, 707–713. [CrossRef]
8. Buzalaf, M.A.R.; Levy, F.M. Autologous platelet concentrates for facial rejuvenation. *J. Appl. Oral Sci.* **2022**, *30*, e20220020. [CrossRef] [PubMed]
9. Zhang, T.; Wang, J.; Le, K.; Guo, Y.; Zhu, B. Platelet-rich fibrin accelerates skin wound healing in pressure injuries: A rat model. *J. Wound Care* **2022**, *31*, 800–804. [CrossRef]
10. Tian, K.; Ye, J.; Zhong, Y.; Jia, Z.; Xu, W.; Gao, S.; Cao, S.; Li, K.; Wu, L. Autologous i-PRF promotes healing of radiation-induced skin injury. *Wound Repair Regen.* **2023**, *31*, 454–463. [CrossRef] [PubMed]
11. Straub, A.; Brands, R.; Borgmann, A.; Vollmer, A.; Hohm, J.; Linz, C.; Müller-Richter, U.; Kübler, A.C.; Hartmann, S. Free Skin Grafting to Reconstruct Donor Sites after Radial Forearm Flap Harvesting: A Prospective Study with Platelet-Rich Fibrin (PRF). *J. Clin. Med.* **2022**, *11*, 3506. [CrossRef]
12. Narayanaswamy, R.; Patro, B.P.; Jeyaraman, N.; Gangadaran, P.; Rajendran, R.L.; Nallakumarasamy, A.; Jeyaraman, M.; Ramani, P.; Ahn, B.C. Evolution and Clinical Advances of Platelet-Rich Fibrin in Musculoskeletal Regeneration. *Bioengineering* **2023**, *10*, 58. [CrossRef] [PubMed]
13. Meza-Mauricio, J.; Furquim, C.P.; Geldres, A.; Mendoza-Azpur, G.; Retamal-Valdes, B.; Moraschini, V.; Faveri, M. Is the use of platelet-rich fibrin effective in the healing, control of pain, and postoperative bleeding in the palatal area after free gingival graft harvesting? A systematic review of randomized clinical studies. *Clin. Oral Investig.* **2021**, *25*, 4239–4249. [CrossRef] [PubMed]
14. Puri, K.; Khatri, M.; Bansal, M.; Kumar, A.; Rehan, M.; Gupta, A. A novel injectable platelet-rich fibrin reinforced papilla reconstruction technique. *J. Indian Soc. Periodontol.* **2022**, *26*, 412–417. [CrossRef] [PubMed]
15. Straub, A.; Utz, C.; Stapf, M.; Vollmer, A.; Kasper, S.; Kübler, A.C.; Brands, R.C.; Hartmann, S.; Lâm, T.T. Investigation of three common centrifugation protocols for platelet-rich fibrin (PRF) as a bio-carrier for ampicillin/sulbactam: A prospective trial. *Clin. Oral Investig.* **2023**, *27*, 5991–5998. [CrossRef] [PubMed]
16. Bartels, L.J.; Sheehy, J.L. Total Obliteration of the Mastoid, Middle Ear, and External Auditory Canal. A Review of 27 Cases. *Laryngoscope* **1981**, *91*, 1100–1108. [CrossRef] [PubMed]
17. Parmekar, S.; Hazarika, P.; Viswanathan, A.; Balakrishnan, R. Mastoid Obliteration Using Temporo-Parietal Fascia Flap-Our Experience. *Indian J. Otolaryngol. Head Neck Surg.* **1997**, *49*, 117–121. [CrossRef]
18. Yung, M. The Use of Temporoparietal Fascial Flap to Eliminate Wound Breakdown in Subtotal Petrosectomy for Chronic Discharging Ears. *Otol. Neurotol.* **2016**, *37*, 248–251. [CrossRef]
19. Bernardeschi, D.; Nguyen, Y.; Smail, M.; Bouccara, D.; Meyer, B.; Ferrary, E.; Sterkers, O.; Mosnier, I. Middle Ear and Mastoid Obliteration for Cochlear Implant in Adults: Indications and Anatomical Results. *Otol. Neurotol.* **2015**, *36*, 604–609. [CrossRef]
20. D'Angelo, G.; Donati, G.; Bacciu, A.; Guida, M.; Falcioni, M. Subtotal Petrosectomy and Cochlear Implantation. *Acta Otorhinolaryngol. Ital.* **2020**, *40*, 450–456. [CrossRef] [PubMed]
21. Cheney, M.L.; Megerian, C.A.; Brown, M.T.; McKenna, M.J. Mastoid Obliteration and Lining Using the Temporoparietal Fascial Flap. *Laryngoscope* **1995**, *105 Pt 1*, 1010–1013. [CrossRef]
22. East, C.A.; Brough, M.D.; Grant, H.R. Mastoid Obliteration with the Temporoparietal Fascia Flap. *J. Laryngol. Otol.* **1991**, *105*, 417–420. [CrossRef]
23. Haginomori, S.; Nonaka, R.; Takenaka, H.; Ueda, K. Canal Wall-Down Tympanoplasty with Soft-Wall Reconstruction Using the Pedicled Temporoparietal Fascial Flap: Technique and Preliminary Results. *Ann. Otol. Rhinol. Laryngol.* **2008**, *117*, 719–726. [CrossRef]

24. Shashank, B.; Bhushan, M. Injectable Platelet-Rich Fibrin (PRF): The Newest Biomaterial and Its Use in Various Dermatological Conditions in Our Practice: A Case Series. *J. Cosmet. Dermatol.* **2021**, *20*, 1421–1426. [CrossRef]
25. Choukroun, J.; Diss, A.; Simonpieri, A.; Girard, M.O.; Schoeffler, C.; Dohan, S.L.; Dohan, A.J.; Mouhyi, J.; Dohan, D.M. Platelet-Rich Fibrin (PRF): A Second-Generation Platelet Concentrate. Part V: Histologic Evaluations of PRF Effects on Bone Allograft Maturation in Sinus Lift. *Oral Surg. Oral Med. Oral Pathol. Oral Radiol. Endod.* **2006**, *101*, 299–303. [CrossRef]
26. Abd El Raouf, M.; Wang, X.; Miusi, S.; Chai, J.; Mohamed Abdel-Aal, A.B.; Nefissa Helmy, M.M.; Ghanaati, S.; Choukroun, J.; Choukroun, E.; Zhang, Y.; et al. Injectable-Platelet Rich Fibrin Using the Low Speed Centrifugation Concept Improves Cartilage Regeneration When Compared to Platelet-Rich Plasma. *Platelets* **2019**, *30*, 213–221. [CrossRef]
27. Zhang, J.; Yin, C.; Zhao, Q.; Zhao, Z.; Wang, J.; Miron, R.J.; Zhang, Y. Anti-Inflammation Effects of Injectable Platelet-Rich Fibrin via Macrophages and Dendritic Cells. *J. Biomed. Mater. Res. A* **2020**, *108*, 61–68. [CrossRef]
28. Bendet, E.; Cerenko, D.; Linder, T.E.; Fisch, U. Cochlear Implantation After Subtotal Petrosectomies. *Eur. Arch. Otorhinolaryngol.* **1998**, *255*, 169–174. [CrossRef] [PubMed]
29. Issing, P.R.; Schönermark, M.P.; Winkelmann, S.; Kempf, H.G.; Ernst, A. Cochlear Implantation in Patients with Chronic Otitis: Indications for Subtotal Petrosectomy and Obliteration of the Middle Ear. *Skull Base Surg.* **1998**, *8*, 127–131. [CrossRef] [PubMed]
30. Leung, R.; Briggs, R.J. Indications for and Outcomes of Mastoid Obliteration in Cochlear Implantation. *Otol. Neurotol.* **2007**, *28*, 330–334. [CrossRef] [PubMed]
31. Altuna, X.; García, L.; Martínez, Z.; de Pinedo, M.F. The Role of Subtotal Petrosectomy in Cochlear Implant Recipients. *Eur. Arch. Otorhinolaryngol.* **2017**, *274*, 4149–4153. [CrossRef]
32. Free, R.H.; Falcioni, M.; Di Trapani, G.; Giannuzzi, A.L.; Russo, A.; Sanna, M. The Role of Subtotal Petrosectomy in Cochlear Implant Surgery—A Report of 32 Cases and Review on Indications. *Otol. Neurotol.* **2013**, *34*, 1033–1040. [CrossRef]
33. Kurkure, R.; Rayamajhi, P.; Castellino, A.; Dharmarajan, S.; Dham, R.; Natarajan, K.; Kameswaran, M. Subtotal Petrosectomy in Cochlear Implant Surgery: Our Experience. *Indian J. Otolaryngol. Head Neck Surg.* **2020**, *72*, 320–325. [CrossRef]
34. Hernández, S.; Ospina, J.C.; Gutiérrez-Gómez, E.; Rodríguez-Ruiz, M.T.; Trujillo, J.G. Alternative Techniques in Cochlear Implant Surgery: Subtotal Petrosectomy. *Am. J. Otolaryngol.* **2020**, *41*, 102338. [CrossRef]
35. Muzaffar, J.; Metcalfe, C.; Colley, S.; Coulson, C. Diffusion-weighted magnetic resonance imaging for residual and recurrent cholesteatoma: A systematic review and meta-analysis. *Clin Otolaryngol.* **2017**, *42*, 536–543. [CrossRef]

audiology research

MDPI

Article

Impact of Cochlear Trauma Degree and Localization on Intracochlear Electrocochleographic Recordings

David Bächinger [1,2], Merlin Schär [1,2], Ahmet Kunut [1,2], Rahel Bertschinger [1,2], Ivo Dobrev [1,2], Leanne Sijgers [1,2], Andreas H. Eckhard [3,4] and Adrian Dalbert [1,2,*]

1 Department of Otorhinolaryngology, Head and Neck Surgery, University Hospital Zurich, 8091 Zurich, Switzerland
2 Faculty of Medicine, University of Zurich, 8032 Zurich, Switzerland
3 Otopathology Laboratory, Department of Otolaryngology, Massachusetts Eye and Ear, Boston, MA 02114, USA
4 Department of Otolaryngology, Head and Neck Surgery, Harvard Medical School, Boston, MA 02115, USA
* Correspondence: adrian.dalbert@usz.ch

Abstract: Background/Objectives: Electrocochleography (ECochG) is a promising tool to monitor preservation of cochlear structures and function during cochlear implant (CI) surgery. However, the interpretation of ECochG signal changes during insertion of the CI electrode array remains controversial. This study investigates the influence of the degree and localization of cochlear trauma on ECochG signal changes using a mouse model. Methods: C57BL/6J-Crl1 mice underwent intracochlear ECochG recordings during the insertion of a platinum–iridium electrode. Results: In case of grade 1 and 2 cochlear trauma, as determined by post-mortem histological analysis, we found that a reduction in intracochlear cochlear microphonic (CM) amplitude correlates more significantly with the location of the trauma than with its severity. The more basally a trauma is located, the larger the CM amplitude drop. Furthermore, the results revealed that grade 1 or 2 trauma was detectable through ECochG before more severe trauma developed. Conclusions: These findings suggest that intracochlear ECochG can serve as a reliable intraoperative tool for detecting early and possibly reversible cochlear trauma, preventing more severe damage and aiding hearing preservation. The results emphasize the need for a nuanced interpretation of CM signal drops, considering trauma location and cochlear structure integrity at the site of trauma and apical to it.

Keywords: electrocochleography; cochlear implant; cochlear trauma; hearing preservation; intracochlear recordings; mouse model

1. Introduction

As cochlear implantation has become a widespread option for hearing rehabilitation not only in deaf patients but also in patients with lesser degrees of sensorineural hearing loss, preserving still-intact cochlear structures and function has become one of the primary objectives during cochlear implant (CI) surgery. Preservation of residual hearing not only allows for improved speech perception with electrical stimulation alone [1] but also enables the implementation of combined electric–acoustic stimulation [2] in selected cases. Furthermore, it addresses the widespread concern of CI patients to become totally deaf.

To date, approximately 50% of CI recipients experience a loss of residual hearing within the first six months after surgery [3]. In combination with further refinement of surgical techniques (e.g., robotics-assisted electrode array insertions) and electrode array design changes, electrocochleography (ECochG) has emerged as a tool that may improve hearing preservation rates in the future. ECochG records responses to acoustic stimuli generated by hair cells as well as neural structures. However, in almost all studies concerning CI and ECochG, the cochlear microphonic (CM) as one of the hair cell components of the ECochG response has been assessed. Previous work in animals has shown that CM amplitude drops can be associated with cochlear trauma during electrode insertion [4–9]. Accordingly, multiple studies in human CI recipients have demonstrated that, on average, such amplitude drops are associated with increased loss of residual hearing after surgery [10–14]. However, it is also evident that not all CM drops during electrode insertion into the cochlea represent cochlear trauma. Changes of the relative contribution to the CM of different cochlear regions as the electrode is advanced into the cochlea can also lead to a decrease of the signal amplitude [15–18].

Whether individual CM drops are trauma related and relevant with regard to structure preservation or not often remains controversial. To address this issue, different approaches have been investigated. By far the most common approach is to rate amplitude drops as relevant or not, based on the extent of the amplitude drop (i.e., depending on the study relevant drops were defined as $\geq$3 dB, $\geq$6 dB or $\geq$30%). Drops exceeding the defined threshold are then rated as trauma related and relevant, while drops below the threshold are not [10–12,19]. However, this approach has two main drawbacks. First, Giardina et al. demonstrated that analyzing phase changes and distortions of the CM alongside amplitude changes improves the accuracy of predictions regarding hearing preservation [15]. Second, there is a lack of understanding of factors influencing the extent of CM drops (e.g., degree of cochlear trauma, intact cochlear structures in the region of trauma, localization of trauma). The prevailing assumption has been that the degree of cochlear trauma is the main influencing factor, but to our knowledge, experimental data confirming this hypothesis is lacking.

Since many factors potentially influencing ECochG signal changes in human CI recipients are not accessible for analysis, this study aimed to determine the influence of the degree and localization of cochlear trauma on intracochlear CM changes in normal hearing C57BL/6 mice. Normal hearing animals were chosen to have a study population as homogenous as possible, although it represents a limitation in terms of translatability to human CI recipients. Mice are a well-suited animal model for cochlear implantation due to the similarity of their auditory system to that of humans [20]. Additionally, the availability of a wide range of genetic models and consequently the future possibility to assess ECochG signals changes also in different inner ear pathologies was further incentive to choose mice as an animal model in this study. We hypothesized that the severity of cochlear trauma and, to a lesser extent, its localization could determine the magnitude of CM amplitude drops.

2. Materials and Methods

All animal experiments adhered to the principles of the 3Rs (Replacement, Reduction, and Refinement) and were performed according to Swiss Animal Welfare laws. All experimental protocols were approved by a named institutional committee (local veterinary authorities, permission number ZH103/2018, Kantonales Veterinäramt, Zurich, Switzerland). The results are reported in accordance with ARRIVE guidelines. Results from eleven ears in eleven female C57BL/6J-Crl1 ("C57BL/6") wild-type mice aged 6 to 8 weeks are reported (including n = 2 control animals). The mice were purchased from Charles River (Freiburg im Breisgau, Germany) and housed in individually ventilated cages at an in-house animal facility. They had unlimited access to a standard chow diet and water ad libitum under a standard 12 h light/dark cycle.

2.1. Surgery

The mice were anaesthetized with an intraperitoneal injection of a mixture of xylazine (12 mg/kg; Rompun, Bayer HealthCare AG, Leverkusen, Germany) and ketamine (80 mg/kg; Narketan, Vétoquinol SA, 34, Magny-Vernois, France). Anesthesia depth was assessed every 15 min by checking the pedal reflex. If reflexes were present, the mice were redosed with ketamine (25 mg/kg).

The left retroauricular region was shaved, the mouse was placed on a heating pad, maintaining an internal temperature of 37.5 °C as monitored via rectal probe. Lidocaine (10 mg/mL; Rapidocain, Sintetica SA, Mendrisio, Switzerland) was injected in the subcutaneous tissue of the left retroauricular region for topical analgesia. Surgical access to the round window was performed using a minimally invasive technique as described previously [21] (Figure 1). Briefly, the left temporal bone was accessed via a retroauricular incision and a blunt dissection of the sternocleidomastoid muscle, the anterior scalene muscle, and the posterior belly of the digastric muscle. Bipolar electrocautery was used for dissection and hemostasis. The auditory bulla was opened using a micro drill with a 0.5 mm burr. The opening was extended until the round window was completely visualized.

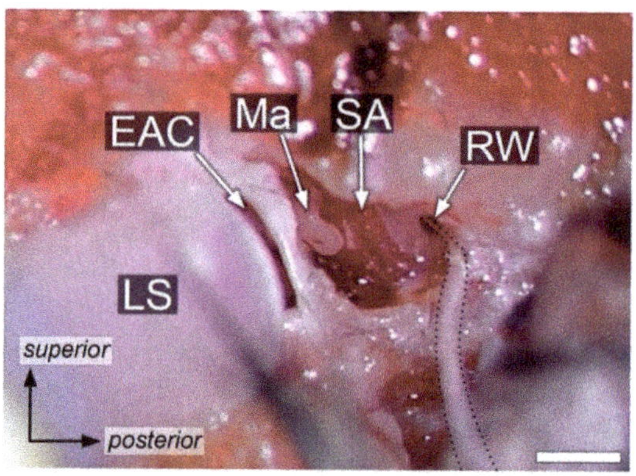

Figure 1. Microscope view following surgical access to the middle ear. The black dashed line outlines the electrode. EAC, external auditory canal; LS, loudspeaker; Ma, malleus; RW, round window; SA, stapedial artery. Scale bar: 1 mm.

The electrode (+) used for intracochlear ECochG recordings was a 25 µm diameter, Teflon-insulated platinum–iridium wire with approximately 50 µm of tip insulation removed. Consequently, the inserted electrode did not closely resemble a CI electrode array. The wire used as intracochlear electrode had a high stiffness and did not behave like a lateral wall or perimodiolar CI electrode. The reason such a stiff wire was used was that it would likely cause cochlear trauma, which was the aim of this study. Due to high stiffness, the electrode could not pass beyond the basal turn. A similar electrode to record ECochG responses and cause intracochlear trauma was used by Adunka et al. [4]. Additionally, a needle electrode was placed in the contralateral neck muscles to provide the inverting input (−), and both inputs were referenced to a needle electrode at the base of the tail (ground). An insert earphone (Biologic Systems, Mundelein, IL, USA) was positioned at the external ear canal for acoustic stimulation. The Navigator Pro stimulation/recording device and the AEP software (Version 7.0.0, Biologic Systems) were used for acoustic stimulation and recording. Tone bursts at 6 or 8 kHz with an intensity of 100 dB SPL were used as acoustic stimuli. These frequencies were chosen to resemble acoustic simulation in human CI recipients in which ECochG recordings are conducted. In human CI recipients, responses can usually only be recorded to low-frequency acoustic stimulation, and by far the most common frequency used for ECochG recordings is 0.5 kHz. In mice, the tonotopic regions of 6 and 8 kHz are comparable to the tonotopic region of 0.5 kHz in humans [22]. Recordings during insertion were conducted with only one frequency. Responses to 500 stimuli with alternating starting phases were recorded. The recorded data were exported from the AEP software using the AEP to ASCII software (Version 1.0, Biologic Systems). For post-processing, MATLAB (Version 24.1, MathWorks Inc., Natick, MA, USA) and GraphPad Prism (Version 10.4.2, GraphPad Software Inc., La Jolla, CA, USA) were used. The CM was derived by subtracting the averages of 500 responses with alternating starting phases. By subtracting both response curves with alternating starting phases, neural responses with the same polarity in both response curves are canceled out, whereas hair cell responses with different polarity in both response curves remain. A Fast Fourier Transform (FFT) was performed on the CM response to determine the peak-to-peak amplitude of each CM curve at the acoustic stimulation frequency. The amount of CM amplitude drop was defined as the difference between the last two ECochG recordings.

The round window membrane was incised, and the recording electrode was inserted in 25 μm to 50 μm steps using a manual micromanipulator (M3301, World Precision Instruments, Friedberg, Germany). At each step, the insertion was paused for the duration of the ECochG recordings. The stepwise insertion was continued up to an insertion depth where a visually detectable drop in the CM signal amplitude or resistance with further insertion occurred. In control animals, the surgical access to the round window was carried out as described above. The platinum–iridium electrode was then placed on the closed round window membrane and two ECochG recordings were conducted within a 30 min interval.

2.2. Histological Analysis

After completion of measurements, the animals were sacrificed during anesthesia. The platinum–iridium electrode was cut at the round window and fixed using cyanoacrylate glue. For tissue fixation, the thoracic cavity was opened, and a cannula was inserted in the left cardiac ventricle for transcardial perfusion with 10 mL phosphate buffered saline (PBS), followed by 10 mL of 10% neutral buffered formalin (catalog no. 15738-01, Lucerna-Chem AG, Luzern, Switzerland). The mice were then decapitated, and soft tissues were removed from the outer surface of the skull using a sharp scalpel. The cranial part of the skull was opened to remove the cerebrum, while the cerebellum was left in situ. The specimens were then immersed in 10% neutral buffered formalin for 24 h on a countertop shaker. After fixation, specimens were decalcified in a formic acid decalcifier for 10 days (RDF mild decalcifier, catalog no. EAA-1000-00A, CellPath Ltd., Newtown, UK). The specimens were then dehydrated in a graded series of ethanol solutions (50%, 70%, 95%, and 100%), embedded in paraffin and sectioned at 4 μm using an HM 355S Automatic Microtome (Thermo Fisher Scientific, Waltham, MA, USA). Specimens were sectioned without removing the electrodes in order to avoid removal artefacts. Sections were collected on SuperFrost Plus slides (Thermo Fisher Scientific), dried on a heating plate at 37 °C overnight and stored at room temperature. The specimens were stained with hematoxylin and eosin. Images were acquired using a Leica DMI6000 microscope (Leica, Wetzlar, Germany) and processed with Adobe Photoshop software (Version 25.0, Adobe Systems, San Jose, CA, USA). The insertion depth was measured from the round window to the tip of the electrode.

Histological trauma was rated on scale from 0 to 4 [23]: 0 represents no observable trauma; 1, elevation of the basilar membrane; 2, rupture of the basilar membrane; 3, electrode in the scala vestibuli; and 4, severe trauma such as fracture of the osseous spiral lamina or modiolus or tear of stria vascularis.

2.3. Micro-Computed Tomography

Micro-computed tomography (μCT; Skyscan 1176, Bruker Corp., Billerica, MA, USA) scans were conducted after completion of the above-described fixation process. The three-dimensional volumes of the cochlear structures and the inserted electrodes were reconstructed from the μCT-images using Amira software (version 6.5, Thermo Fisher Scientific Inc., Waltham, MA, USA). The insertion depth was measured from the round window to the tip of the electrode.

2.4. Statistical Analyses

Statistical analyses were conducted using GraphPad Prism (GraphPad Software Inc., La Jolla, CA, USA). Linear regression analyses were performed to determine the correspondence between the insertion depth of the electrode according to histological and μCT findings as well as to correlate the degree and the localization of cochlear trauma with CM amplitude changes.

3. Results

In both control animals (M1C, M2C), no amplitude differences in the CM curve at 6 and 8 kHz could be detected between the two recordings (Figure 2).

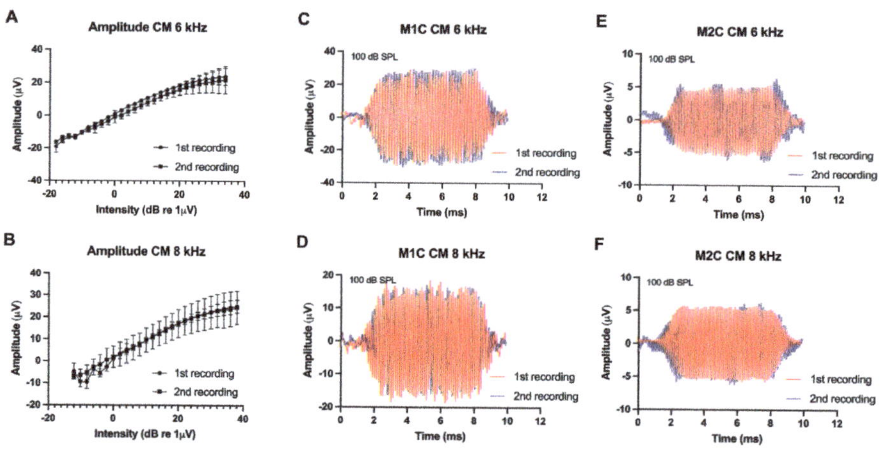

Figure 2. (**A**,**B**) show the mean CM curve amplitudes at different intensities at 6 and 8 kHz in control animals in both recordings (bars are standard error of the mean). (**C**–**F**) display the CM responses at 100 dB SPL at 6 and 8 kHz in both control animals.

ECochG recordings during stepwise insertion of the electrode were performed in nine animals. The chosen frequency for acoustic stimulation was 8 kHz for $n = 1$ (M1) and 6 kHz for $n = 8$. Mean amplitude of the first CM response at the round window was 31.7 dB re 1 μV ($n = 9$, range 13.2 dB re 1 μV to 45.4 dB re 1 μV). Seven recordings showed a CM drop (mean amplitude drop 14.6 dB ($n = 7$), range 36.5 dB to 5.6 dB). Figure 3 shows two examples of CM responses at different stages of insertion. In both animals, a drop of the CM was detectable. In all animals, except M6, a CM amplitude increase was detectable during insertion of the electrode. However, it has to be noted that the amplitude increase in M5 was only minimal with 0.8 dB (Figure 3A). In M6, an amplitude drop occurred with the first insertion step; therefore, only a shallow insertion of 0.7 mm was achieved (Figure 3B). This finding was associated with very basally located cochlear trauma in the histological assessment. In two animals, the insertion was stopped due to resistance and buckling of the electrode outside of the cochlea without an associated CM drop (M7, M9). Mean insertion depth for all insertions was 1.2 mm (range 0.7 mm to 1.8 mm), which means that 10 to 29% of the cochlea were covered by the electrode and that the tonotopic region of 6 and 8 kHz, which lays between 60 to 70% of the distance from the round window, was not reached in any animal [22]. With an insertion depth of 1.2 mm, the characteristic frequency of approximately 20 kHz is reached. Histological, radiological, and electrophysiological findings are summarized in Table 1.

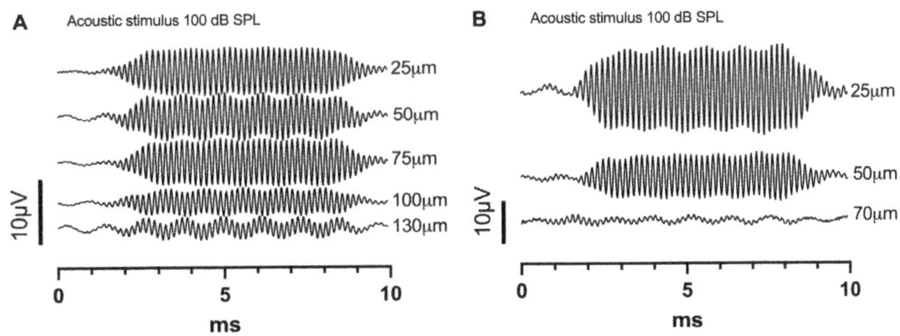

Figure 3. Examples of CM responses at different insertion steps are displayed. The CM amplitude drops were 9 μV ((**A**), M5) and 27 μV ((**B**), M6). These changes were associated with a histological trauma grade 2 at an insertion depth of 130 μm in M5 and grade 1 at an insertion depth of 70 μm in M6.

Table 1. μCT stands for micro-computed tomography; NA, not applicable.

Animal	Histology	Histological Trauma Grade	μCT	Insertion Depth (mm)	Cochlear Microphonic Amplitude First Recording (dB re 1 μV)	Last Recording (dB re 1 μV)	Amplitude Change (dB)
M1	Yes	4	No	1.7	37.8	12.3	−36.5
M2	No	NA	Yes	0.9	13.2	19.1	−10
M3	Yes	1	Yes	1.3	33.8	37	−6.3
M4	Yes	1	Yes	1.3	35.8	36.5	−5.6
M5	Yes	2	Yes	1.4	31	22.1	−9
M6	Yes	1	Yes	0.7	26	−1.5	−27
M7	Yes	2	Yes	1.1	30.5	34.9	0
M8	Yes	2	Yes	1.1	45.4	35.5	−8
M9	Yes	2	Yes	1.8	32.2	35.5	3

Histology and μCT (Figure 4A) could be assessed in eight animals each. A strong correlation was observed between insertion depths estimated by histology and μCT-images when the insertion depth could be reliably assessed by both modalities (linear regression, $r^2 = 0.94$, $p < 0.01$, $n = 6$, Figure 4B).

Histological trauma (grade 0–4) could be assessed in eight animals. In one animal, due to difficulties during preparation of the histological specimen, the histological sections could not be interpreted. Histological trauma was classified as grade 1 in three animals, grade 2 in four animals, and grade 4 in one animal (Table 1, Figure 5). All histological trauma was localized in the region where the tip of the stiff electrode got in contact with cochlear structures and insertion was stopped. No widespread trauma or secondary sites with cochlear trauma were detected.

The degree of histological trauma showed no correlation with the magnitude of the CM amplitude drop (linear regression, $r^2 = 0.23$, $p = 0.22$, $n = 8$, Figure 6A). However, the localization of intracochlear trauma showed a significant correlation with the amount of CM amplitude drop in case of trauma grade 1 or 2. Basally located intracochlear trauma was associated with significantly larger CM amplitude drops (linear regression, $r^2 = 0.63$, $p = 0.03$, $n = 7$, Figure 6B).

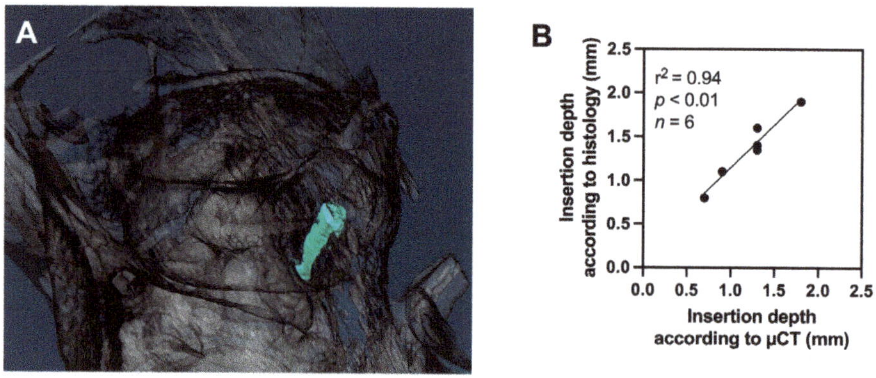

Figure 4. (**A**) displays an exemplary three-dimensional reconstruction of µCT-images. The electrode wire is shown in cyan blue. (**B**) shows the strong correlation between insertion depth estimation according to histological results and µCT-images.

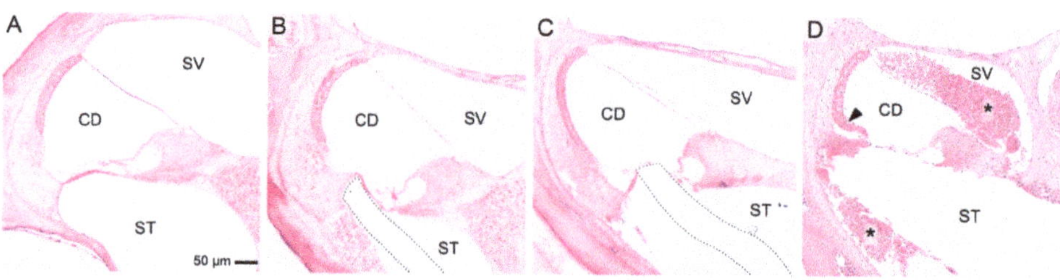

Figure 5. Example of microscope images of histologic trauma in the middle cochlear turn. (**A**) Normal cochlear morphology in a control animal. (**B**) Grade 1 trauma with elevation of the basilar membrane. (**C**) Grade 2 trauma with rupture of the basilar membrane. (**D**) Grade 4 trauma featuring a fracture of the osseous spiral lamina and a tear of the stria vascularis (black arrowhead). Note the extensive intracochlear bleeding (black asterisks). The dotted line outlines the electrode tract. CD, cochlear duct; ST, scala tympani; SV, scala vestibuli.

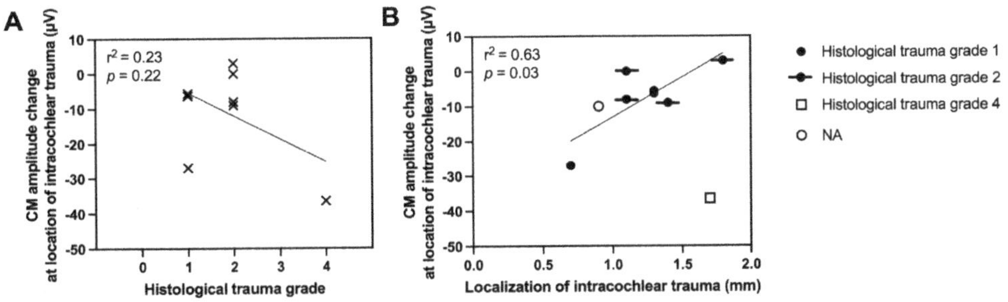

Figure 6. (**A**) Correlation between degree of histological trauma and the amount of CM amplitude drop. (**B**) Correlation between localization of intracochlear trauma and amount of amplitude drop. In the case of intracochlear trauma grade 1–2, the localization of the intracochlear trauma showed a significant correlation with the CM amplitude drop. Basally located intracochlear trauma was associated with larger CM amplitude drops. NA stands for not applicable.

4. Discussion

The aim of this study was to determine factors influencing the magnitude of the CM amplitude drops observed in intracochlear ECochG recordings during electrode insertion. To correlate CM response changes with histological findings and minimize confounding factors, such as varying presurgical cochlear health, we conducted this study using normal hearing C57BL/6 mice. Our results reveal for the first time that the magnitude of the CM amplitude drop in cochlear trauma grades 1 and 2 is significantly correlated with the intracochlear location of trauma, while the degree of trauma—at least in case of grade 1 and 2 traumata—does not show such a correlation. Previous animal studies have primarily examined the relationship between cochlear trauma and the presence of an CM amplitude drop, without addressing the magnitude of these drops [4–9]. In concordance with these studies, seven out of nine animals with cochlear trauma exhibited a decrease of the CM amplitude in the study presented here. However, the correlation between localization of trauma and CM changes have never been previously explored.

The underlying mechanism for the detected correlation between trauma location and magnitude of the CM amplitude drops in cochlear trauma grade 1 and 2 remains unclear. However, defining a specific magnitude of the CM amplitude drop as a relevant indicator for cochlear trauma may be questionable, as both the occurrence and magnitude of amplitude drops are largely determined by the location of the trauma and its relation to still intact cochlear structures. Small drops may still indicate significant trauma that might not be detected by such an approach. A promising method to overcome this limitation and to gain frequency- and location-specific information about cochlear trauma could be multi-frequency and -locational ECochG recordings [16,24].

The mouse cochlea has proven to be a suitable model for the human cochlea. Structurally, the mouse cochlea is similar to the human cochlea and many genes affecting hearing in humans also cause hearing loss in mice, often with similar disease progression [25]. In this study, 6 to 8 kHz sinusoid tone bursts were used as acoustic stimuli. The tonotopic region for these frequencies in mice lays between 60 to 70% of the distance from the round window. In humans, the tonotopic region of 0.5 kHz—the frequency usually used for ECochG recordings in human CI recipients—is located in a similar location [26]. Due to the stiff wire used as a recording electrode in this study, the tonotopic region of the acoustic stimulus was not reached. Similarly, in human CI recipients, the tonotopic region of 0.5 kHz is not reached by most commercially available electrode arrays. However, it must be noted that the coverage of the cochlea by CI electrodes in humans is usually far more than in this study. In this study, only 10–29% of the mouse cochlea were covered. Consequently, the cochlear trauma described here can generally be seen as basally located trauma.

In this cohort, grade 4 cochlear trauma was observed in only one case, based on histological findings, which included a fracture of the spiral osseous lamina, disruption of the stria vascularis, and extensive intracochlear bleeding. This severe trauma was associated with an immediate and large decrease of the CM response, implying that more severe cochlear trauma with intracochlear bleeding is likely to result in substantial and immediate CM drops, even when the trauma occurs in more apical cochlear regions as in this case. However, no definitive conclusions can be drawn from this single instance. Further research with larger samples of severe trauma cases, as well as studies correlating specific trauma mechanisms (e.g., trauma to stria vascularis, to basilar membrane) with electrophysiological response patterns, is needed to advance this research field.

The results presented here suggest that grade 1 and 2 cochlear trauma can typically be detected by ECochG before more severe cochlear trauma occurs. Following the study protocol, insertion was stopped as soon as a noticeable decrease of the CM amplitude was visually observed—analogous to ECochG assessments performed in human CI recipients during surgery. This finding underscores the potential of ECochG as a valuable tool for intraoperative monitoring during cochlear implantation in the future, as it seems capable of detecting early trauma and, in some cases, potentially reversible damage, provided that intact cochlear structures remain at or apical to the trauma site.

Limitations

Due to the design of the study with a stiff electrode inserted into the cochlea, some degree of cochlear trauma was detectable in all animals. Therefore, the research question of which CM drops represent cochlear trauma and which do not cannot be addressed. From the presented results, only some conclusions regarding factors influencing the amount of CM drops in the case of cochlear trauma can be drawn. Furthermore, due to the stiff character of the electrode, insertions beyond the basal turn were not possible. Consequently, the investigated cochlear trauma in this study only represents basal trauma. Further studies will need to investigate if ECochG changes with deeper insertions show similar characteristics.

This study was conducted in normal hearing animals, which represents a major difference compared to the highly pathological cochlea in CI recipients. Therefore, the results cannot be directly translated to human CI recipients. However, the principal mechanism that intact cochlear structures apical to the trauma site are silenced and that therefore the site of cochlea trauma and its relation to intact cochlear structures influences CM changes during insertion seems applicable to human CI recipients.

A further limitation is the absence of auditory threshold testing (e.g., auditory brainstem responses) to confirm the assumed normal hearing status of the animals before the study procedure. However, extended cochlear pathology before electrode insertion that would influence the reported study outcome seems unlikely in the chosen study animals. Additionally, in future studies, correlating ECochG changes and auditory threshold testing may allow a conclusive assessment between ECochG changes and acute hearing changes.

The fact that the insertion was stopped when an amplitude drop of the CM response was detectable and that the drop at the same time was the primary dependent variable in the analysis represents a methodological conflict. However, this approach was chosen as it reflects how ECochG responses are most often used in the operating theatre with human CI recipients. The incentive was to find out what histological and μCT findings are present in the moment the first ECochG drop occurred.

5. Conclusions

The location of cochlear trauma and its relation to still-intact cochlear structures have influence on the occurrence and on the magnitude of the CM amplitude drops during electrode insertion. When intact cochlear structures are present, early detection of cochlear trauma is possible. If the insertion is stopped upon detecting signal decrease, severe cochlear trauma (grade 3 or 4) seems to be rare. These findings suggest that applying this approach to cochlear implantation in human CI recipients could enhance hearing preservation during cochlear implant surgeries.

Author Contributions: D.B. and A.D. designed this research. I.D. participated in preparing the experiments. D.B., A.K., R.B. and A.D. performed the experiments. M.S., I.D. and L.S. participated in data analysis. D.B., A.H.E. and A.D. wrote the manuscript and prepared the figures. All authors contributed substantially to this research and reviewed the manuscript. All authors have read and agreed to the published version of the manuscript.

Funding: This research was funded by the Vontobel-Stiftung (80002, Zürich, Switzlerland) and Cochlear Ltd. (IIR-2308).

Institutional Review Board Statement: The animal study protocol was approved by a named institutional committee (local veterinary authorities, permission number ZH103/2018, 16 January 2020, Kantonales Veterinäramt, Zurich, Switzerland) for studies involving animals.

Informed Consent Statement: Not applicable.

Data Availability Statement: The raw data supporting the conclusions of this article will be made available by the authors on request.

Conflicts of Interest: This manuscript has received research grants from the Vontobel-Stiftung and Cochlear Ltd. The sponsors had no role in the design, execution, interpretation, or writing of the study. The authors declare no conflicts of interest.

References

1. Dalbert, A.; Huber, A.; Baumann, N.; Veraguth, D.; Roosli, C.; Pfiffner, F. Hearing Preservation After Cochlear Implantation May Improve Long-term Word Perception in the Electric-only Condition. *Otol. Neurotol.* **2016**, *37*, 1314–1319. [CrossRef] [PubMed]
2. Gantz, B.J.; Turner, C.; Gfeller, K.E.; Lowder, M.W. Preservation of hearing in cochlear implant surgery: Advantages of combined electrical and acoustical speech processing. *Laryngoscope* **2005**, *115*, 796–802. [CrossRef] [PubMed]
3. Van Abel, K.M.; Dunn, C.C.; Sladen, D.P.; Oleson, J.J.; Beatty, C.W.; Neff, B.A.; Hansen, M.; Gantz, B.J.; Driscoll, C.L. Hearing preservation among patients undergoing cochlear implantation. *Otol. Neurotol.* **2015**, *36*, 416–421. [CrossRef] [PubMed]
4. Adunka, O.F.; Mlot, S.; Suberman, T.A.; Campbell, A.P.; Surowitz, J.; Buchman, C.A.; Fitzpatrick, D.C. Intracochlear recordings of electrophysiological parameters indicating cochlear damage. *Otol. Neurotol.* **2010**, *31*, 1233–1241. [CrossRef]
5. Campbell, A.P.; Suberman, T.A.; Buchman, C.A.; Fitzpatrick, D.C.; Adunka, O.F. Correlation of early auditory potentials and intracochlear electrode insertion properties: An animal model featuring near real-time monitoring. *Otol. Neurotol.* **2010**, *31*, 1391–1398. [CrossRef]
6. Choudhury, B.; Adunka, O.F.; Demason, C.E.; Ahmad, F.I.; Buchman, C.A.; Fitzpatrick, D.C. Detection of intracochlear damage with cochlear implantation in a gerbil model of hearing loss. *Otol. Neurotol.* **2011**, *32*, 1370–1378. [CrossRef]
7. Ahmad, F.I.; Choudhury, B.; De Mason, C.E.; Adunka, O.F.; Finley, C.C.; Fitzpatrick, D.C. Detection of intracochlear damage during cochlear implant electrode insertion using extracochlear measurements in the gerbil. *Laryngoscope* **2012**, *122*, 636–644. [CrossRef]
8. DeMason, C.; Choudhury, B.; Ahmad, F.; Fitzpatrick, D.C.; Wang, J.; Buchman, C.A.; Adunka, O.F. Electrophysiological properties of cochlear implantation in the gerbil using a flexible array. *Ear Hear.* **2012**, *33*, 534–542. [CrossRef]
9. Choudhury, B.; Adunka, O.F.; Awan, O.; Pike, J.M.; Buchman, C.A.; Fitzpatrick, D.C. Electrophysiologic consequences of flexible electrode insertions in gerbils with noise-induced hearing loss. *Otol. Neurotol.* **2014**, *35*, 519–525. [CrossRef]
10. Kim, J.S. Electrocochleography in Cochlear Implant Users with Residual Acoustic Hearing: A Systematic Review. *Int. J. Environ. Res. Public Health* **2020**, *17*, 7043. [CrossRef]

11. Trecca, E.M.C.; Riggs, W.J.; Mattingly, J.K.; Hiss, M.M.; Cassano, M.; Adunka, O.F. Electrocochleography and Cochlear Implantation: A Systematic Review. *Otol. Neurotol.* **2020**, *41*, 864–878. [CrossRef] [PubMed]
12. Yin, L.X.; Barnes, J.H.; Saoji, A.A.; Carlson, M.L. Clinical Utility of Intraoperative Electrocochleography (ECochG) During Cochlear Implantation: A Systematic Review and Quantitative Analysis. *Otol. Neurotol.* **2021**, *42*, 363–371. [CrossRef] [PubMed]
13. Lenarz, T.; Buechner, A.; Gantz, B.; Hansen, M.; Tejani, V.D.; Labadie, R.; O'Connell, B.; Buchman, C.A.; Valenzuela, C.V.; Adunka, O.F.; et al. Relationship Between Intraoperative Electrocochleography and Hearing Preservation. *Otol. Neurotol.* **2022**, *43*, e72–e78. [CrossRef] [PubMed]
14. O'Leary, S.; Mylanus, E.; Venail, F.; Lenarz, T.; Birman, C.; Di Lella, F.; Roland, J.T.; Gantz, B.; Beynon, A.; Sicard, M.; et al. Monitoring Cochlear Health With Intracochlear Electrocochleography During Cochlear Implantation: Findings From an International Clinical Investigation. *Ear Hear.* **2023**, *44*, 358–370. [CrossRef]
15. Giardina, C.K.; Brown, K.D.; Adunka, O.F.; Buchman, C.A.; Hutson, K.A.; Pillsbury, H.C.; Fitzpatrick, D.C. Intracochlear Electrocochleography: Response Patterns During Cochlear Implantation and Hearing Preservation. *Ear Hear.* **2019**, *40*, 833–848. [CrossRef]
16. Dalbert, A.; Sijgers, L.; Grosse, J.; Veraguth, D.; Roosli, C.; Huber, A.; Pfiffner, F. Simultaneous Intra- and Extracochlear Electrocochleography During Electrode Insertion. *Ear Hear.* **2021**, *42*, 414–424. [CrossRef]
17. Sijgers, L.; Pfiffner, F.; Grosse, J.; Dillier, N.; Koka, K.; Röösli, C.; Huber, A.; Dalbert, A. Simultaneous Intra- and Extracochlear Electrocochleography During Cochlear Implantation to Enhance Response Interpretation. *Trends Hear.* **2021**, *25*, 2331216521990594. [CrossRef]
18. Bester, C.; Dalbert, A.; Collins, A.; Razmovski, T.; Gerard, J.M.; O'Leary, S. Electrocochleographic Patterns Predicting Increased Impedances and Hearing Loss after Cochlear Implantation. *Ear Hear.* **2023**, *44*, 710–720. [CrossRef]
19. Weder, S.; Bester, C.; Collins, A.; Shaul, C.; Briggs, R.J.; O'Leary, S. Real Time Monitoring During Cochlear Implantation: Increasing the Accuracy of Predicting Residual Hearing Outcomes. *Otol. Neurotol.* **2021**, *42*, e1030–e1036. [CrossRef]
20. Claussen, A.D.; Vielman Quevedo, R.; Mostaert, B.; Kirk, J.R.; Dueck, W.F.; Hansen, M.R. A mouse model of cochlear implantation with chronic electric stimulation. *PLoS ONE* **2019**, *14*, e0215407. [CrossRef]
21. Soken, H.; Robinson, B.K.; Goodman, S.S.; Abbas, P.J.; Hansen, M.R.; Kopelovich, J.C. Mouse cochleostomy: A minimally invasive dorsal approach for modeling cochlear implantation. *Laryngoscope* **2013**, *123*, E109–E115. [CrossRef] [PubMed]
22. Ou, H.C.; Harding, G.W.; Bohne, B.A. An anatomically based frequency-place map for the mouse cochlea. *Hear. Res.* **2000**, *145*, 123–129. [CrossRef] [PubMed]
23. Eshraghi, A.A.; Yang, N.W.; Balkany, T.J. Comparative study of cochlear damage with three perimodiolar electrode designs. *Laryngoscope* **2003**, *113*, 415–419. [CrossRef] [PubMed]
24. Skarżyński, P.H.; Lorens, A.; Walkowiak, A.; Polak, M.; Skarżyński, H. Multi-Frequency Intraoperative Monitoring of Hearing Preservation during Cochlear Implantation. *Life* **2022**, *12*, 636. [CrossRef]
25. Avraham, K.B. Mouse models for deafness: Lessons for the human inner ear and hearing loss. *Ear Hear.* **2003**, *24*, 332–341. [CrossRef]
26. Greenwood, D.D. A cochlear frequency-position function for several species—29 years later. *J. Acoust. Soc. Am.* **1990**, *87*, 2592–2605. [CrossRef]

MDPI AG
Grosspeteranlage 5
4052 Basel
Switzerland
Tel.: +41 61 683 77 34

Audiology Research Editorial Office
E-mail: audiolres@mdpi.com
www.mdpi.com/journal/audiolres

www.ingramcontent.com/pod-product-compliance
Lightning Source LLC
Chambersburg PA
CBHW061601210926
51850CB00009B/2177
* 9 7 8 3 7 2 5 8 5 1 3 1 7 *